# Dynamic Radiology of the Abdomen

## Normal and Pathologic Anatomy

Third Edition

Morton A. Meyers

# Dynamic Radiology of the Abdomen

## Normal and Pathologic Anatomy

### Third Edition

With 1061 Illustrations, 14 in Full Color

Springer-Verlag
New York Berlin Heidelberg
London Paris Tokyo

Morton A. Meyers, M.D.
Professor and Chairman
Department of Radiology
School of Medicine
State University of New York at Stony Brook
Stony Brook, New York 11794, USA

Library of Congress Cataloging-in-Publication Data
Meyers, Morton A.
    Dynamic radiology of the abdomen: normal and pathologic anatomy/
Morton A. Meyers.—3rd ed.
        p.      cm.
    Includes bibliographies and index.
    ISBN 0-387-96624-2
    1. Abdomen—Diseases—Diagnosis.   2. Abdomen—Radiography.
I. Title.
    [DNLM: 1. Abdomen—anatomy & histology.   2. Abdomen—radiography.
WI 900 M615d]
RC944.M48 1988
617'.5507572—dc19
DNLM/DLC
for Library of Congress                                          87-28453

Typeset by Bi-Comp, Inc., York, Pennsylvania.
Printed and bound by Arcata Graphics/Halliday Lithograph, West Hanover, Massachusetts.
Printed in the United States of America.

9 8 7 6 5 4 3 2 1

ISBN 0-387-96624-2 Springer-Verlag New York Berlin Heidelberg
ISBN 3-540-96624-2 Springer-Verlag Berlin Heidelberg New York

There are some things which cannot be learned quickly, and time, which is all we have, must be paid heavily for their acquiring. They are the very simplest things; and, because it takes a man's life to know them, the little new that each man gets from life is very costly and the only heritage he has to leave.

ERNEST HEMINGWAY (1898–1961)
Death in the Afternoon

# Foreword to First Edition

Few books present so fresh an approach and so clear an exposition as does *Dynamic Radiology of the Abdomen: Normal and Pathologic Anatomy.*

This well-documented, clearly written, and beautifully illustrated book details the answers not only to "what is it?" but also "how?" and "why?" Such fundamental information regarding the pathogenesis of disease within the abdomen reinforces and simplifies accurate radiologic analysis. The characteristic radiologic features of intraabdominal diseases are shown to be easily identified, expanding the practical application of the term "pattern recognition." It certainly is of practical value in daily clinical experience and will be of considerable help for further advances.

The traditional *dissectional* method of learning anatomy disturbs the intimate relationships of structures. The *sectional* anatomy presented in this book is the framework for understanding the findings in conventional radiology—in plain films and routine contrast studies—as well as in ultrasonography and computed tomography of the abdomen.

This is not just a review of others' experiences, but a crystallization of the author's contributions over the past several years. Dr. Meyers' concept of dynamic circulation within the peritoneal cavity is a breakthrough in our understanding of the spread of intraabdominal disease, particularly abscesses and malignancies. Peritoneography, the opacification of the largest lumen in the body, offers a potential yield of vast diagnostic information. The precise definition of the three extraperitoneal spaces represents a charting of previously unexplored territory. Awareness of the renointestinal and duodenocolic relationships, the spread of pancreatitis along mesenteric planes, and the pathways of extrapelvic spread of disease again underscores the practical importance of anatomic features. The approach to the mesenteric and antimesenteric borders of the small bowel and to the haustral pattern of the colon adds a new dimension to the interpretation of abdominal radiology.

This book confirms Dr. Meyers' reputation as one of the authorities in normal and pathologic radiologic anatomy of the abdomen.

1976

RICHARD H. MARSHAK, M.D.
Clinical Professor of Radiology
Mount Sinai School of Medicine
New York City

# Foreword to First Edition

Dr. Morton A. Meyers indeed has developed a dynamic text relating to radiologic aspects of abdominal disease. But this statement, with its emphasis on radiology, is misleading. This book is an important reading source for surgeons. Dr. Meyers' observations have not been confined to those arising from a purely radiologic study of the abdomen. The inclusion of observations based on injection studies both in the cadaver and *in vivo* has given this work a noteworthy comprehensiveness.

The insights provided by both the atlas of full-page color anatomic cross sections of the abdomen and pelvis and the excellent anatomic–radiologic correlations found in the text make the book indispensable. The atlas establishes the basis for intimate anatomic relationships which are then applied to the practical areas of clinical diagnosis and treatment of intraabdominal pathology. Presentations of these diagnostic and therapeutic considerations are enhanced by illustrated discussions relative to the new techniques of ultrasonography and computed tomography.

Dr. Meyers' presentation of this timely information is valuable, but what makes this book invaluable is the vast personal experience he is able to bring to it. This is not "just another" book purporting to give us something *new* in this important field. I believe the special approach given to this subject by Dr. Meyers is truly innovative. The radiologist and surgeon looking for the latest techniques in angiography for the diagnosis and treatment of massive bleeding from the gastrointestinal tract will not find it here. What they will find is major help in the understanding of, and indeed, therapeutic approach to a number of common intraabdominal problems, including infection and malignancy.

1976

LLOYD M. NYHUS, M.D., F.A.C.S.
Warren H. Cole Professor
and Chairman, Department of Surgery
The Abraham Lincoln School of Medicine
University of Illinois at the Medical Center
Chicago, Illinois

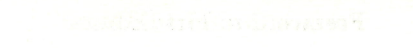

# Preface to Third Edition

The clinical insights and rational system of diagnostic analysis stimulated by an appreciation of the dynamic intraabdominal relationships outlined in previous editions of *Dynamic Radiology of the Abdomen: Normal and Pathologic Anatomy* have been universally adopted. Spanish and Japanese editions have encouraged more widespread applications of the principles which in turn have led to further contributions to our understanding of the features of spread and localization of intraabdominal diseases.

The basic aims in writing this book have not changed from those cited in the Preface to the First Edition. To satisfy these aims, special attention has been given to updating and revision with the addition of new material covering advances in the six years since the publication of the Second Edition. This edition contains over 230 new illustrations. Some nonessential material has been eliminated and several illustrations have been judiciously rearranged. Many of the Second Edition's illustrations have been replaced with better images and improved line drawings. The presentation of new material is amply supported by highly selected images, including particularly computed tomography (CT) and a few relevant magnetic resonance images. As in previous editions, although a few of the illustrations may not be of the very highest quality, the reader will understand they have been carefully selected for the particular abnormality or dynamic principle demonstrated.

Advances in appreciation of normal anatomic relationships and variants include the lobar anatomy of the liver, the structural relationships of the porta hepatis and its contents, and the developmental distortion of the adrenal glands in association with certain renal anomalies.

Developments in understanding the intraperitoneal spread of infections include the CT anatomy of the lesser sac, ligamentous demarcations of subphrenic abscesses, and the spread of abscesses following surgical transection of anatomic ligamentous barriers. Concepts of the pathways of dissemination of malignancies have been highly expanded by identification of the peritoneal ligaments and mesenteries as avenues for direct spread; indeed as bridging structures between what has been conventionally thought of as extraperitoneal and intraperitoneal tissues, these lead to a unifying concept of the subperitoneal space of the abdomen. Further advances in the understanding of the intraperitoneal spread of malignancies include the illumination of seeded perihepatic and subdiaphragmatic metastases and of certain aspects of lymphatic permeation.

Numerous major developments have also refined our precise evaluation of the extraperitoneal fascia and spaces. Among these are further discrete identification of the landmarks and insertions of the renal fascia and their anatomic demarcation of spaces; the appearance and causes of thickening of the renal fascia; the composition of the posterior renal fascia into two layers and the consequences of pancreatitis with its extension to produce the Grey-Turner sign; bridging renal septa; further features of spread through the anterior pararenal space; CT features of uriniferous perirenal pseudocyst; and rupture of abdominal aortic aneurysms.

The references have been considerably expanded and yet carefully selected, citing both classic articles and recent contributions. A lengthy index with cross-references provides immediate access to the detailed material presented.

Many persons have contributed importantly to the Third Edition and I thank them sincerely. I wish to express my particular appreciation to Michael Oliphant, M.D. and Alfred S. Berne, M.D., Crouse-Irving Memorial Hospital, State University of New York, Syracuse, New York and to Michiel Feldberg, M.D., Ph.D., of the University of Utrecht, The Netherlands. They have offered selfless cooperation and the stimulating pleasure of sharing intellectual enthusiasms. I submit this third manuscript to Springer-Verlag, confident that their skills will produce another edition of high technical quality.

1988                                                          MORTON A. MEYERS, M.D.

# Preface to First Edition

This book provides a systematic application of anatomic and dynamic principles to the practical understanding and diagnosis of intraabdominal diseases. Anatomic sections and injection studies form a basis for understanding the characteristic features of many common and uncommon diseases and their spread and localization in the abdomen. These relationships and specific criteria provide a rational system for accurate radiologic analysis in plain films, conventional contrast studies, ultrasonography, and computed tomography (CT). This information leads to the uncovering of clinically deceptive diseases, the evaluation of the effects of disease, the anticipation of complications, and the determination of the appropriate diagnostic and therapeutic approaches.

The introductory atlas presents full-color anatomic cross-sections of the abdomen and pelvis, complemented by labeled tracings, and detailed CT scans at corresponding levels. The sections, which are approximately 3.8 cm (1.5 in.) thick, were obtained from fresh cadavers frozen in dry ice for 48 hours, in order to maintain the true intimate anatomic relationships. The accompanying text of the atlas stresses normal gross relationships, common variants, and the basis of their radiologic identification, particularly in plain films. The subsequent chapters deal with the diagnosis and the pathways of spread of infection, malignancies, and traumatic and inflammatory effusions within the intra- and extraperitoneal spaces. Emphasis is placed on the specific localizing features based on the anatomic planes and recesses and the dynamics of extension of disease. Sagittal and coronal as well as horizontal anatomic sections support the findings in conventional radiologic procedures, ultrasonography, and computed tomography throughout. Correlation with the clinical findings and management underscores the value of the radiologic observations. Diagnostic criteria which are easily applied are established for the characteristic features of specific disease processes ranging from localized abscesses to disseminated metastases.

Many of the insights detailed in this book have been made only in the past few years. The application of peritoneography as a clinical diagnostic study, for example, first indicated the dynamic circulation of fluid states within the peritoneal recesses and permitted an insight into the spread of infection and malignancies. Similarly, the significance of the anatomic and radiologic definition of the extraperitoneal spaces, the small bowel mesentery and other peritoneal reflections, the haustral contours of the large intestine, and the contiguity of certain organ relationships has only recently been appreciated.

1976                                                        MORTON A. MEYERS, M.D.

# Contents

# Color Plates

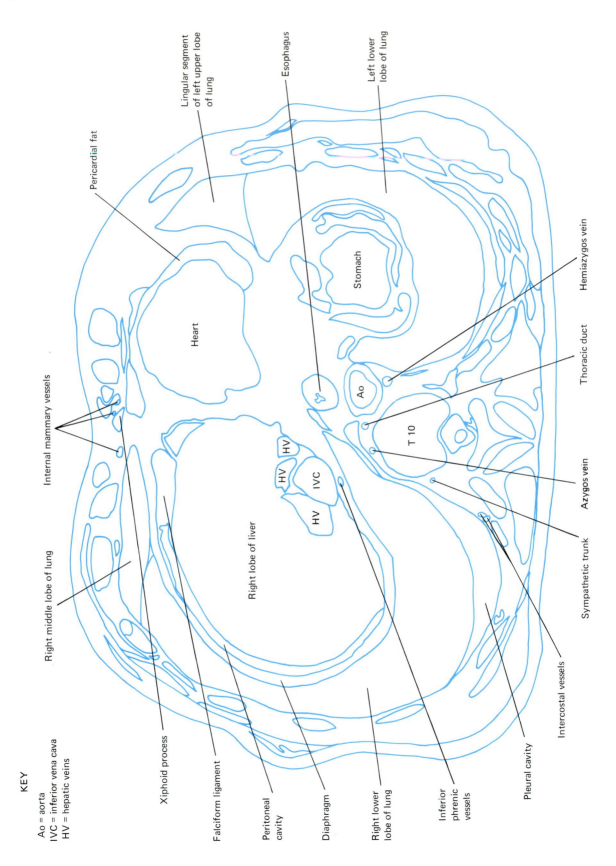

KEY

Ao = aorta
IVC = inferior vena cava
HV = hepatic veins

Pericardial fat

Lingular segment
of left upper lobe
of lung

Esophagus

Left lower
lobe of lung

Hemiazygos vein

Thoracic duct

Stomach

Heart

Ao

T 10

Azygos vein

Internal mammary vessels

HV
HV

HV
IVC

Right lobe of liver

Sympathetic trunk

Right middle lobe of lung

Intercostal vessels

Xiphoid process

Falciform ligament

Peritoneal
cavity

Diaphragm

Right lower
lobe of lung

Inferior
phrenic
vessels

Pleural cavity

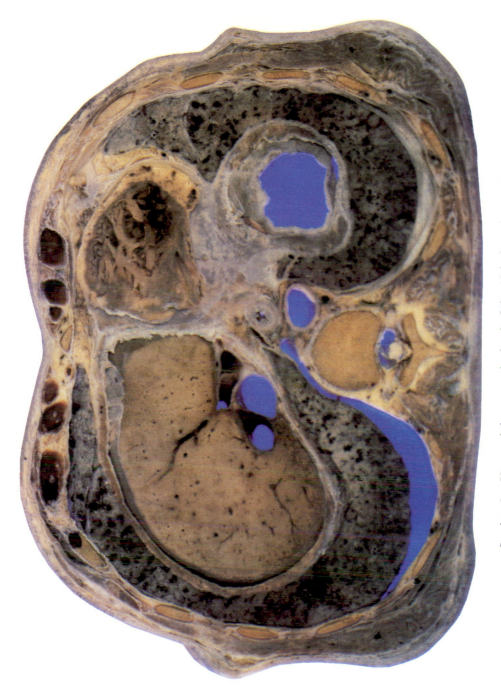

**Section 1.** Upper abdomen at the level of the 10th thoracic vertebra.

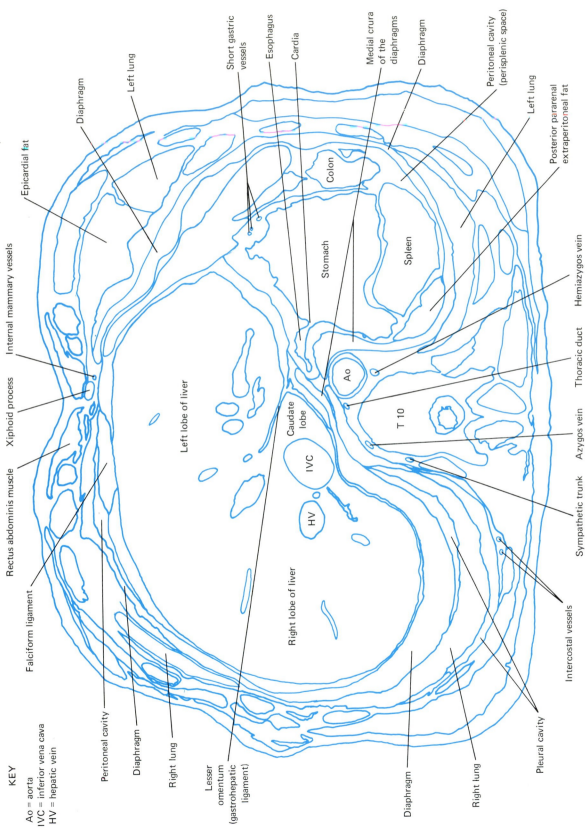

KEY

Ao = aorta
IVC = inferior vena cava
HV = hepatic vein

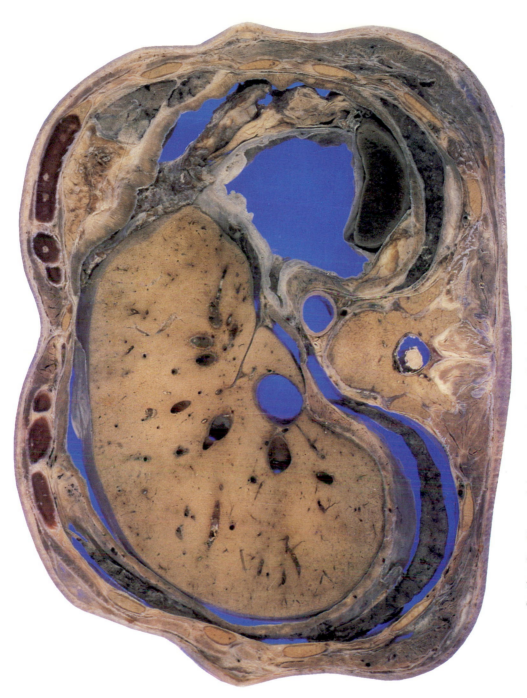

**Section 2.** Upper abdomen at the level of the lower border of the 10th thoracic vertebra.

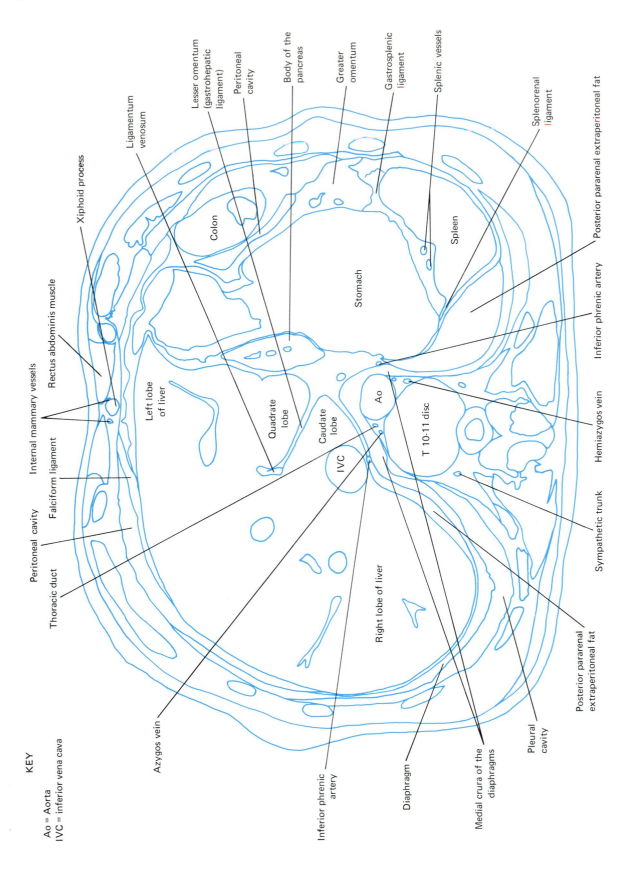

KEY

Ao = Aorta
IVC = inferior vena cava

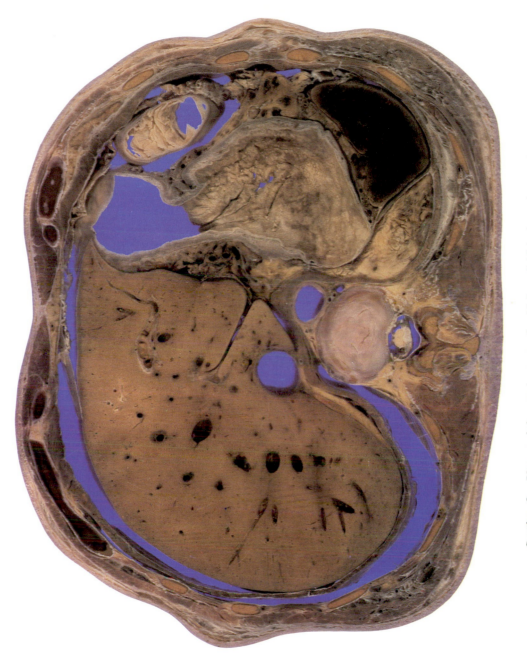

**Section 3.** Upper abdomen between the 10th and 11th thoracic vertebrae.

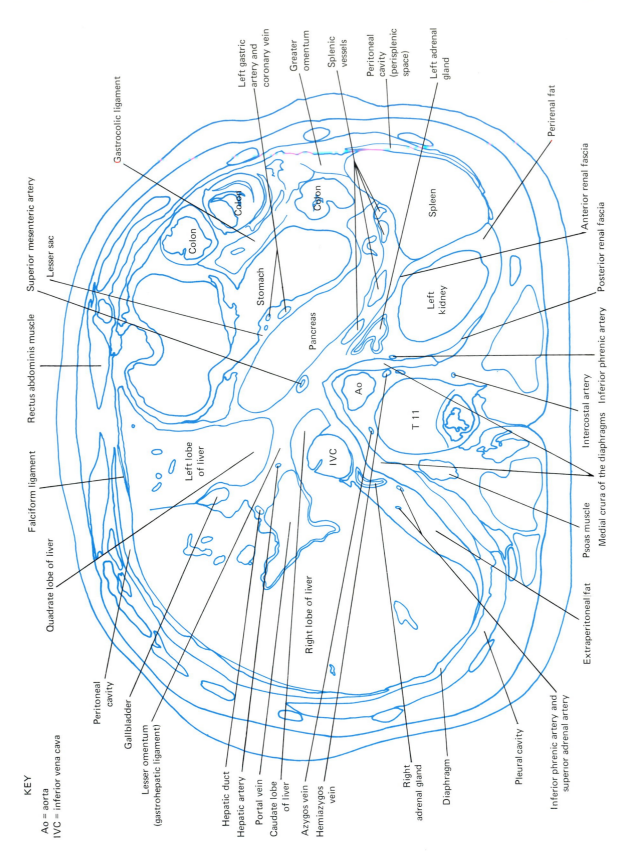

KEY

Ao = aorta
IVC = inferior vena cava

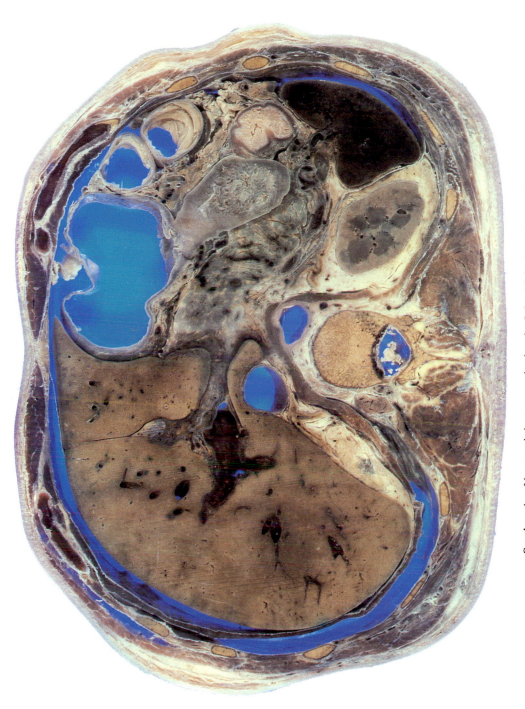

**Section 4.** Upper abdomen at the level of the 11th thoracic vertebra.

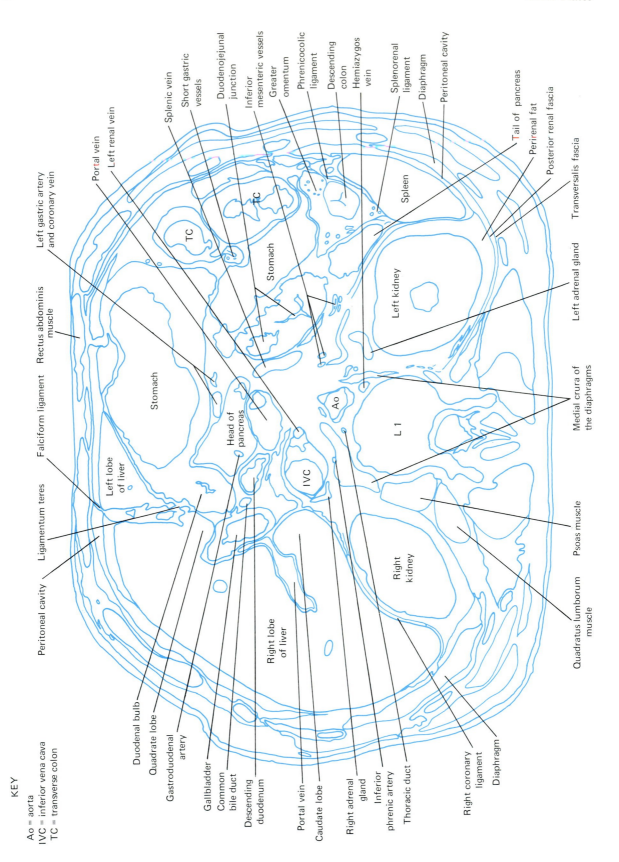

KEY

Ao = aorta
IVC = inferior vena cava
TC = transverse colon

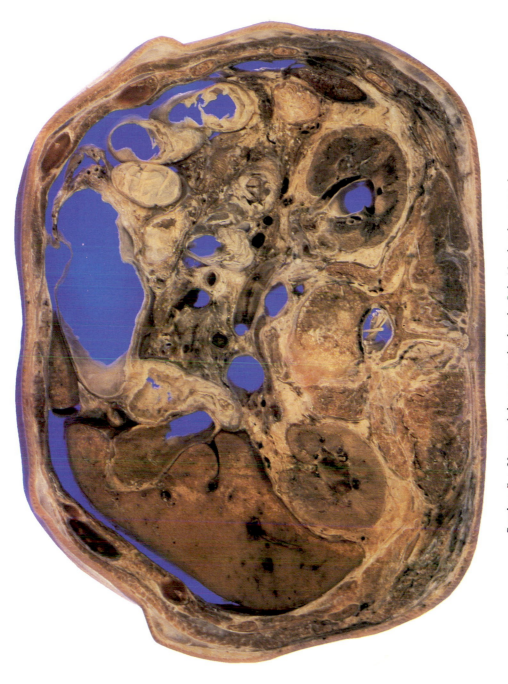

**Section 5.** Upper abdomen at the level of the 1st lumbar vertebra.

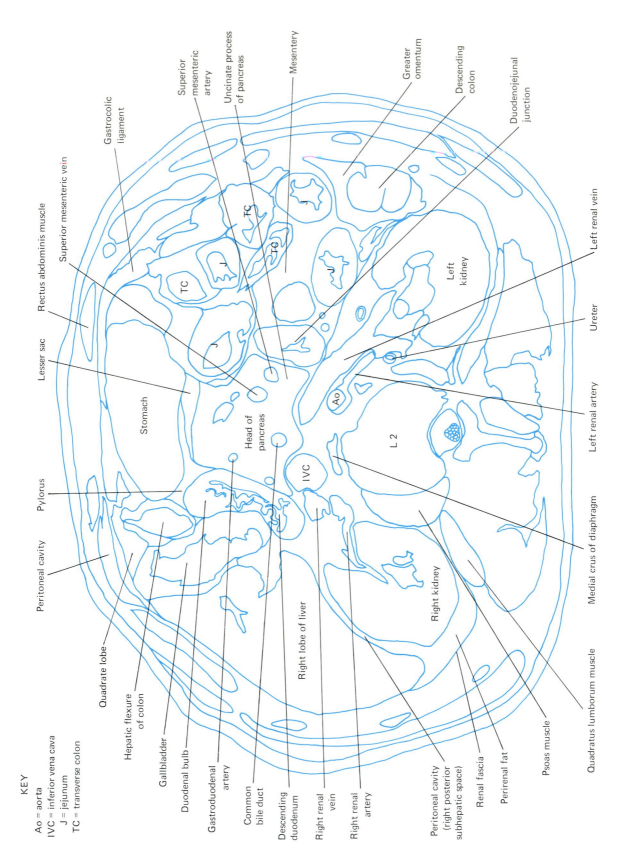

KEY

Ao = aorta
IVC = inferior vena cava
J = jejunum
TC = transverse colon

Gastrocolic ligament

Superior mesenteric artery

Uncinate process of pancreas

Mesentery

Greater omentum

Descending colon

Duodenojejunal junction

Rectus abdominis muscle

Superior mesenteric vein

Left renal vein

Lesser sac

Left kidney

Stomach

Ureter

Head of pancreas

Left renal artery

Ao

L 2

IVC

Peritoneal cavity

Pylorus

Medial crus of diaphragm

Quadrate lobe

Right lobe of liver

Right kidney

Hepatic flexure of colon

Gallbladder

Duodenal bulb

Gastroduodenal artery

Common bile duct

Descending duodenum

Right renal vein

Right renal artery

Peritoneal cavity (right posterior subhepatic space)

Renal fascia

Perirenal fat

Psoas muscle

Quadratus lumborum muscle

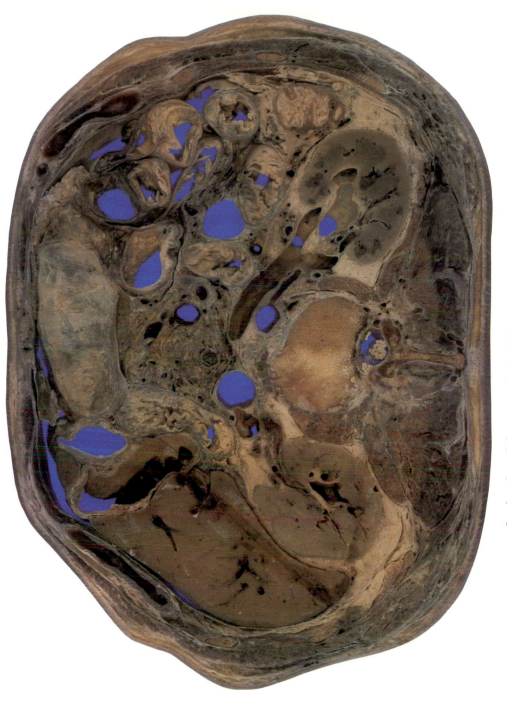

**Section 6.** Abdomen at the level of the 2nd lumbar vertebra.

KEY

IVC = inferior vena cava
Ao = aorta
TC = transverse colon
J = jejunum

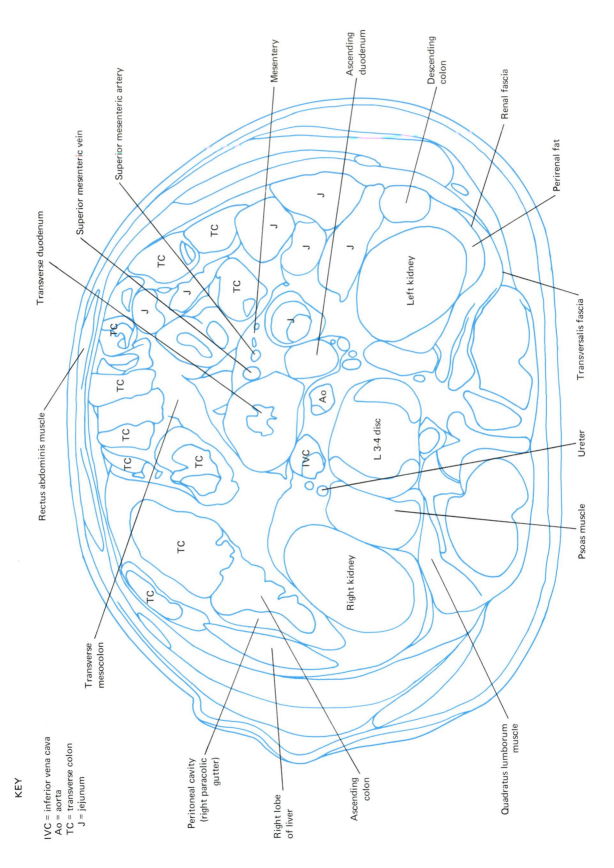

Mesentery

Ascending duodenum

Descending colon

Renal fascia

Perirenal fat

Superior mesenteric artery

Superior mesenteric vein

Transverse duodenum

Transversalis fascia

Rectus abdominis muscle

Ureter

Psoas muscle

Transverse mesocolon

Quadratus lumborum muscle

Peritoneal cavity (right paracolic gutter)

Right lobe of liver

Ascending colon

TC

J

J

J

J

J

J

J

J

TC

TC

TC

TC

TC

TC

TC

TC

TC

TC

TC

Left kidney

Ao

L 3-4 disc

IVC

Right kidney

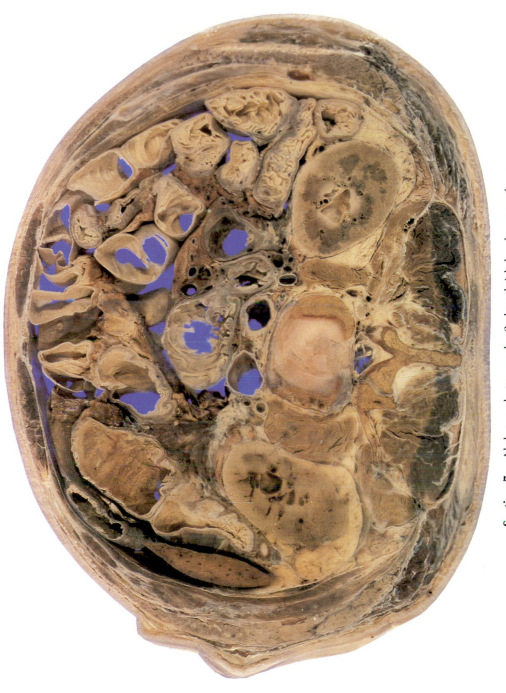

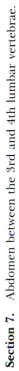

**Section 7.** Abdomen between the 3rd and 4th lumbar vertebrae.

KEY

Ao = aorta
IVC = inferior vena cava
J = jejunum
I = ileum
TC = transverse colon

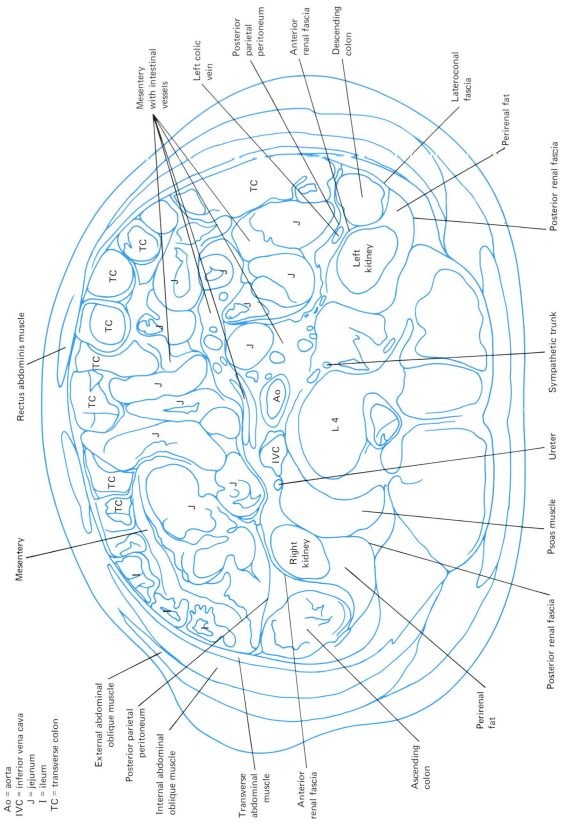

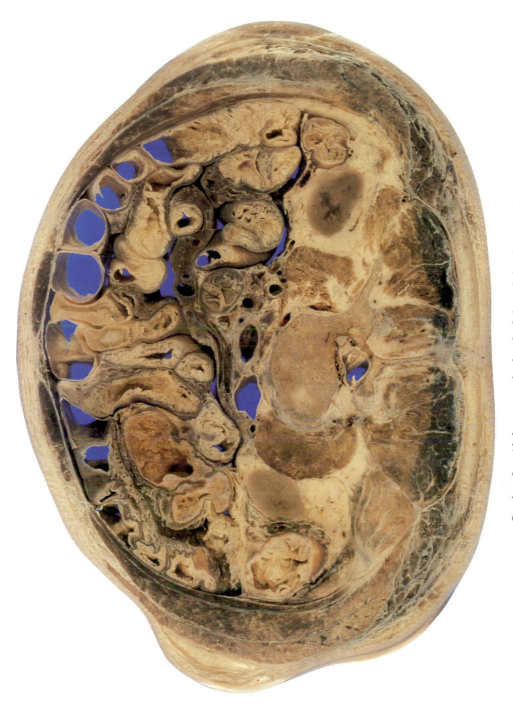

**Section 8.** Abdomen at the level of the 4th lumbar vertebra.

KEY

I = ileum
TC = transverse colon
SC = sigmoid colon

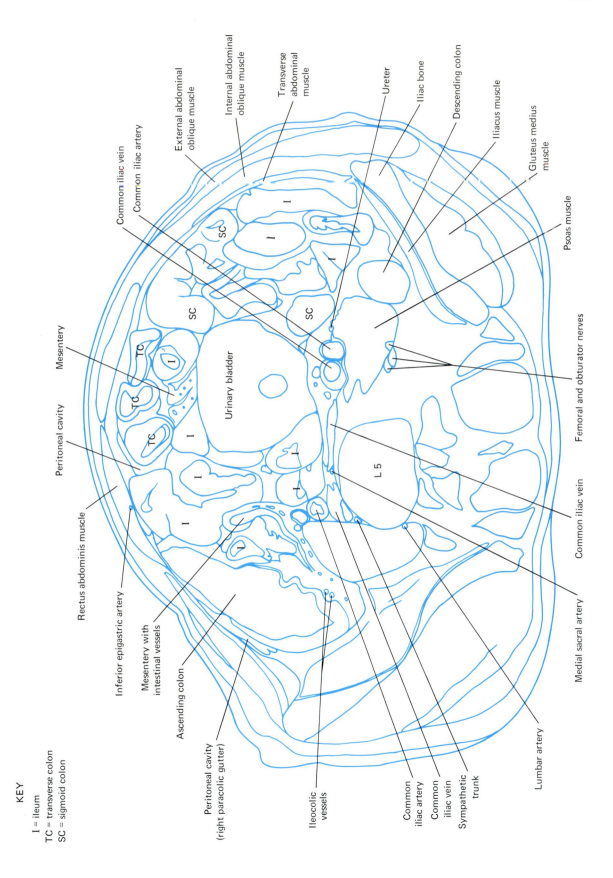

External abdominal oblique muscle

Internal abdominal oblique muscle

Transverse abdominal muscle

Ureter

Iliac bone

Descending colon

Iliacus muscle

Gluteus medius muscle

Common iliac vein

Common iliac artery

Psoas muscle

Mesentery

Peritoneal cavity

Femoral and obturator nerves

Urinary bladder

L 5

Common iliac vein

Rectus abdominis muscle

Medial sacral artery

Inferior epigastric artery

Mesentery with intestinal vessels

Ascending colon

Peritoneal cavity (right paracolic gutter)

Ileocolic vessels

Common iliac artery

Common iliac vein

Sympathetic trunk

Lumbar artery

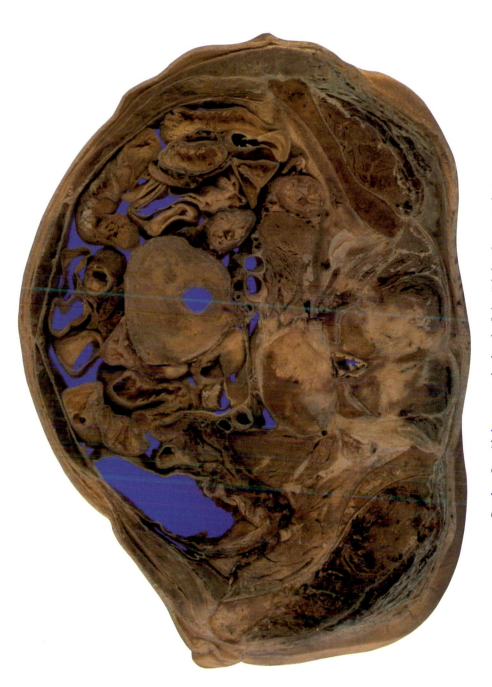

**Section 9.** Abdomen at the level of the 5th lumbar vertebra.

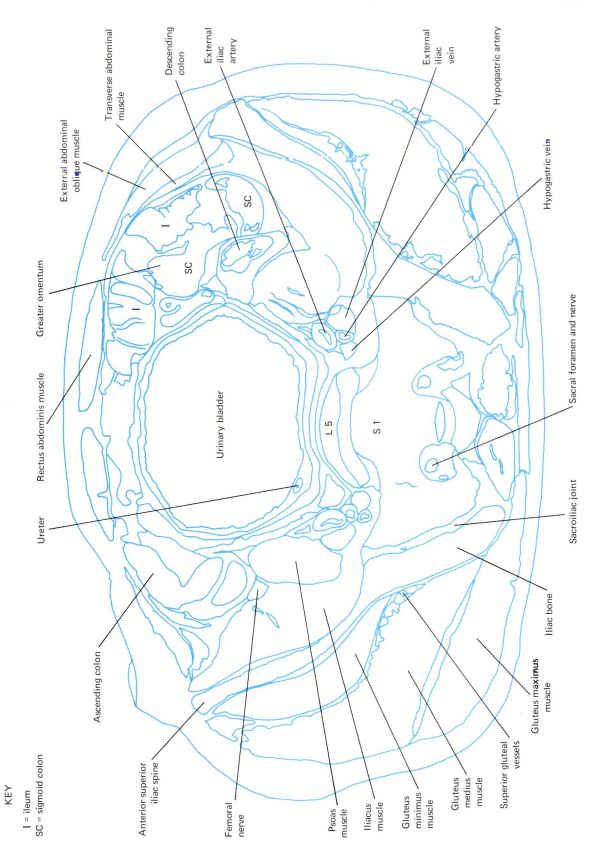

KEY

I = ileum
SC = sigmoid colon

External abdominal oblique muscle

Transverse abdominal muscle

Descending colon

External iliac artery

External iliac vein

Hypogastric artery

Hypogastric vein

Greater omentum

Rectus abdominis muscle

Ureter

Ascending colon

Anterior superior iliac spine

Femoral nerve

Psoas muscle

Iliacus muscle

Gluteus minimus muscle

Gluteus medius muscle

Superior gluteal vessels

Gluteus maximus muscle

Iliac bone

Sacroiliac joint

Sacral foramen and nerve

Urinary bladder

L 5

S 1

SC

SC

I

I

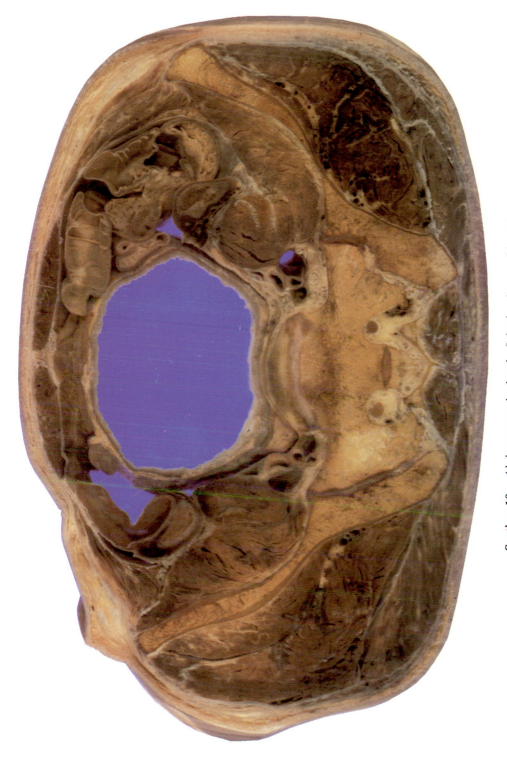

**Section 10.** Abdomen at the level of the lumbosacral junction.

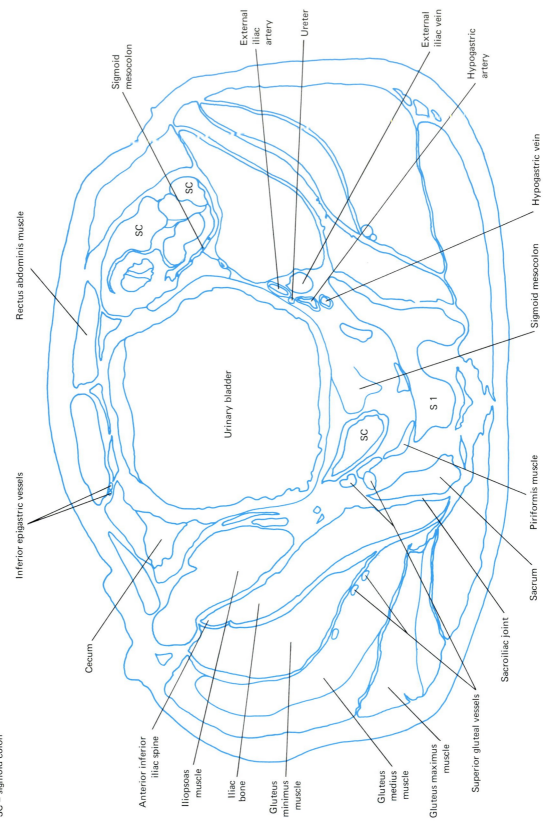

KEY

SC = sigmoid colon

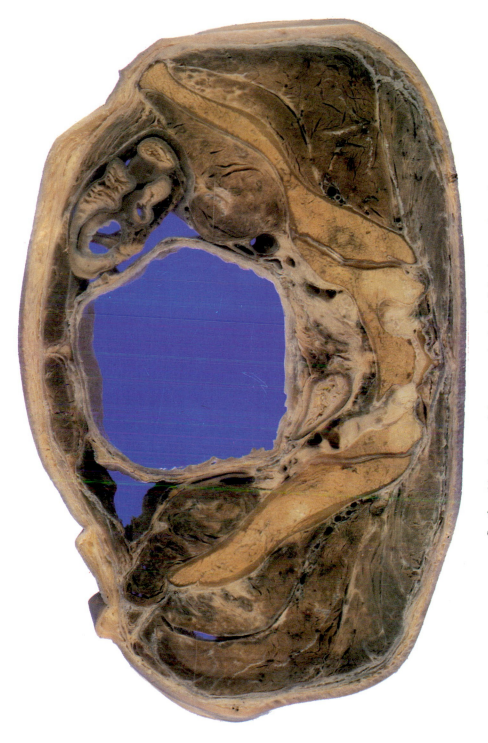

**Section 11.** Lower abdomen at the level of the 1st sacral vertebra.

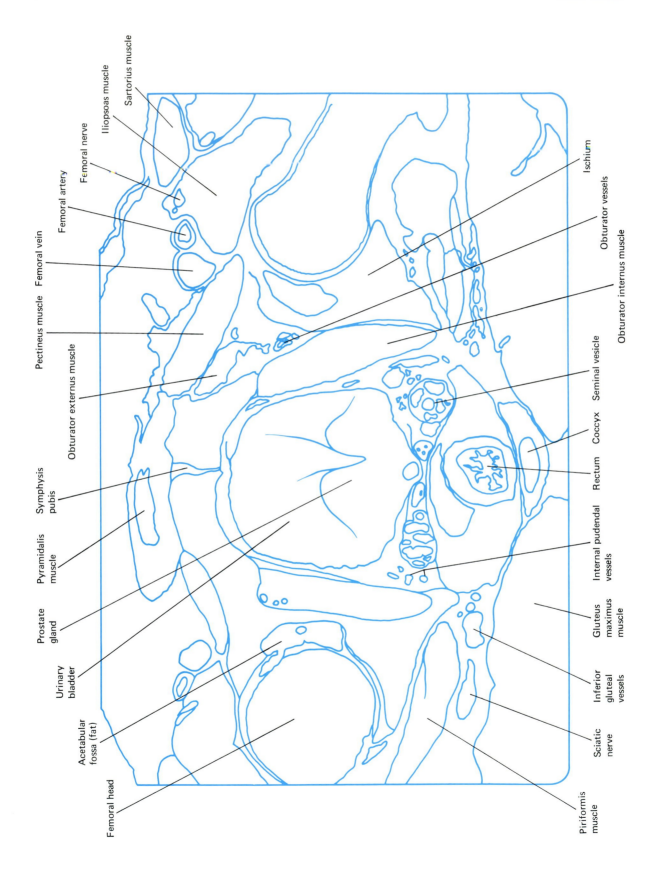

Sartorius muscle

Iliopsoas muscle

Femoral nerve

Femoral artery

Femoral vein

Pectineus muscle

Obturator externus muscle

Symphysis pubis

Pyramidalis muscle

Prostate gland

Urinary bladder

Acetabular fossa (fat)

Femoral head

Ischium

Obturator vessels

Obturator internus muscle

Seminal vesicle

Coccyx

Rectum

Internal pudendal vessels

Gluteus maximus muscle

Inferior gluteal vessels

Sciatic nerve

Piriformis muscle

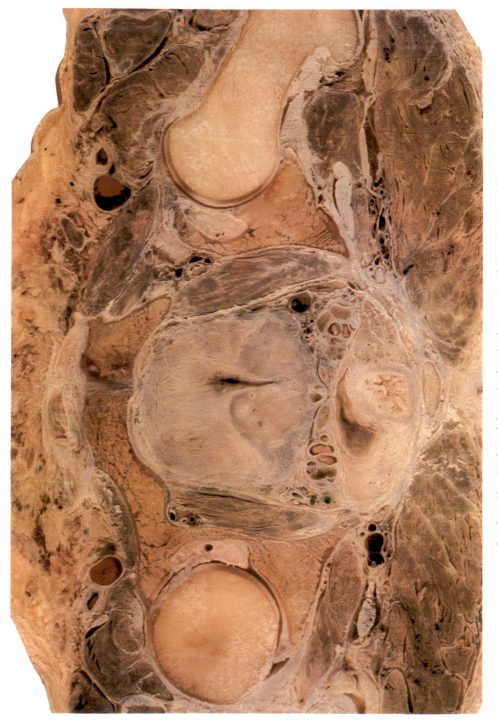

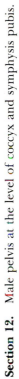

**Section 12.** Male pelvis at the level of coccyx and symphysis pubis.

# 1 Normal Anatomic Relationships and Variants

## General Introduction

A basic knowledge of normal anatomic relationships and variants is essential to understanding the effects of pathologic processes. Fundamental considerations include constant anatomic landmarks, variations in positions of structures, relationships maintained and bounded by peritoneal and fascial attachments, distribution of intra- and extraperitoneal fat providing the contrasting interfaces of organ and viscus contours, and governance of the configuration of the hollow viscera by specific anatomic characteristics and general physical laws.

Figure 1–1 illustrates that the image one first sees is determined by the relationship established between individual features.[1] In a similar manner, clinical and radiologic diagnosis is based on the extraction of a set of features characteristic of a particular process. Deviation from the normal, however, must be recognized before a lesion can be suspected.

Figure 1–2 and 1–3 and the atlas in color of transverse anatomic sections included in this chapter (pp. 1–25) provide a detailed overview of the complex anatomic relationships within the abdomen. The accompanying text and illustrations further stress normal radiographic features. Cadavers, frozen in dry ice for 48 hours, were sectioned into horizontal slices approximately 3.8 cm (1.5 in.) thick with a band saw (Sections 1 through 12). Tracings of the anatomic sections, appropriately labeled, are included to facilitate identification. The clarity of the features demonstrated in the anatomic sections readily provide correlation with the structures now identifiable by computed tomography.

## The Diaphragm

Whereas the peripheral portion of the diaphragm consists of muscle fibers, the central portion is tendinous.

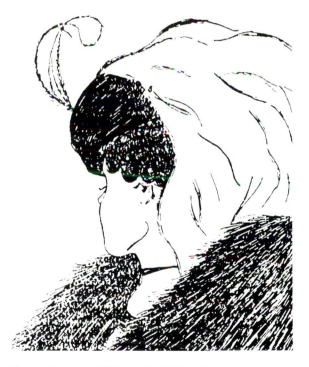

**Fig. 1–1. W. E. Hill's "My Wife and My Mother-in-law."**
Both images are present in the drawing. The viewer first sees either an old woman or a young lady. The old woman's prominent nose in profile is the young woman's chin. This drawing illustrates that perception is determined by the relationships.

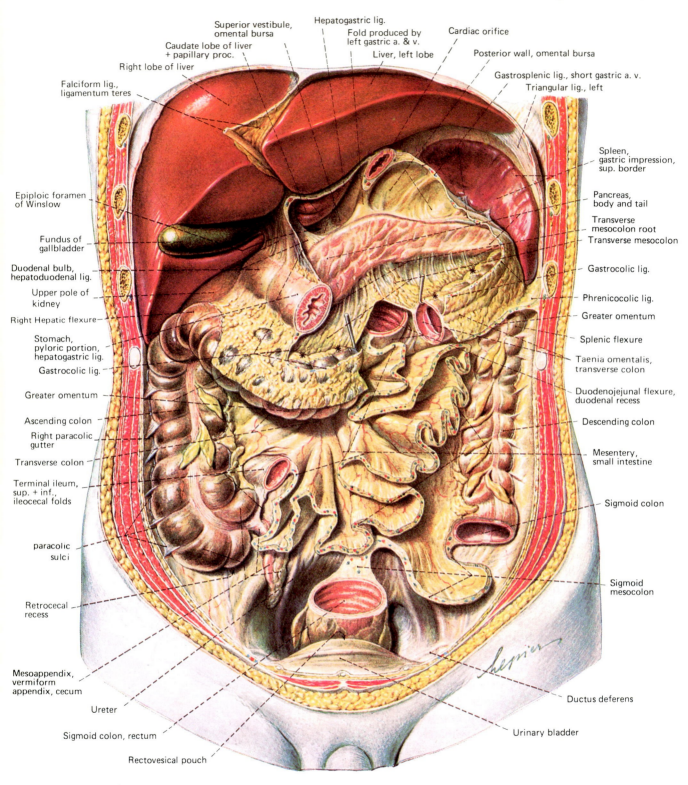

**Fig. 1—2. Abdominal viscera.**
The stomach has been removed from the cardia to the pylorus, revealing the lesser sac (omental bursa) and structures on the posterior wall. (From Sobotta, Courtesy of Urban & Schwarzenberg)

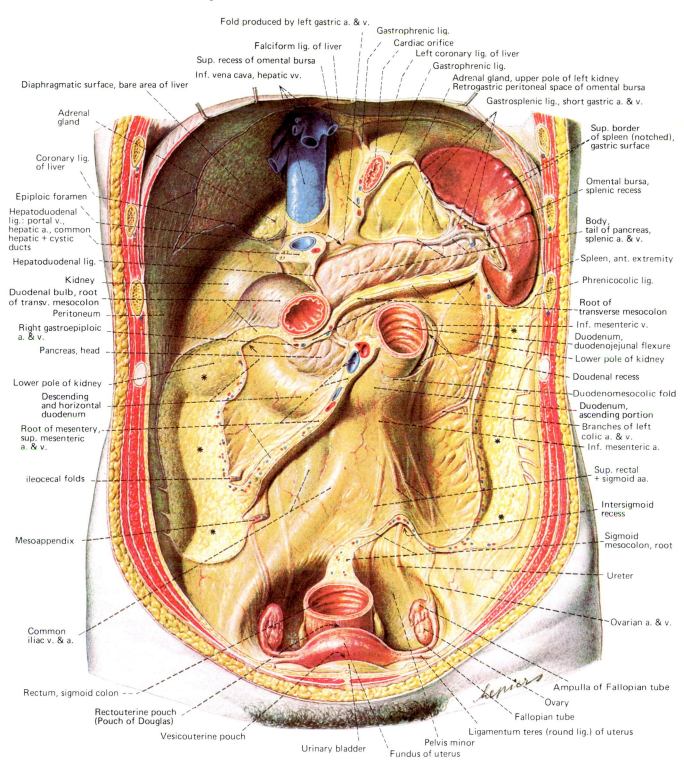

Fold produced by left gastric a. & v.
Gastrophrenic lig.
Falciform lig. of liver
Cardiac orifice
Sup. recess of omental bursa
Left coronary lig. of liver
Inf. vena cava, hepatic vv.
Gastrophrenic lig.
Adrenal gland, upper pole of left kidney
Retrogastric peritoneal space of omental bursa
Diaphragmatic surface, bare area of liver
Gastrosplenic lig., short gastric a. & v.
Adrenal gland
Sup. border of spleen (notched), gastric surface
Coronary lig. of liver
Omental bursa, splenic recess
Epiploic foramen
Hepatoduodenal lig.: portal v., hepatic a., common hepatic + cystic ducts
Body, tail of pancreas, splenic a. & v.
Hepatoduodenal lig.
Spleen, ant. extremity
Kidney
Phrenicocolic lig.
Duodenal bulb, root of transv. mesocolon
Root of transverse mesocolon
Peritoneum
Inf. mesenteric v.
Right gastroepiploic a. & v.
Duodenum, duodenojejunal flexure
Pancreas, head
Lower pole of kidney
Lower pole of kidney
Doudenal recess
Descending and horizontal duodenum
Duodenomesocolic fold
Duodenum, ascending portion
Root of mesentery, sup. mesenteric a. & v.
Branches of left colic a. & v.
Inf. mesenteric a.
ileocecal folds
Sup. rectal + sigmoid aa.
Intersigmoid recess
Mesoappendix
Sigmoid mesocolon, root
Ureter
Common iliac v. & a.
Ovarian a. & v.
Ampulla of Fallopian tube
Rectum, sigmoid colon
Ovary
Rectouterine pouch (Pouch of Douglas)
Fallopian tube
Vesicouterine pouch
Ligamentum teres (round lig.) of uterus
Pelvis minor
Urinary bladder
Fundus of uterus

**Fig. 1–3. Retroperitoneum of an adult female.**
(From Sobotta, Courtesy of Urban & Schwarzenberg)

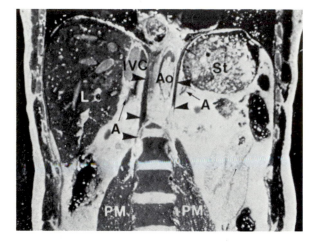

**Fig. 1-4. Coronal section showing relationships of aorta to diaphragm.**
The aortic hiatus is behind the diaphragm and then the aorta (Ao) passes into the abdomen surrounded by the diaphragmatic crura (arrowheads). Note the relationships of the crura to the psoas muscles (PM) and that the right crus descends lower than the left. IVC = inferior vena cava, L = liver, St = stomach, A = adrenal gland. (Courtesy of Manual Viamonte, Jr, MD, Mt. Sinai Hospital, Miami Beach, Fla.)

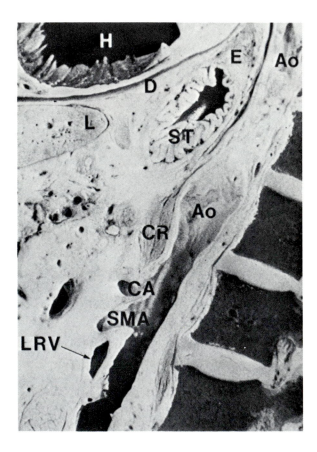

There are three large openings in the diaphragm. The aortic hiatus is not strictly an apperture, because the aorta passes posterior to the diaphragm and is surrounded by the crura (Figs. 1–4 and 1–5). The esophageal hiatus is located in the muscular portion of the diaphragm at the level of T10. The vena caval opening is situated in the tendinous portion at the level of T8.

The medial lumbocostal arch surrounds the psoas major muscle and the lateral lumbocostal arch surrounds the quadratus lumborum muscle. The two crura are tendinous; the right crus extends approximately to L3, and the left extends approximately to L2[2] (Figs. 1–4 and 1–6).

# The Liver

The lobar anatomy of the liver in many textbooks and atlases is based on the external configuration and divides the liver classically into four lobes: right, left, quadrate, and caudate. However, surgical considerations dictate that lobar divisions should be based on ductal and vascular anatomy.[3–7]

The *true* right lobe lies to the right of a plane through the fossa of the gallbladder and the sulcus of the inferior vena cava. The *true* left hepatic lobe lies to the left of the plane, and includes the quadrate and left "lobes"; the quadrate lobe, between the fossa of the gallbladder and the ligamentum teres, represents the medial segment of the left lobe of the liver, whereas what has been referred to in the past as the left "lobe" in fact represents the lateral segment of the true left hepatic lobe[3,4] (Fig. 1–7). The two lobes are separated from each other by the porta hepatis. The caudate lobe, located between the fossa of the inferior vena cava and the ligamentum venosum, cannot be included en-

◁—————————————————————

**Fig. 1–5. Left parasagittal section showing relationships of aorta to diaphragm.**
The aorta (Ao) passes posterior to the diaphragm (D) behind the esophagus (E), seen here entering the stomach (ST). In its upper portion, the abdominal aorta is surrounded by the diaphragmatic crura (CR) which descend and join each other just above the origin of the celiac axis (CA). H = heart, L = left lobe of liver, SMA = superior mesenteric artery, LRV = left renal vein.

**Fig. 1–6. Diaphragmatic crura shown in coronal plane by magnetic resonance imaging.**
Note the relationships of the crura (arrowheads) to the lumbar vertebral bodies and psoas muscles (PM).

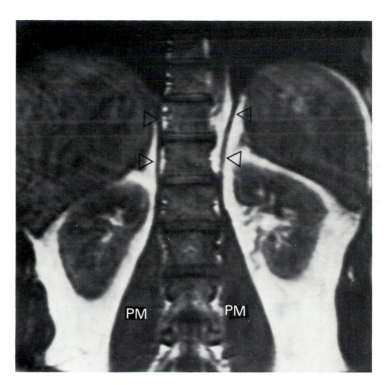

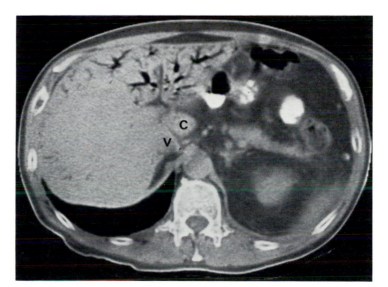

**Fig. 1–7. Anatomic division of left lobe of liver.**
On computed tomography, air in the portal venous system has risen into the medial (quadrate lobe) and lateral segments of the left lobe of the liver. C = caudate lobe, V = inferior vena cava.

tirely in either true hepatic lobe; although highly variable, its vascular and ductal supply most frequently come from both the right and left lobar systems.[3]

Figure 1–8 illustrates the lobar anatomy of the liver as indicated by its ligaments and fissures. Fat associated with the ligamentum teres may be identifiable on plain films[8] (Figs. 1–9 and 1–10).

The *right lobe* is much larger than the left and extends from its domed surface near the diaphragm to its inferior visceral surface which faces posteriorly and has complex relationships to several intraperitoneal and extraperitoneal structures. The anterior third of the inferior surface of the right lobe is indented by the hepatic flexure of the colon. A fossa for the right kidney lies posterior to the colonic impression.

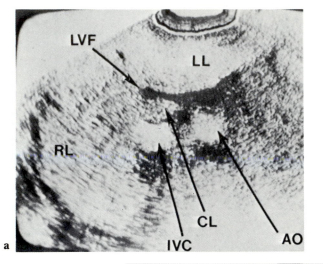

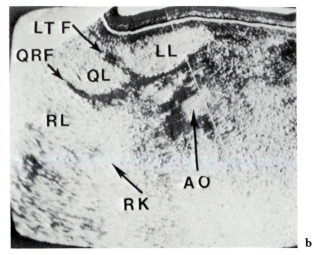

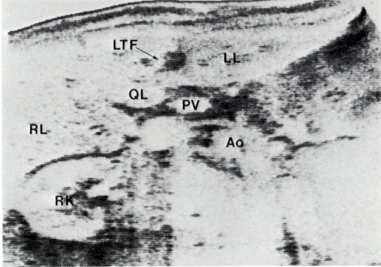

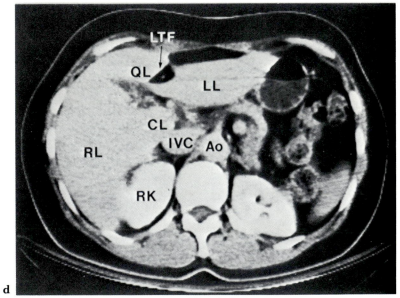

**Fig. 1–8**

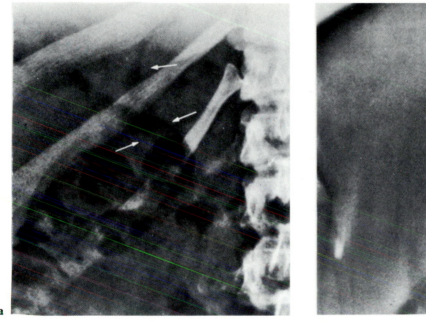

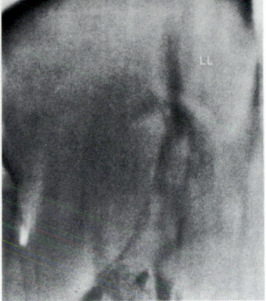

a                                                                          b

**Fig. 1–9. Plain film identification of ligamentum teres.**
**(a)** Plain film. Fatty radiolucent streaks (arrows) project within the liver shadow.
**(b)** Intravenous cholangiogram. The lucent shadows are distinct from the common hepatic and common bile ducts. The medial one outlines a portion of the left lobe (LL) of the liver.

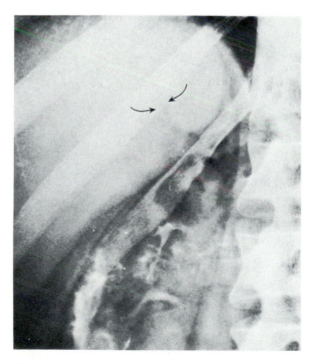

◁————————————————————————

**Fig. 1–8. Ligaments and fissures of the liver.**
**(a)** Transverse sonogram demonstrates the fissure for the ligamentum venosum (LVF) separating the left lobe (LL) from the caudate lobe (CL) which is situated just anterior to the inferior vena cava (IVC). RL = right lobe, Ao = aorta. (From Parulekar SG: Ligaments and fissures of the liver: Sonographic anatomy. Radiology 130: 409–411, 1979)
**(b)** The fissure for the ligamentum teres (LTF) separates the left lobe (LL) from the quadrate lobe (QL) which in turn is separated by a fissure (QRF) from the right lobe (RL). Ao = aorta, RK = right kidney. (Courtesy of SG Parulekar, MBBS, Mt. Sinai Hospital, Cleveland, Ohio)
**(c and d)** Sonogram and CT in two different patients show the ligamentum teres within its fissure separating the lateral segment of the left lobe (LL) from the quadrate lobe (QL). Note that in the CT scan the umbilical vein can be seen within the ligamentum teres. CL = caudate lobe, RL = right lobe, Ao = aorta, IVC = inferior vena cava, PV = portal vein, RK = right kidney.

**Fig. 1–10. Plain film identification of ligamentum teres.**
Lucent fat within its fissures identifies the position of the ligamentum teres (arrows), separating the medial and lateral segments of the left lobe of the liver.

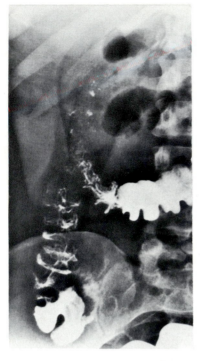
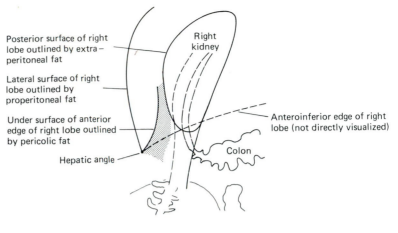

Posterior surface of right
lobe outlined by extra –
peritoneal fat

Right
kidney

Lateral surface of right
lobe outlined by
properitoneal fat

Under surface of anterior
edge of right lobe outlined
by pericolic fat

Anteroinferior edge of right
lobe (not directly visualized)

Hepatic angle

Colon

Fig. 1–11. Plain film visualization of the liver as determined by anatomic relationships.

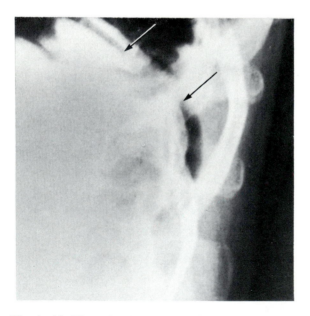

Fig. 1–12. The reflections of the right coronary ligament (arrows) suspending the right lobe of the liver are outlined by free intraperitoneal air in the lateral view.
The inferior leaf is at the level of the 12th rib. The nonperitonealized bare area of the posterior surface of the right lobe lies between the reflections of the ligament.

The gallbladder lies just under the anterior-inferior edge of the liver. Medial to the gallbladder lie the first and second portions of the duodenum. The gallbladder cannot be seen on plain films because it is not invested by or adjacent to any significant adipose tissue, but its position may be inferred from the gas-containing hepatic flexure or duodenal bulb.

The *quadrate lobe,* the segment between the gallbladder fossa and the ligamentum teres, is in relation to the pyloric end of the stomach, the superior portion of the duodenum, and the transverse colon.

The *caudate lobe* posteriorly lodges the inferior vena cava against the bare area of the liver. A process of the caudate lobe forms the upper border of the epiploic foramen of Winslow and thus faces the superior recess of the lesser sac.

A common variant in females is a Riedel's lobe, a conspicuous inferior tonguelike extension of the right lobe of the liver. Normally, the lower edge of the right lobe of the liver does not cross the right psoas margin or extend below the iliac crest.

The nature of plain film visualization of the shadow of the liver's lower edge appears to be dependent on body habitus and the interfaces presented to the roentgen beam,[9] but the ana-

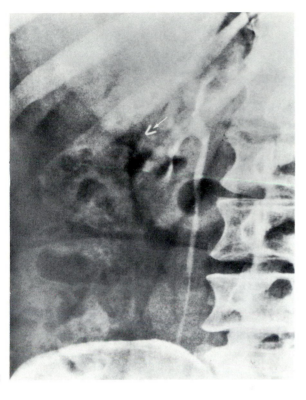

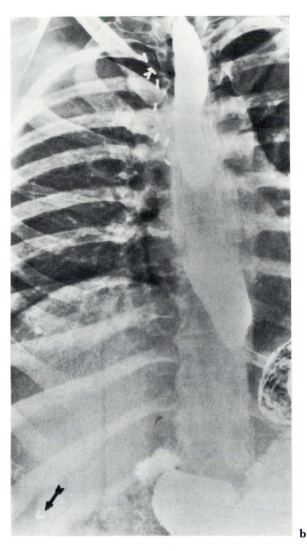

**Fig. 1–13. The inferior extent of the right pleural space in relationship to the abdominal viscera.**
This is shown by the presence of a surgical clip (arrow) which has gravitated to the posterior costophrenic sulcus following an intrathoracic operation.
**(a)** Intravenous urogram, oblique view.
**(b)** Upper GI series, prone view.

tomic relationships of the right lobe of the liver in the main determine the image. These are illustrated in Figure 1–11. The anteroinferior edge of the liver, which can be clinically palpated, is generally not directly visualized radiographically but only indirectly by its known relationship to the hepatic flexure of the colon. Occasionally, sufficient omental and pericolic fat may exist to outline it only along its lateral margin.[9] The posterior aspect of the right lobe, in relationship to the kidney, and the hepatic angle abut the extraperitoneal adipose tissue, accounting for visualization of their contours which present as a soft tissue–fat interface.[10] The peritoneal cavity extends between the right kidney and the visceral surface of the right lobe of the liver as the hepatorenal fossa (right posterior subhepatic space, or Morison's pouch). The

posterior parietal peritoneum reflects to form the right coronary ligament which suspends the liver intraperitoneally (Fig. 1–12).

It is important to recognize that the pleural cavity posteriorly extends downward to come into relationship with the bare area of the liver, the upper portion of the right kidney, and the posterior subhepatic space (Fig. 1–13). Although the pleura extends in front as low as the seventh costal cartilage, posteriorly the costophrenic sulcus reaches as low as the twelfth rib and at times even to the transverse process of L1.

The *porta hepatis* separates the quadrate lobe in front from the caudate lobe and process behind. It transmits the portal vein, the hepatic artery, and the hepatic duct.[11] The vascular and ductal structures of the liver course within the

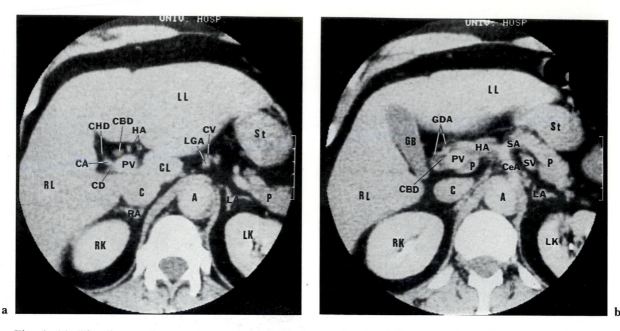

**Fig. 1–14. The three primary components of the hepatoduodenal ligament shown by computed tomography.**

**(a)** At the level of the porta hepatis, the common bile duct (CBD) is anterolateral, the hepatic artery (HA) anteromedial, and the portal vein (PV) posterior. CHD = common bile duct, CD = cystic duct, CA = cystic artery, RL = right liver lobe, LL = left liver lobe, CL = caudate lobe, A = aorta, C = inferior vena cava, RK = right kidney, LK = left kidney, RA = right adrenal, LA = left adrenal, P = pancreas, St = stomach, LGA = left gastric artery, CV = coronary vein.

**(b)** More caudally, the common bile duct has assumed a more posterior relationship. GB = gallbladder, GDA = gastroduodenal artery, CeA = celiac artery, SA = splenic artery, SV = splenic vein.

free edge of the lesser omentum. The portal vein is normally the largest structure and runs posteriorly in the hepatoduodenal ligament. The common hepatic or common bile duct lies in the anterior lateral aspect of the ligament, and the hepatic artery lies in the anterior medial region of the ligament (Fig. 1–14). A fibrofatty sheath of tissue invaginates the liver parenchyma from the porta hepatis and continues along the course of the portal vein, hepatic artery, and bile duct branches.

More caudally, the hepatic artery courses medially in the same anteroposterior plane and joins the celiac artery. The portal vein moves to a more anterior position before receiving the major tributaries, i.e., the splenic and superior mesenteric veins. The common bile duct courses in a progressively posterior position terminating along the posterior lateral aspect of the head of the pancreas.

As shown in Fig. 1–15, the precise level of the porta may occasionally be determined on plain films. Extraperitoneal fat extends into the liver hilus, enveloping the common bile duct and its

ramifications in a sleevelike fashion. This periductal fat may produce a striking tubular radiolucent shadow which characteristically projects within the liver anterior to the upper pole of the right kidney and superior to the duodenal bulb, with a gentle lateral convexity and branching in its upper segment.[12] The portal vein may occasionally be seen in a similar manner (Fig. 1–16).

The *left lobe* is smaller and more flattened than the right. It comes into its fullest dimensions superiorly in the epigastrium. Above, it is molded by the diaphragm. A tuberosity from its under surface fits into the concavity of the lesser curvature of the stomach, and the lobe may then extend anterior to the stomach for a variable distance into the left upper quadrant. Inferiorly, it typically becomes abruptly attenuated. The area of the left lobe of the liver has been best evaluated radiologically as the space anterior to the stomach on lateral views during an upper gastrointestinal series. Plain film identification is generally impossible, although occasionally an apical lordotic projection may permit it to be viewed tangentially (Fig. 1–17).

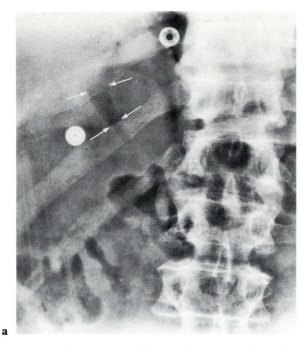

a

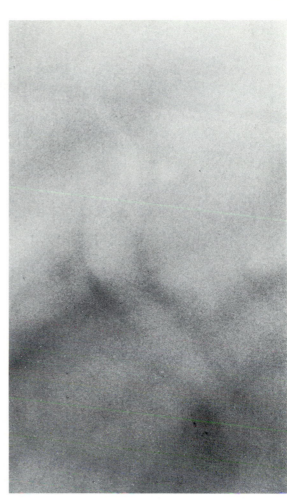

b

**Fig. 1—15. Location of porta hepatis indicated by periductal fat.**
(a) Plain film. A curved tubular radiolucent band (arrows) projects within the liver shadow over the upper renal pole.
(b) Intravenous cholangiography with tomography confirms sleevelike lucent periductal fat paralleling the contours of the common hepatic and common bile ducts. Extraperitoneal fat outlining the visceral border of the liver is continuous with the periductal hilar fat.
(From Govoni and Meyers[12])

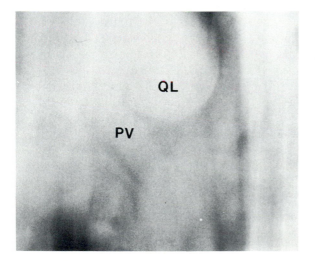

**Fig. 1—16. Perivascular fat outlining the portal vein within the porta hepatis.**
Tomogram of right upper quadrant demonstrates visualization of portal vein (PV) as tubular density outlined by fat in porta hepatis. QL = quadrate lobe.

**Fig. 1—17. The left lobe of the liver (LL) is seen in an apical lordotic projection.**
S = stomach, Sp = spleen.

# The Spleen

The spleen lies deep in the left upper quadrant between the fundus of the stomach and the diaphragm. Although it is an intraperitoneal organ, its extremely posterior position explains why only considerable enlargement allows it to become clinically palpable through the anterior

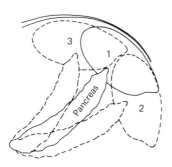

**Fig. 1–18. Positions of the spleen and axes of insertion of the tail of the pancreas.**
Schematic frontal view. The spleen is usually obliquely oriented (1) but may be vertical (2), or, rarely, horizontal (3). The tail of the pancreas inserts within the splenic hilus.

abdominal wall. Generally, the main axis of the spleen is obliquely oriented between the lateral cusp of the diaphragm and the posterolateral abdominal wall (Fig. 1–18). Some variability exists, however. At times, the spleen is vertical, extending inferiorly in the flank. Rarely, it is horizontal between the gastric fundus and the diaphragm, radiologically simulating a mass widening the gastrophrenic interval.

The anterior notched border of the spleen separates its diaphragmatic and visceral surfaces. On plain films, this border can be visualized by virtue of the fatty contrast provided by the greater omentum (Fig. 1–19). At times, as the distal portion of the mesenteric transverse colon insinuates itself between the greater curvature of the stomach and the medial aspect of the spleen, the anterior notched border is indicated by a characteristic scalloping of the colonic surface (Fig. 1–20). The medial visceral surface of the spleen faces the posterior wall of the stomach anteriorly and the upper part of the left kidney posteriorly. The hilum of the spleen receives the reflections of its supporting mesenteries, the gastrosplenic and splenorenal ligaments (Figs. 1–21 and 1–22). On plain films, the

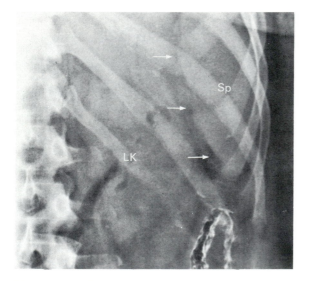

**Fig. 1–19. The anterior notched border of the spleen** (Sp) (arrows).
This is seen because of intraperitoneal fat. The posteromedial border of the spleen is in intimate relationship to the lateral border of the left kidney (LK), both of which are seen because of extraperitoneal fat.

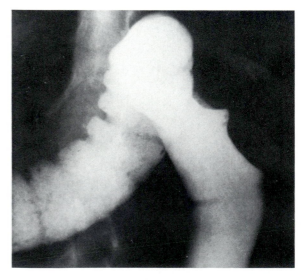

**Fig. 1–20. The anterior notched border of the spleen.**
This margin produces scalloped indentations on the distal transverse colon.

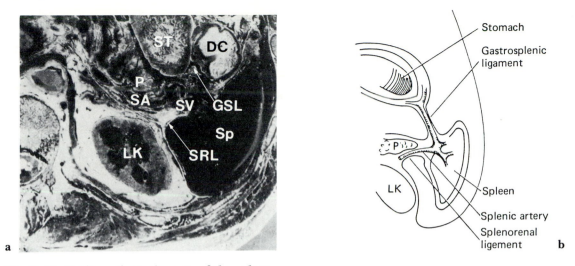

a

b

**Fig. 1–21. Peritoneal attachments of the spleen.**
**(a)** Transverse anatomic section demonstrates gastrosplenic ligament (GSL), within which course the short gastric and left gastroepiploic vessels, and the splenorenal ligament (SRL) which envelops the pancreatic tail and the proximal splenic vein (SV) and splenic artery (SA). Sp = spleen, ST = stomach, P = pancreas, DC = descending colon, LK = left kidney.
**(b)** Transverse drawing illustrates the intraperitoneal suspension of the spleen by the gastrosplenic and splenorenal ligaments.

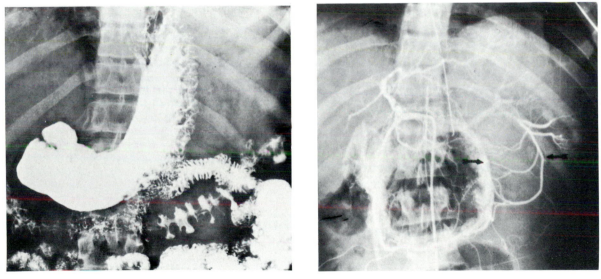

a

b

**Fig. 1–22. Hematoma in gastrosplenic ligament.**
**(a)** Upper GI series shows irregular scalloping of greater curvature of stomach with the appearance of prominent rugal pattern. These features are due to the effects of blood within the gastrosplenic ligament.
**(b)** Celiac arteriogram documents stretching and separation of the short gastric vessels (arrows) from hematoma within the gastrosplenic ligament.

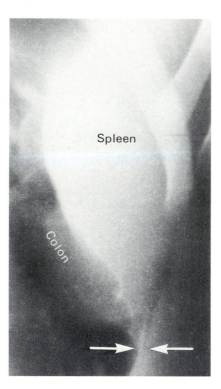

**Fig. 1–23. The phrenicocolic ligament** (arrows). On this plain film, this ligament is seen as a striplike density subtending the splenic angle at the level of the anatomic splenic flexure of the colon. (From Meyers[13])

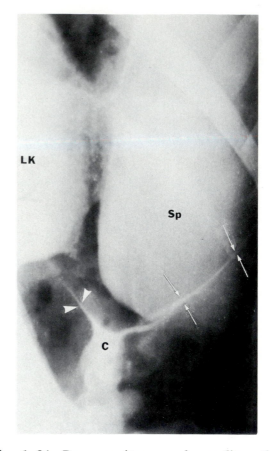

**Fig. 1–24. Prone peritoneography outlines the phrenicocolic ligament** (arrows). This structure supports the spleen (Sp) as it extends from the splenic flexure of the colon (C) to the left diaphragm and is in continuity with the gastrosplenic ligament (arrowheads) seen on end. The close relationship of the posterior margin of the spleen to the left kidney (LK) is shown. (From Meyers[14])

posteromedial border of the spleen can be visualized by virtue of the contrast provided by extraperitoneal fat, against which this intraperitoneal organ abuts.[10] The inferior tip, referred to as the splenic angle, extends downward to the level of the anatomic splenic flexure of the colon where it tends to be supported by the phrenicocolic ligament. Occasionally, this peritoneal reflection can be seen on plain films of the abdomen[13] (Fig. 1–23), and its dimensions and relationships have been clearly shown *in vivo* by peritoneography[14] (Fig. 1–24).

Accessory spleens, reported in 10–31% of cases in autopsy series,[15] are usually located in the splenic hilum or along the splenic vessels or associated ligaments (Figs. 1–25 and 1–26). Most remain small nodules but following a splenectomy, residual splenic tissue can undergo compensatory enlargement[16] (Fig. 1–27). Their identification can be easily verified with $^{99m}$Tc sulfur colloid scintigraphy.

## The Pancreas

The head of the pancreas is cradled by the descending duodenum, its body lies in the bed of the stomach, and the tail is near the spleen, creating complex anatomic relationships as the pancreas crosses the upper abdomen. The head, in particular, and the body of the pancreas are situated well in front of the midcoronal plane of the body. This relatively anterior position of the pancreas is often surprising if one assumes that extraperitoneal organs are necessarily posterior in the abdomen. The uncinate process is an extension of the head of the pancreas which lies

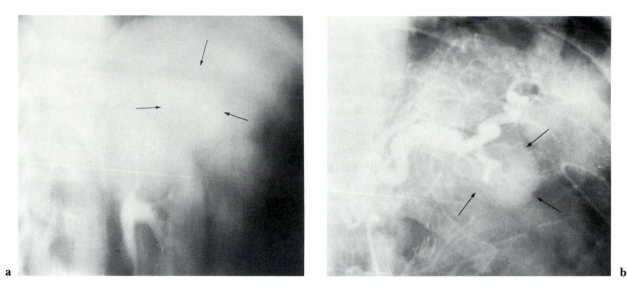

**a**
**b**

**Fig. 1–25. Accessory spleen.**
**(a)** Oblique nephrotomogram demonstrates a soft-tissue mass (arrows) anterolateral to the upper pole of the left kidney.
**(b)** Selective splenic arteriogram documents the arterial supply to the accessory spleen (arrows).

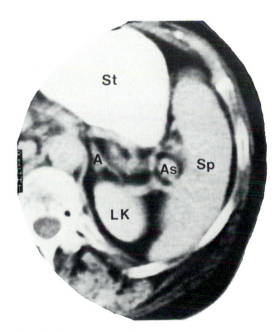

**Fig. 1–26. Accessory spleen.**
CT scan demonstrates nodule of accessory spleen (As) in the hilus of the spleen (Sp) within the branching of the splenic artery. LK = left kidney, A = adrenal gland, St = stomach.

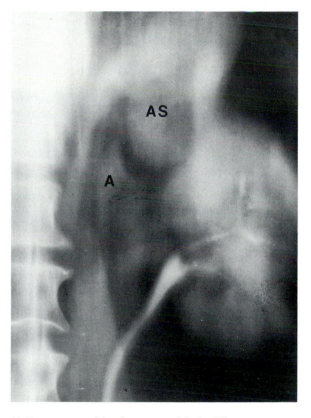

**Fig. 1–27. Hypertrophied residual accessory spleen.**
Nephrotomogram in a postsplenectomy patient shows lateral deviation of the left kidney and demonstrates the soft-tissue mass of an accessory spleen (AS), presumably hypertrophied. The accessory spleen was further verified by arteriography and a splenic scan. The normal left adrenal gland (A) is also identified.

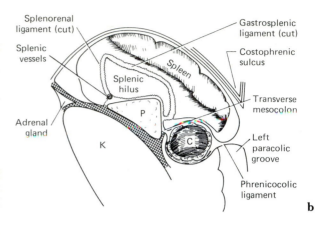

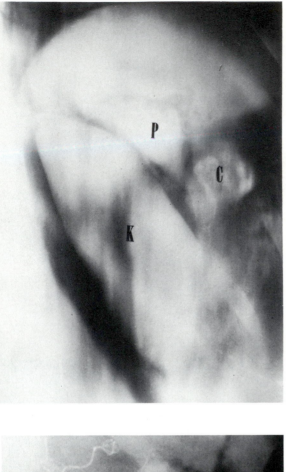

a

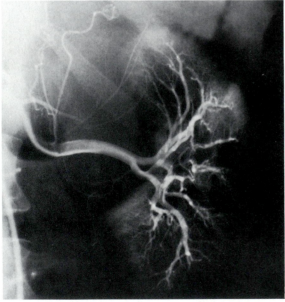

**Fig. 1–28. Relationships of the tail of the pancreas.**
(**a** and **b**) Retroperitoneal pneumography with tomography in the left posterior oblique position illustrates the tail of the pancreas (P) ventral to the upper half of the left kidney (K) as it inserts within the splenic hilus. The splenic flexure of the colon (C) is outlined by some residual barium.

**Fig. 1–29. Displacement of left kidney by pancreatic pseudocyst.**
Selective renal arteriogram demonstrates lateral displacement of upper renal pole with compression of its parenchyma. These changes are due to a pseudocyst of the tail of the pancreas.

posterior to the superior mesenteric vessels and anterior to the aorta. An insufficient amount of adjacent extraperitoneal fat prevents plain film visualization of the pancreas.

The duodenojejunal junction serves as a useful demarcation between the body and the tail of the pancreas. The tail curves posteriorly to cross the left kidney, usually in its upper part (Fig. 1–28). It then enters the splenic hilus, being ensheathed within the splenorenal ligament. It is important to recognize that since it is here incorporated within a mesenteric reflection, the extreme tip of the pancreatic tail is, by definition, an intraperitoneal structure. These intimate anatomic relationships of the pancreatic tail are essential in understanding the effects of pancreatic lesions on the left kidney[17,18] (Fig. 1–29) and spleen[22] (Figs. 1–30, 1–31, and 1–32).

Postmortem and *in vivo* studies have documented considerable variation in the size, shape, and position of the pancreas. Its course across the abdomen may be oblique, sigmoid, transverse, or horseshoe-shaped.[19,20] Much of this variation appears to be related not only to the descent of some organs with age because of the

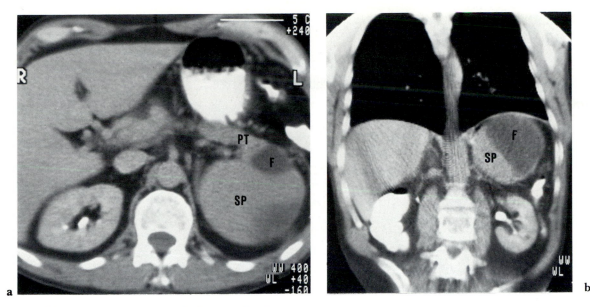

**Fig. 1–30. Intrasplenic pancreatic fluid collection.**
**(a)** Computed tomography shows a pancreatic fluid collection (F) in pancreatic tail (PT) extending into the spleen (SP).
**(b)** Direct coronal CT section demonstrates this intrasplenic fluid clearly.
(Reproduced from Feldberg MAM: Computed Tomography of the Retroperitoneum. Martinus Nijhoff, The Hague, 1983)

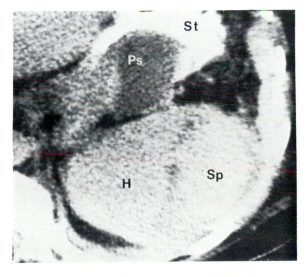

**Fig. 1–31. Subcapsular hematoma of the spleen secondary to pancreatic pseudocyst.**
CT scan demonstrates a large subcapsular hematoma (H) extending from the medial aspect of the spleen (Sp). This is a consequence of a pseudocyst (Ps) of the tail of the pancreas, here shown indenting the posterior wall of the opacified stomach (St), extending into the hilum of the spleen.

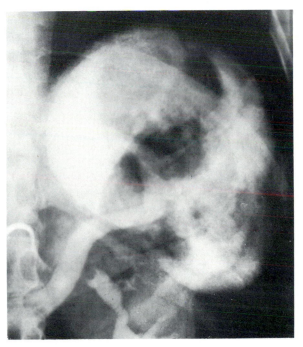

**Fig. 1–32. Intrasplenic pancreatic pseudocyst.**
Venous phase of selective splenic arteriogram demonstrates a large spherical defect in the splenic opacification secondary to a pseudocyst extending from the tail of the pancreas. (From Farman et al[22])

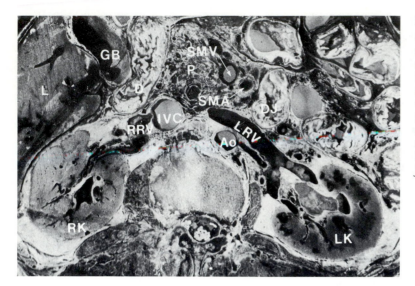

**Fig. 1–33. Anatomic cross-section showing the relationships of the right renal vein (RRV) and left renal vein (LRV).**
RK = right kidney, LK = left kidney, Ao = aorta, IVC = inferior vena cava, P = pancreas, SMA = superior mesenteric artery, SMV = superior mesenteric vein, D = descending duodenum, GB = gallbladder, L = liver, DJ = duodenojejunal junction.

laxity of supporting structures, but to the axis of insertion of the tail of the pancreas as dictated by the position of the spleen (Fig. 1–18). As a gross landmark, however, the longitudinal axis of the pancreas can be projected along a line from the mid-descending duodenum to the central area between the spleen's posteromedial contour and anterior notched border. The pancreas is a mobile organ, moving with respiration more than its craniocaudal dimension.[21]

# The Kidneys and Adrenal Glands

## Kidneys

The anatomic features of the kidneys related to the renal capsule, perirenal fat, renal fascia, and adjacent segments of the gastrointestinal tract—features that underlie diagnostic radiologic criteria in a spectrum of clinical lesions—are detailed in Chapters 4 and 5.

The renal veins present a significant difference in course and relationships. Whereas the right renal vein assumes a direct short course to the inferior vena cava, the left renal vein courses transversely anterior to the aorta and posterior to the superior mesenteric artery and vein to its junction with the inferior vena cava (Fig. 1–33). The "nutcracker" effect of the aorta and superior mesenteric artery on the left renal vein may be a factor contributing to the increased incidence of varicoceles on the left side in males.

## Adrenal Glands

Apart from their suprarenal position, the right and left adrenal glands have important differences in gross morphology and relationships.[23]

The right adrenal is roughly triangular in shape. It lies deep to the nonperitonealized (bare) area of the right lobe of the liver laterally and deep to the inferior vena cava medially (Figs. 1–4 and 1–34). Posteromedially the gland is near the diaphragm. Inferiorly, it has only a

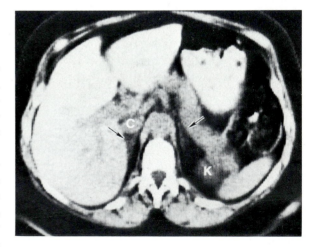

**Fig. 1–34. Normal adrenal glands (arrows) shown bilaterally by computed tomography.**
Note their normal outline, shape, and position. On the right, the gland lies just behind the inferior vena cava (C). On the left, the gland projects anterior to the kidney (K).

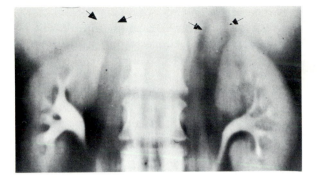

**Fig. 1–35. Relationships of adrenal glands to the kidneys.**
Nephrotomogram. The adrenal glands (arrows) can be identified in size, shape, and position. Note that the right is completely suprarenal in position, but the left extends downward along the medial aspect of the upper renal pole and has a mildly convex medial border.

loose attachment to the upper pole of the kidney.

The left adrenal is closely adjacent to the upper medial border of the kidney, at times extending anteriorly to the level of the renal hilus (Figs. 1–34 and 1–35). It thus presents typically a semilunar contour, concave laterally facing the kidney and convex medially. Anteriorly, the gland is in relationship to the tail of the pancreas and the posterior parietal peritoneum of the lesser sac, and posteriorly, to the lumbar insertions of the diaphragm.

Although the adrenal glands arise in intimate anatomic relation to the kidneys, their separate embryologic origin means that their development is generally unaffected by common renal anomalies. In congenital renal hypoplasia and crossed renal ectopia, the adrenals mature fully and develop in their normal position.[23,24] (Figs. 1–36 and 1–37). When a kidney is congenitally absent from a renal fossa, however, the adrenal gland assumes the shape of a paraspinal disc and appears as a linear structure on a cross-

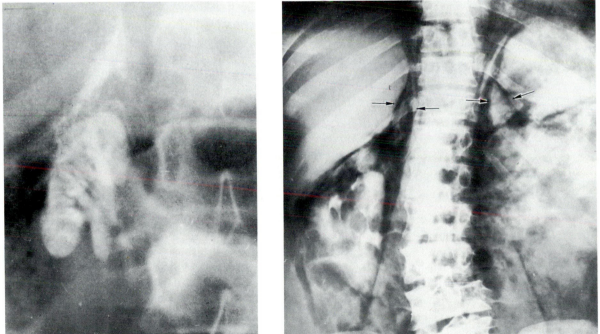

1-36                                                                    1-37

**Fig. 1–36. Normal adrenal gland associated with congenital renal hypoplasia.**
Capillary phase of selective renal arteriogram shows a normal-sized adrenal despite the kidney maturing in size no longer than the height of the adjacent vertebral body. (From Meyers et al[24])

**Fig. 1–37. Normal adrenal glands (arrows) in presence of crossed fused renal ectopia.**
Intravenous urography with retroperitoneal pneumography shows that there is congenital fusion of both kidneys on the right. Despite this, the adrenal glands (arrows) have developed to their normal positions and size. (From Meyers[23])

sectional CT image.[25] Presumably this occurs because indentation fails to take place as the ascending kidney impacts on the large, globular fetal adrenal in normal development.

The adrenal glands are fixed superiorly to Gerota's fascia. Erect films may thus be helpful in distinguishing an adrenal tumor from a renal mass. The kidney may descend sufficiently to be clearly separated from the adrenal lesion, which remains fixed in position (Fig. 1–38).

Based on an understanding of the normal corticomedullary relationships in the different parts of the gland, it can be appreciated that the shape alone of an adrenal tumor may reliably indicate its nature[26] (Fig. 1–39). The medulla resides within the base of the gland and the major portion of the cortex lies in the apex; in fact, the apex of the adrenal gland is composed of cortical tissue only. The apical sign of pheochromocytoma and the wedge sign of adrenocortical adenoma may be seen on plain films or tomograms, but more often is demonstrated on nephrotomograms or in the capillary phase of arteriograms. It can also be documented occasionally by computed tomography.

# The Gastrointestinal Tract

The *stomach* should be considered three-dimensionally. Rather than lying in one plane of the body, this organ is normally rotated about both the vertical and horizontal axes of the abdomen. In this way, the greater curvature of the stomach represents a portion of its anterior wall and the lesser curvature a portion of its posterior wall. The fundus lies quite posteriorly in the left upper quadrant, whereas the distal body and antrum course anteriorly. The first and second portions of the duodenum are then redirected posteriorly.

The *jejunum* and *ileum* are supported by the small bowel mesentery. The root of this mesentery extends for a distance of only about 15 cm from the region of the duodenojejunal junction to the cecocolic junction. Jejunal loops, therefore, are most commonly seen in the left upper quadrant and ileal loops in the lower midabdomen and right lower quadrant. A common variant is nonrotation of the small bowel, wherein jejunal loops are suspended from the mesentery in the right midabdomen.

The *large intestine* has complex anatomic relationships as it courses through the abdomen. The cecum may be completely extraperitoneal, but is often suspended intraperitoneally. This is particularly common in females, the extreme of which is seen as the "mobile" cecum. This lack of fixation also explains why volvulus of the cecum is more common in females than males. The ascending colon is extraperitoneal up to the anterior hepatic flexure, which marks the beginning of the transverse mesocolon. This peritoneal reflection permits the transverse colon to be suspended anteriorly in the abdomen. At the level of the anatomic splenic flexure, the large intestine penetrates the posterior parietal peritoneum to continue as the extraperitoneal descending colon. The sigmoid mesocolon reflects obliquely off the level of the left sacroiliac joint to suspend the redundant sigmoid loops anteriorly. The large intestine then penetrates the peritoneum at S2–S4 to continue as the subperitoneal rectum.

Gas in the intestinal tract provides a natural contrast of the luminal contours. Its normal distribution and localization is a consequence primarily of the effects of gravity and its relationship to hydrostatic pressure. In the supine position, gas rises and fills the distal pars media and antrum of the stomach, the cecum and proximal ascending colon, the transverse colon and often the splenic flexure, and the distal descending and sigmoid colon. In the prone position, gas enters the gastric fundus, the duodenal bulb and often the descending duodenum, the distal ascending colon, hepatic flexure, the proximal descending colon, and the rectum. At times, advantage may be taken of such localization by intentionally positioning a patient to demonstrate optimally a particular area or lesion.

Normal variability in the position of portions of the bowel and their relationship to each other are determined largely by body habitus and differences in mesenteric attachments. In a tall, thin female the stomach may be J-shaped and the transverse colon may curve into the lower abdomen or pelvis. In contrast, a short, stocky male typically has a stomach horizontally oriented in the upper abdomen with the duodenal bulb directed posteriorly, accompanied by a straight and high transverse colon. Individual differences in length of their major peritoneal reflections—the greater (gastrocolic ligament)

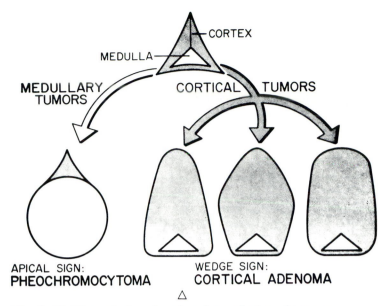

**Fig. 1–39. The apical and wedge signs of adrenal tumors.**
In pheochromocytomas, which arise from the medulla in the basal portion, the uninvolved apex containing most of the adrenal gland's cortical tissue may be clearly visualized.

Cortical adenomas tend to produce proportionately greater enlargement in upper third of the gland in the tissue of origin, yielding a wedge-shaped outline. (From Meyers[26])

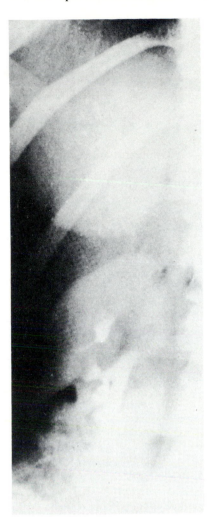

◁
**Fig. 1–38. Attachment of adrenal superiorly to Gerota's fascia.**
Erect view during intravenous urography permits the kidney to fall, clearly outlining a large adrenal carcinoma containing flecks of calcifications. (From Meyers[23])

and lesser (gastrohepatic and hepatoduodenal ligaments) omenta and the transverse mesocolon—which are somewhat related to body habitus, and their increased laxity with age result in variability. Nevertheless, the greater curvature of the stomach maintains a generally parallel, if not close, relationship to the superior aspect of the transverse colon. Any localized increase should be viewed with suspicion.

## The Extraperitoneal Planes and Tissues

The extraperitoneal region is anatomically divided by well-defined fascial extensions into three compartments.[27,28] These are discussed in detail in Chapter 4. The *anterior pararenal space* contains little fat, explaining why the outlines of the major extraperitoneal portions of the alimentary tract within it (ascending and descending colon, the entire duodenal loop, and the pancreas) are not directly seen on plain films. The central *perirenal space* contains abundant fat and permits visualization of the kidneys and, occasionally, the adrenal glands. The most dorsal extraperitoneal compartment, the *posterior pararenal space*, contains no major organs, but its properitoneal fat continues laterally around the flanks, where it is visualized radiographically as the "flank stripe."

The lateral borders of the psoas muscles are normally seen because of extraperitoneal fat, but different portions of it contribute to visualization of specific segments.[27,28] In its upper portion at the level of the kidneys, the psoas muscles are seen because of the contrast provided by perirenal fat. The lower portions, however, are visualized because they are outlined by posterior pararenal fat.

Extraperitoneal fat also outlines the inferior contours of the diaphragms. At times, it may appear radiologically as a strikingly lucent, thin subdiaphragmatic crescent and should not be mistaken for free intraperitoneal air or other abnormalities. The same fat can be traced medially where it permits plain film visualization of the medial crura of the diaphragms.

In the pelvis, subperitoneal fat frequently outlines the dome of the urinary bladder. Its identification on plain films may be very helpful in distinguishing a true supravesical soft-tissue mass from a distended urinary bladder. Visualization of the levator ani and obturator internus muscles bordering the bony pelvis is common.

# References

1. Meyers MA, Oliphant M: Pitfalls and Pickups in Plain-Film Diagnosis of the Abdomen. Current Problems in Radiology. Year Book Medical, Chicago, Vol. IV, No. 2, pp. 1–37, March–April 1974
2. Shin MS, Berland LL: Computed tomography of retrocrural spaces: Normal, anatomic variants, and pathologic conditions. AJR 145: 81–86, 1985
3. Goldsmith NA, Woodburne RT: The surgical anatomy pertaining to liver resection. Surg Gynecol Obstet 105: 310–318, 1957
4. Healey JE Jr, Schroy PC: Anatomy of the biliary duct within the human liver: Analysis of the prevailing pattern of branchings and the major variations of the biliary ducts. Arch Surg 66: 599–616, 1953
5. Michels NA: Newer anatomy of the liver and its variant blood supply and collateral circulation. Am J Surg 112: 337–347, 1966
6. Pagani JJ: Intrahepatic vascular territories shown by computed tomography. The value of CT in determining resectability of hepatic tumors. Radiology 147: 173–178, 1983
7. Sexton CS, Zeman RK: Correlation of computed tomography, sonography, and gross anatomy of the liver. AJR 141: 711–718, 1983
8. Haswell DM, Berne AS, Schneider B: Plain film recognition of the ligamentum teres hepatis. Radiology 114: 263–267, 1975
9. Gelfand DW: Anatomy of the liver, Rad Cl N Am 18: 187–194, 1980
10. Whalen JP, Berne AS, Riemenschneider PA: The extraperitoneal perivisceral fat pad. I. Its role in the roentgenologic visualization of abdominal organs. Radiology 92: 466–472, 1969
11. Weinstein JB, Heiken JP, Lee JKT, et al: High resolution CT of the porta hepatis and hepatoduodenal ligament. Radiographics 6(1): 55–73, 1986
12. Govoni AF, Meyers MA: Pseudopneumobilia. Radiology 118. 526, 1976
13. Meyers MA: Roentgen significance of the phrenicocolic ligament. Radiology 95: 539–545, 1970
14. Meyers MA: Peritoneography: Normal and pathologic anatomy. Am J Roentgenol Rad Ther Nucl Med 117: 353–365, 1973
15. Curtis GM, Moritz D: The surgical significance of the accessory spleen. Ann Surg 123: 276–298, 1946
16. Beahrs JR, Stephens DH: Enlarged accessory spleens: CT appearance in postsplenectomy patients. AJR 135: 483–486, 1980
17. Atkinson GO, Clements JL Jr, Milledge RD, et al: Pancreatic disease simulating urinary tract disease. Clin Radiol 24: 185–191, 1973
18. Marshall S, Lapp M, Schutte JW: Lesions of the pancreas mimicking renal disease. J Urol 93: 41–45, 1965
19. Kreel L, Sandin B, Slavin G: Pancreatic morphology: A combined radiological and pathological study. Clin Radiol 24: 154–161, 1973
20. Varley PF, Rohrmann CA Jr, Silvis SE, et al: The normal endoscopic pancreatogram. Radiology 118: 295–300, 1976
21. Kivisaari L, Makela P, Aarimaa M: Technical note/pancreatic mobility: An important factor in pancreatic computed tomography. J Computer Assist Tomogr 6(4): 854–856, 1982
22. Farman J, Dallemand S, Schneider M, et al: Pancreatic pseudocysts involving the spleen. Gastrointest Radiol 1: 339–343, 1977
23. Meyers MA: Diseases of the Adrenal Glands: Radiologic Diagnosis. Charles C Thomas, Springfield, Ill., 1963
24. Meyers MA, Friedenberg R, King M, et al: Significance of the renal capsular arteries. Br J Radiol 40: 949–956, 1967
25. Kenney PJ, Robbins GL, Ellis DA, et al: Adrenal glands in patients with congenital renal anomalies: CT appearance. Radiology 155: 181–182, 1985
26. Meyers MA: Characteristic radiographic shapes of pheochromocytomas and adrenocortical adenomas. Radiology 87: 889–891, 1966
27. Meyers MA: Acute extraperitoneal infection. Semin Roentgenol 8: 445–464, 1973
28. Meyers MA, Whalen JP, Peele K, et al: Radiologic features of extraperitoneal effusions: An anatomic approach. Radiology 104: 249-257, 1972

# 2 Intraperitoneal Spread of Infections

## General Introduction

A remarkable change in the epidemiology of subphrenic and subhepatic abscesses has occurred over the last several decades. In the past, the most common causes included perforations of anterior gastric or duodenal ulcers and rupture of a gangrenous appendix. Today, 60–71% of such abscesses are postoperative and are particularly frequent following gastric and biliary tract operations and colonic surgery.[1–3] Many of the cases of postoperative abscesses are secondary to anastomotic leaks.[4] More prompt diagnosis currently in conditions such as peptic ulcer and appendicitis, leading to earlier surgical intervention, results in an increasing proportion of postoperative abscesses. The bacterial flora generally consist of multiple strains of aerobic and anaerobic organisms. The aerobes include particularly *E. coli, Streptococcus, Klebsiella,* and *Proteus;* and the anaerobes *Bacteroides* and cocci.[2]

Paralleling this epidemiologic change has been a change in the clinical presentation. The fulminating course described classically is no longer generally seen, and today abscesses most often present in an insidious fashion, typically consisting of mild abdominal pain, malaise, and a slight fever. Later, the patient may develop a mass, referred pain to the shoulder, and subcostal or flank pain. The clinical spectrum is illustrated by this analogy:

> It can rapidly build up a crater of sepsis giving the patient an acute illness with a clear cut diagnosis . . . on the other hand, it may linger apparently quiescent, causing only a slight fever, only to erupt unexpectedly some weeks or months later. Finally, it may be like Vesuvius, apparently extinct, apart from occasional rumbles, making its presence felt only by causing ill health.[5]

Early radiologic identification and localization of an intraabdominal abscess are of extreme importance, since morbidity and mortality increase with delay in treatment. Diagnosis can be most prompt and accurate when there is an understanding of the intraperitoneal routes of spread of contaminated material.

## Anatomic Considerations

### The Posterior Peritoneal Attachments

Figure 2–1 shows the roots of the mesenteric attachments of the intraperitoneal segments of bowel and Figure 2–2 illustrates the reflections of the peritoneum from the posterior abdominal wall deep to the bowel, liver, and spleen. The *transverse mesocolon* constitutes the major barrier dividing the abdominal cavity into supra- and inframesocolic compartments. The obliquely oriented *root of the small bowel mesentery* further divides the inframesocolic compartment into two spaces of unequal size: (a) the smaller *right infracolic space* bounded inferiorly by the junction of the mesentery with the attachment of the ascending colon, and (b) the larger *left infracolic space,* which is open anatomically toward the pelvis.

The *pelvis* is the most dependent part of the peritoneal cavity in either the supine or erect position. It is anatomically continuous with both paracolic gutters, the peritoneal recesses lateral

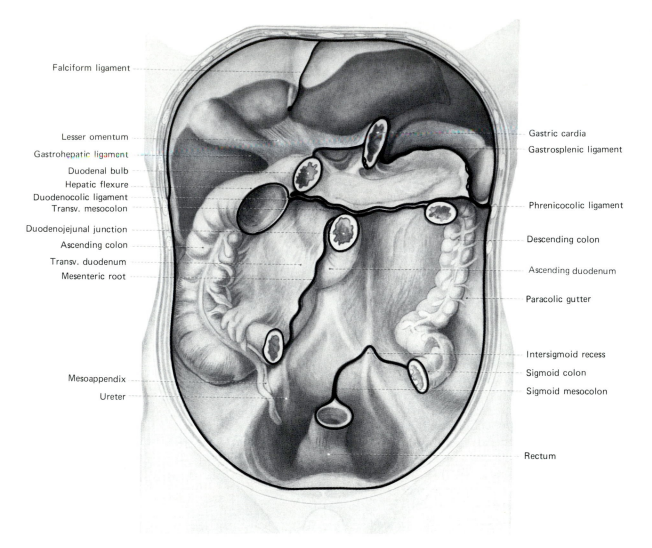

Falciform ligament

Lesser omentum
Gastrohepatic ligament
Duodenal bulb
Hepatic flexure
Duodenocolic ligament
Transv. mesocolon
Duodenojejunal junction
Ascending colon
Transv. duodenum
Mesenteric root

Mesoappendix
Ureter

Gastric cardia
Gastrosplenic ligament

Phrenicocolic ligament

Descending colon

Ascending duodenum

Paracolic gutter

Intersigmoid recess
Sigmoid colon
Sigmoid mesocolon

Rectum

**Fig. 2–1. The peritoneal investment of the extraperitoneal segments of the alimentary tract.**
The mesenteric portions of the gut have been removed, including the stomach, small bowel, transverse colon, and sigmoid colon.

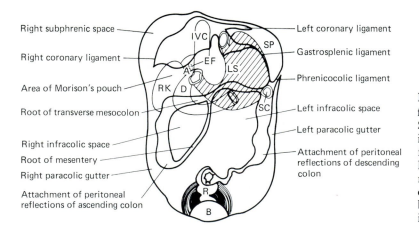

Right subphrenic space
Right coronary ligament
Area of Morison's pouch
Root of transverse mesocolon
Right infracolic space
Root of mesentery
Right paracolic gutter
Attachment of peritoneal reflections of ascending colon

Left coronary ligament
Gastrosplenic ligament
Phrenicocolic ligament
Left infracolic space
Left paracolic gutter
Attachment of peritoneal reflections of descending colon

**Fig. 2–2. Posterior peritoneal reflections and recesses.**
SP = spleen, LS = lesser sac, IVC = inferior vena cava, EF = epiploic foramen of Winslow, RK = right kidney, D = duodenum, A = adrenal gland, SC = splenic flexure, of colon, R = rectum, B = urinary bladder. The removed stomach is indicated. (Modified from Meyers[6])

to the ascending and descending colon. The *right paracolic gutter* is wide and deep and is continuous superiorly with the right subhepatic space and its posterosuperior extension deep to the liver, which is surgically known as *Morison's pouch*.[7] The *right subhepatic space* is anatomically continuous with the *right subphrenic space* around the lateral edge of the *right coronary ligament* of the liver. In contrast, the *left paracolic gutter* is narrow and shallow and is interrupted from continuity with the *left subphrenic space* (perisplenic or left perihepatic space) by the *phrenicocolic ligament*, which extends from the splenic flexure of the colon to the left diaphragm.

## Detailed Anatomy of the Right Upper Quadrant

Since Barnard's original classification[8] in 1908, a great deal of confusion in the definition and true anatomic location of right upper quadrant abscesses has arisen. All pus accumulations in the supramesocolic compartment tended to be termed "subphrenic abscesses," but this is misleading because only some of the abscesses lie immediately below the diaphragm. In 1938, Ochsner and DeBakey[9] cited the right posterior subphrenic space as the most frequent site of infection. This recess is now recognized as actually subhepatic in position. In 1955, Harley[10] helped to clarify the topography:

> My view is that the subphrenic region extends from the diaphragm to the transverse colon and mesocolon. It is divided into the suprahepatic and infrahepatic compartments by the liver. The suprahepatic compartment is divided into right and left portions by the falciform ligament and the infrahepatic compartment is similarly divided by the ligamentum teres and ligamentum venosum.

The key to the problem lies in the locations of the ligamentous attachments of the liver. A generation of surgeons schooled on "keyhole" incisions had believed that the right lobe of the liver is suspended superiorly from the diaphragm by the right coronary ligament. Although pointed out by Mitchell[11] in 1940, it was not until 1966 that Boyd clearly defined the coronary ligament as actually suspending the right lobe of the liver from the parietes *posteriorly*.[12,13] In this way, the peritoneal recess around the right lobe of the liver is grossly compartmentalized into a subphrenic space and a subhepatic space (Fig. 2–3).

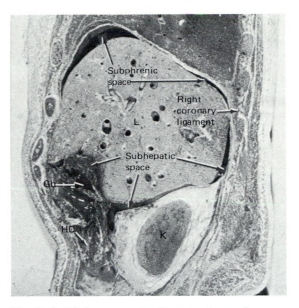

**Fig. 2–3. Right parasagittal anatomic section.** The right coronary ligament suspends the liver from the diaphragm posteriorly and divides the peritoneal cavity around the right lobe into a subphrenic space and a subhepatic space. Gb = gallbladder, HC = hepatic flexure of the colon, K = right kidney.

## The Right Subhepatic Space

Underlying the visceral surface of the right lobe of the liver, the right subhepatic space is composed of two compartments (Figs. 2–4 and 2–5):

1. The *anterior subhepatic space* is limited inferiorly by the beginning of the transverse colon and mesocolon.
2. The *posterior subhepatic space* lies in close relationship to the posterior parietal peritoneum overlying the right kidney. It projects upward in the form of a recess between the renal impression of the liver in front and the upper pole of the right kidney behind. The posterosuperior extension of the right subhepatic space to its margination above by the right coronary ligament is known anatomically as the *hepatorenal fossa* and clinically as *Morison's pouch*.

Morison's pouch is of great significance in the spread and localization of intraperitoneal infections since it is the lowest part of the right paravertebral groove when the body is in the supine position. Figures 2–6 and 2–7 illustrate its important anatomic relationships. Inferiorly, it is bounded by the hepatic flexure of the colon

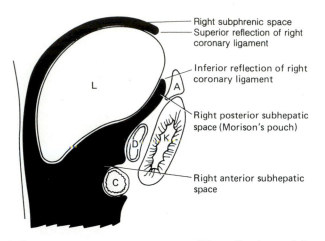

**Fig. 2–4. Right parasagittal diagram.**
The right subhepatic space is comprised of anterior and posterior (Morison's pouch) compartments and is anatomically continuous with the right subphrenic space. The reflections of the coronary ligament mark the site of the nonperitonealized "bare area" of the liver (L). K = right kidney, A = adrenal gland, D = descending duodenum, C = transverse colon.

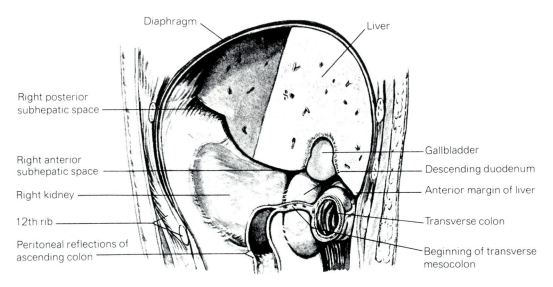

**Fig. 2–5. Right parasagittal anatomic drawing, viewed from the right.**
The relationships of the right anterior and posterior subhepatic spaces are shown.

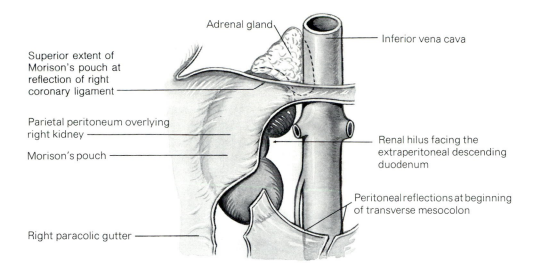

**Fig. 2–6. Frontal view of the anatomic relationships of Morison's pouch facing the deep visceral surface of the right lobe of the liver.**

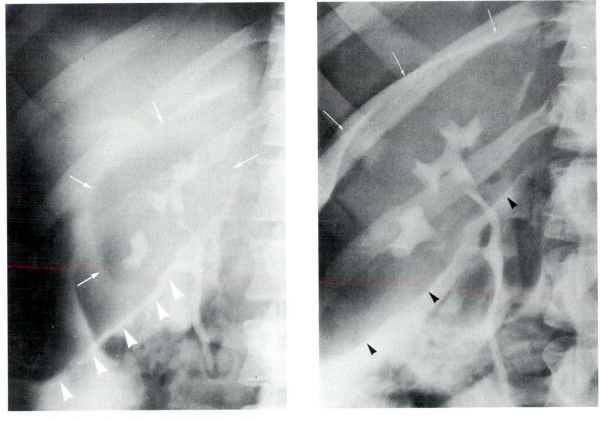

a                                                                                                                                b

**Fig. 2–7. Visceral surface of right lobe of liver.**
**(a)** Supine peritoneography. Positive-contrast medium parallels the posteroinferior edge of the liver (arrowheads). Gas within Morison's pouch outlines the contours of the renal fossa on the posterior surface of the liver (arrows).
**(b)** Prone peritoneography. The inferior reflection of the coronary ligament, immediately below the bare area of the liver marking the superior extent of Morison's pouch, is outlined (upper arrows). Note that here it corresponds to the level of the 11th posterior rib. Positive-contrast medium also pools along the notched anteroinferior border of the liver (arrowheads). (**a** and **b,** from Meyers[14])

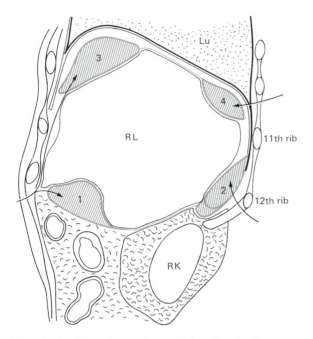

**Fig. 2–8. The four sites of localized abscesses around the right lobe of the liver.**
(See Fig. 2–3.) (1) Anterior subhepatic, (2) posterior subhepatic, (3) anterior subphrenic, (4) posterior subphrenic. The surgical approaches to the spaces are indicated. Lu = lung, RL = right lobe of liver, RK = right kidney. (After Boyd[12])

and the peritoneal reflections at the beginning of the transverse mesocolon and medially by the second portion of the duodenum as it descends anterior to the hilus of the kidney. Laterally, it communicates deep to the liver around the margin of the right coronary ligament with the subphrenic space above and the right paracolic gutter in the flank.

Although these two compartments communicate freely anatomically, they are frequently separated by the development of pyogenic membranes (Fig. 2-8).

## The Right Subphrenic Space

The right subphrenic space is a large continuous compartment extending over the diaphragmatic surface of the right lobe of the liver to its margination posteriorly and inferiorly by the right coronary ligament. No true anatomic separation into anterior and posterior subphrenic spaces actually occurs, but such compartmentalization of abscesses frequently takes place by the formation of pyogenic membranes (Fig. 2–8).

The falciform ligament separates the right and left subphrenic spaces. Mitchell[11] has stressed that the region below and on either side

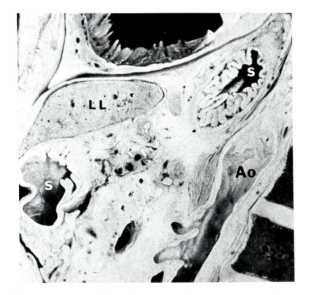

**Fig. 2–9. Sagittal section through the left lobe of the liver.**
The smaller left lobe (LL) of the liver lies anterior to the stomach (S), including both its upper fundic and distal body portions. Ao = aorta.

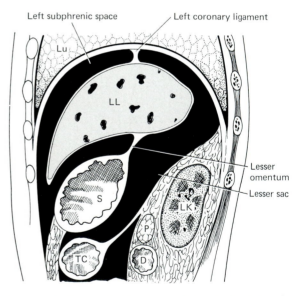

**Fig. 2–10. Parasagittal section through the left lobe of the liver.**
At this level, the perihepatic spaces are freely continuous. The lesser sac is a distinctly separate space. D = duodenum, LK = left kidney, LL = left lobe of liver, Lu = lung, P = pancreas, S = stomach, TC = transverse colon. (After Boyd[12])

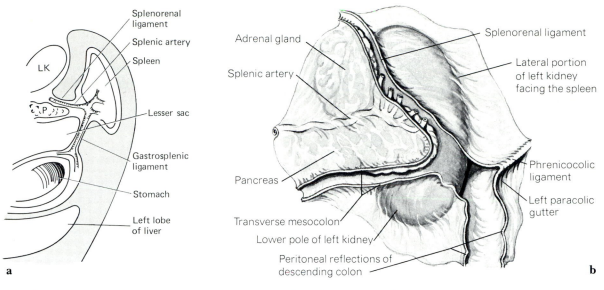

**Fig. 2–11. Peritoneal attachments and recesses of the left upper quadrant.**
**(a)** Diagram of horizontal section. The intraperitoneal spaces around the left lobe of the liver and the spleen are freely continuous (gray area). The perisplenic space is bounded by the splenorenal and gastrosplenic ligaments. LK = left kidney, P = tail of pancreas.
**(b)** Frontal drawing (spleen removed). The phrenicocolic ligament partially bridges the junction between the perisplenic space and the left paracolic gutter. The lesser sac resides above the transverse mesocolon and medial to the splenorenal ligament.

of the free margin of the falciform ligament resembles a delta in which the two subphrenic and the right subhepatic spaces communicate.

## The Left Subphrenic Space

The suspending coronary ligament of the left lobe of the liver, unlike the right, is attached superiorly, almost in the center of the abdomen and more anteriorly than the right coronary and triangular ligaments.[11,15,16] It is quite small and usually insignificant for the margination of abscess cavities. The anatomic spaces surrounding the left lobe of the liver are thus freely communicating (Figs. 2–9 and 2–10). Generally, therefore, the whole left side should be considered as one potential abscess area[12,13,15] (Fig. 2–10). The mesenteric attachments of the left upper quadrant, i.e., the splenorenal ligament, the gastrosplenic ligament, and the lesser omentum, aided by the development of inflammatory adhesions, may serve to compartmentalize abscesses to the immediate subphrenic (between the diaphragm and the gastric fundus), subhepatic (between the visceral surface of the liver

and the stomach), or perisplenic areas (Fig. 2–11).

A structure of particular significance in the left upper quadrant of the abdomen is the phrenicocolic ligament[17] (Figs. 2–11b through 2–13). This is a strong, falciform peritoneal fold that extends from the anatomic splenic flexure of the colon to the diaphragm at the level of the 11th rib. Older literature refers to it also as the "sustentaculum lienis," since it is in immediate inferior relationship to and serves the purpose of supporting the spleen at its tip. Its importance in limiting the spread of infection is based on the anatomic fact that it separates partially the perisplenic space from the left paracolic gutter.

## The Lesser Sac

During fetal life, the development of the dorsal mesogastrium and the rotation of the stomach cut off a bay of peritoneum, the lesser sac (omental bursa), from the rest of the peritoneal cavity. The narrow inlet is known as the epiploic foramen (foramen of Winslow).

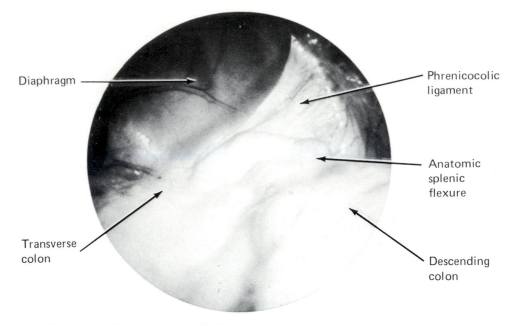

Diaphragm

Phrenicocolic
ligament

Anatomic
splenic
flexure

Transverse
colon

Descending
colon

**Fig. 2–12. The phrenicocolic ligament as seen *in vivo* by peritoneoscopy.**

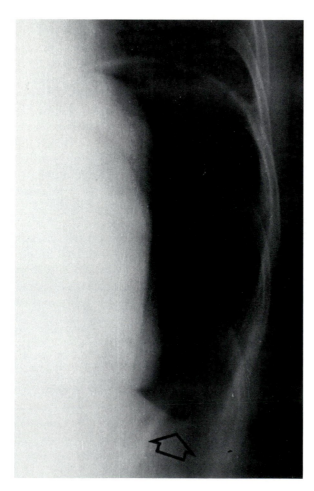

The lesser sac (Figs. 2–10, 2–11a, 2–14, and 2–15) lies behind the lesser omentum, the stomach and duodenal bulb, and the gastrocolic ligament. It is bounded inferiorly by the transverse colon and the mesocolon, although a well-defined inferior recess persists in a few individuals between the anterior and posterior reflections of the greater omentum (Fig. 2–16). The lesser sac is defined posteriorly chiefly by most of the pancreas; to the right, the caudate lobe of the liver projects into the sac. A prominent oblique fold of peritoneum raised from the posterior abdominal wall by the left gastric artery often divides the lesser sac into two compartments—a smaller medial compartment to the right with a superior recess dorsal to the medial segment of the left hepatic lobe and a larger lateral compartment to the left inferiorly (Fig. 2–15).

On the left, the lesser sac is bounded by the splenic attachments—the gastrosplenic ligament in front and the splenorenal ligament behind (Fig. 2–11a). On the right side, the space extends just to the right of the midline where it

◁────────────────────────────────

**Fig. 2–13. The phrenicocolic ligament** is seen (arrow) partially subtending the left subphrenic (perisplenic) space in a case of free intraperitoneal air. Decubitus projection. The liver and spleen have fallen to the right. (From Meyers[17])

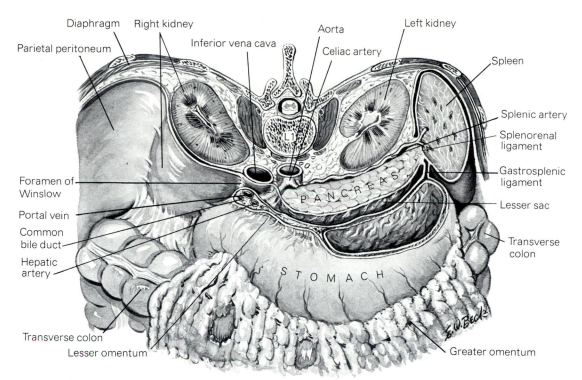

**Fig. 2–14. The lesser sac and its relationships.**
The foramen of Winslow is generally only large enough to admit the introduction of one finger, but *in vivo* it represents merely a potential communication between the greater and lesser peritoneal cavities.

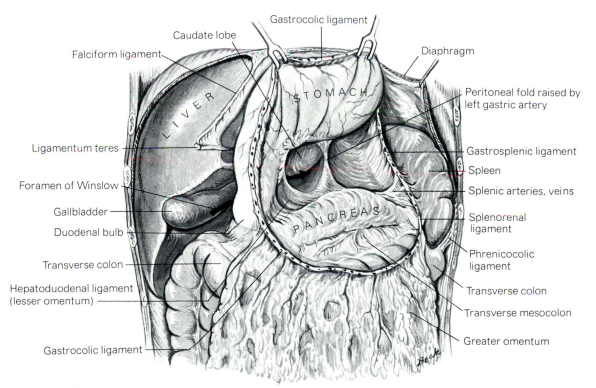

**Fig. 2–15. The lesser sac and its relationships, shown with the stomach upraised.**
Foramen of Winslow (see arrow).

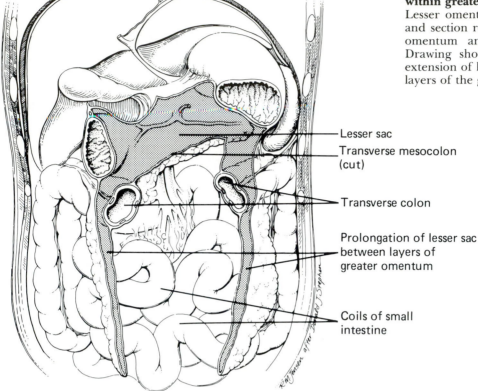

Lesser sac

Transverse mesocolon (cut)

Transverse colon

Prolongation of lesser sac between layers of greater omentum

Coils of small intestine

**Fig. 2–16. Extent of lesser sac within greater omentum.**
Lesser omentum and stomach cut and section removed from greater omentum and transverse colon. Drawing shows potential inferior extension of lesser sac between the layers of the greater omentum.

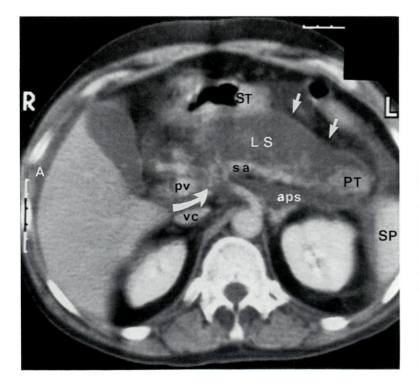

**Fig. 2–17. CT anatomy of the lesser sac.**
Fluid in the lesser sac (LS) behind the stomach (ST) is bounded anteriorly by the gastrocolic ligament (white arrows) and communicates via the epiploic foramen (curved arrow) between the inferior vena cava (vc) and portal vein (pv) with ascitic fluid (A) in the greater peritoneal cavity. Deep to the splenic artery (sa) and pancreatic tail (PT), there is associated fluid within the anterior pararenal space (aps) extending to the angle of the spleen (SP).

communicates, at least potentially, behind the free edge of the lesser omentum with the right subhepatic space via the slitlike foramen of Winslow (Fig. 2–15).

The ultrasonographic features of the lesser sac have been described,[18,19] but it is computed tomography which clearly demonstrates the anatomic characteristics *in vivo*[20–22] (Figs. 2–17 to 2–19).

# Radiologic Features

## The Spread and Localization of Intraperitoneal Abscesses

I have documented that the spread of infection within the peritoneal cavity is governed by (1) the site, nature, and rapidity of outflow of the escaping visceral contents; (2) mesenteric partitions and peritoneal recesses; (3) gravity; (4) intraperitoneal pressure gradients; and (5) the position of the body.[6,14,17,23]

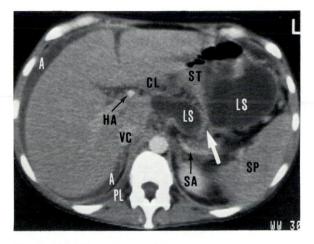

**Fig. 2–18. CT anatomy of the lesser sac.** Identification of landmarks enhanced by intraperitoneal fluid. The lesser sac (LS) is divided into two compartments by a peritoneal fold (arrow) enclosing the left gastric artery as it passes from the posterior abdominal wall to reach the lesser curvature of the stomach (ST). Differentiation between ascites fluid (A) and intrapleural fluid (PL) is clear. CL = caudate lobe of liver, HA = hepatic artery, SA = splenic artery, SP = spleen, VC = vena cava. (Reproduced from Feldberg[55])

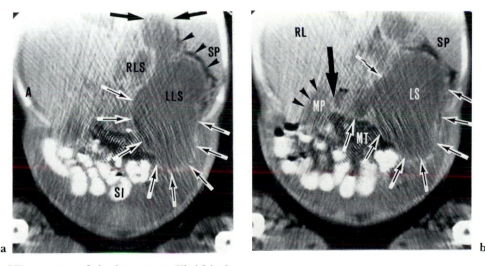

**Fig. 2–19. CT anatomy of the lesser sac. Fluid in lesser sac.**
**(a)** Direct coronal image demonstrates extent of right (RLS) and left (LLS) compartments of the lesser sac. LSS is larger and its inferior recess (black-white arrows) may extend between anterior and posterior leaves of greater omentum. Superiorly the left part of the lesser sac extends to a level below the apex of the diaphragm (black arrows). The greater omentum (arrowheads) is compressed between the lesser sac and the spleen (SP). A = ascites around liver, SI = opacified small intestine.
**(b)** The lesser sac (LS) communicates with Morison's pouch (MP) through the epiploic foramen of Winslow (black arrow). MT = mesentery of small intestine.
(Reproduced from Feldberg[55])

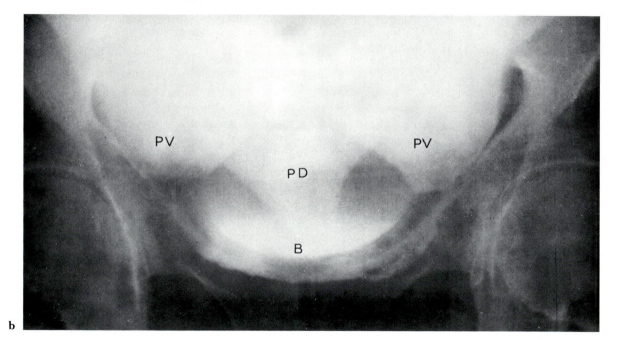

**Fig. 2–20. Fluid accumulation in pelvic recesses.**
**(a)** A small amount of contrast medium introduced into the peritoneal cavity immediately gravitates to the pelvis, filling out the central pouch of Douglas (PD) and then the lateral paravesical fossae (PV).
**(b)** In another patient, erect view shows a larger amount of intraperitoneal contrast medium distending the midline pouch of Douglas (PD) and the lateral paravesical fossae (PV). The urinary bladder (B) is opacified.

**Table 2–1.** Radiologic–anatomic classification of intraperitoneal abscesses[a]

| Supramesocolic | Inframesocolic |
|---|---|
| Right subphrenic | Pelvic |
| Anterior | Paracolic |
| Posterior | Right |
| Right subhepatic | Left |
| Anterior | Infracolic |
| Posterior (Morison's pouch) | Right |
| Left subphrenic | Left |
| Lesser sac | |

[a] Modified from Meyers MA, Whalen JP.[23]

The dynamic pathways of flow of intraperitoneal fluid *in vivo* have been established in a series of adult patients by peritoneography.[6,14] The peritoneal reflections and recesses provide watersheds and drainage basins for the spread and localization of infection (Table 2–1).

Intraabdominal abscesses may be radiologically manifested by demonstrating (a) a soft-tissue mass, (b) a collection or pattern of extraluminal gas, (c) viscus displacement, (d) loss of normally visualized structures, (e) fixation of a

**Fig. 2–21. Intraperitoneal fluid drainage into the cul-de-sac.** Computed tomography following the intraperitoneal injection of water-soluble contrast medium demonstrates pooling within the pouch of Douglas (PD) between the rectum (R) and vagina (V). B = urinary bladder.

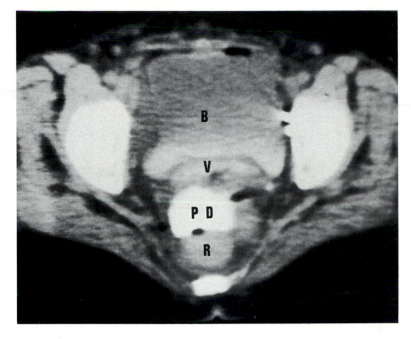

normally mobile organ, or (f) opacification of a communicating sinus or fistulous tract. Secondary signs include scoliosis, elevation or splinting of a diaphragm, localized or generalized ileus, and pulmonary basilar changes. These pathways and localizing features are evident not only by conventional radiologic techniques, but have also been confirmed by ultrasonography,[24,25] isotopic studies,[26] and computed tomography.[27,28] Knowledge of the preferential pathways of spread and subsequent compartmentalization permits the early diagnosis of abscess formation often remote from its site of origin.[6,23]

## Pelvic Abscesses

Fluid introduced into the inframesocolic compartment almost immediately seeks the pelvic cavity, first filling out the central pouch of Douglas (cul-de-sac) and then the lateral paravesical fossae (Fig. 2–20 and 2–21). A small amount in the left infracolic space readily pursues this course, but on the right, it is first arrested at the confluence of the small bowel mesentery with the colon before it overflows into the dependent recesses of the pelvis. This pathway is a function primarily of gravity and explains why the pelvis is the most common site of any residual abscess formation following generalized peritonitis.

Fluid within the pouch of Douglas may be identified easily on supine plain films as a soft-tissue density superior to the urinary bladder (Fig. 2–22), at times with symmetric circular extensions representing further fluid collections within the paravesical fossae.[29] In cases of abdominal trauma, it may be the earliest and most reliable sign of the laceration or rupture of an organ. If doubt exists, a prone film permits the fluid to escape and the radiographic density is lost. Mass displacements by an abscess are seen most easily by extrinsic distortion of the dome of the urinary bladder, by compression on the rectosigmoid junction, or by displacement of the sigmoid colon, usually posteriorly and superiorly (Figs. 2–23 through 2–25). Lateral displacement of sigmoid loops may occur if the abscess extends beyond the midline. A huge abscess may arise out of the pelvis, displacing the intestine superiorly and to the side.

Fluid collections in additional pelvic fossae may be identifiable by CT and ultrasonography.[30]

## Right Subhepatic and Subphrenic Abscesses

From the pelvis, fluid ascends both paracolic gutters. Passage up the shallower left one is slow and weak, and cephalad extension is limited by

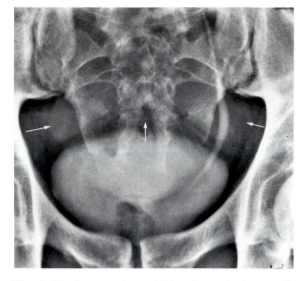

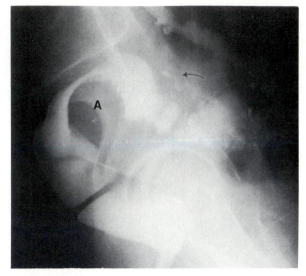

**Fig. 2–22. Intraperitoneal blood** gravitating to the pelvic recesses can be identified as a soft tissue density (arrows) superior to the urinary bladder in this intravenous urogram.

**Fig. 2–24. Pelvic abscess secondary to sigmoid diverticulitis.**
Following perforation of a diverticulum of the sigmoid colon (arrow) in the left lower quadrant, drainage into the pelvis results in an abscess (A) in the pouch of Douglas, shown by its characteristic compression on the rectosigmoid junction.

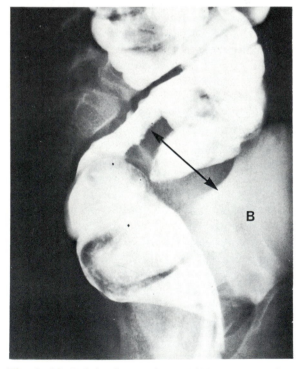

**Fig. 2–23. Pelvic abscess in a child postappendectomy.**
A large soft-tissue mass compresses and separates the rectosigmoid junction and the urinary bladder (B). A redundant sigmoid loop seen in this lateral view projects in this area but is truly off the midline.

the phrenicocolic ligament.[6,17] The major flow from the pelvis is up the right paracolic gutter.[6] It then progresses deep to the inferior edge of the liver into the right subhepatic space, particularly draining into its posterior extension (Morison's pouch) (Figs. 2–26 through 2–31). The right paracolic gutter consistently provides an avenue of spread for exudates. Abscess formation may coalesce in the anterior subhepatic space (Fig. 2–32), but this is unusual. Fluid preferentially seeks first the most dependent recess of Morison's pouch. This is formed by the triangular groove between the lateral aspect of the descending duodenum and the underlying right kidney, just above the beginning of the transverse mesocolon (Fig. 2–33). Thereafter, fluid occupies the entire pouch (Figs. 2–33 through 2–36). This drainage pathway from the pelvis is so constant that if the right paracolic groove can be referred to as a "gutter," then the "sewer" into which it preferentially drains its contaminated material is clearly Morison's pouch.

Intraperitoneal fluid lateral to the liver may be radiographically noted by identifying the lateral margin of the liver which becomes medially displaced (Hellmer's sign[31]) (Figs. 2–37 and 2–38). The appreciable difference in density is sec-

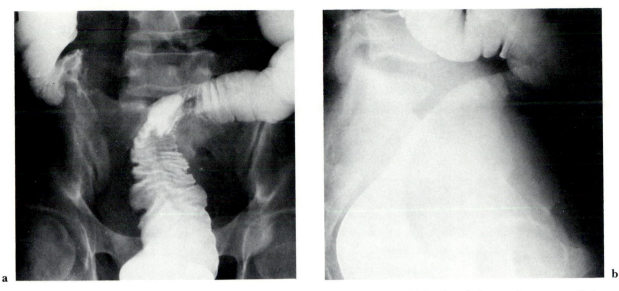

a

b

**Fig. 2–25. Large pelvic abscess** drains from an appendiceal abscess which also deforms the caput of the cecum. Gravitational flow is clearly indicated in the frontal (**a**) and lateral (**b**) views, with the large pelvic abscess displacing the rectum posteriorly against the sacral hollow. (From Meyers[6])

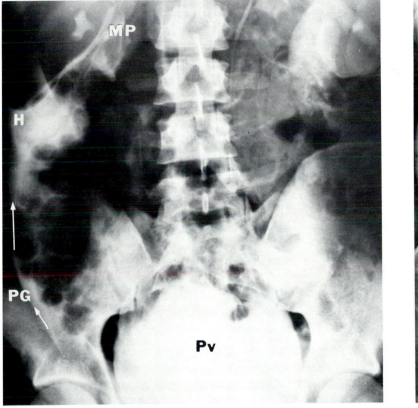

2-26

2-27

**Fig. 2–26. Preferential spread up right paracolic gutter.**
Peritoneography in a patient demonstrates that contrast material, after first filling the pelvis (Pv), then extends directly up the right paracolic gutter (PG). It then outlines the hepatic angle (H) and progresses preferentially into Morison's pouch (MP). (From Meyers[6])

**Fig. 2–27. Contrast medium injected through a misplaced cystotomy tube** (T) whose tip is outside the urinary bladder. The fluid proceeds up the right paracolic gutter (PG) to the subhepatic spaces (SH).

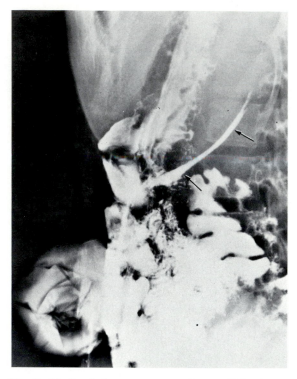

**Fig. 2–28. Leak from anastomotic site** following an ileotransverse colostomy. Extravasation seeks the right subhepatic space (arrows).

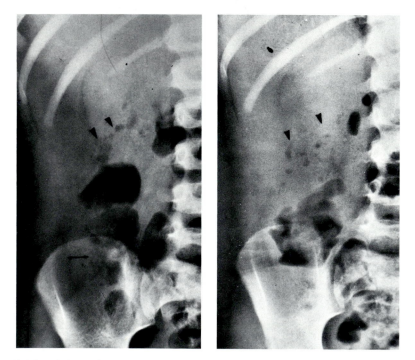

**Fig. 2–29. Appendicitis with perforation.**
Right paracolic fluid results in a density (arrow) that displaces the ascending colon medially. Gaseous exudate (arrowheads) progresses beneath the edge of the liver toward Morison's pouch.

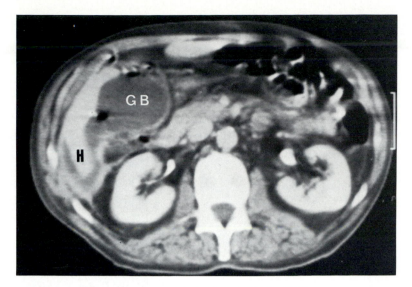

**Fig. 2–30. Infected fluid in Morison's pouch and right paracolic gutter.**
Secondary to perforation of the gallbladder (GB) from emphysematous cholecystitis, CT demonstrates fluid pooling in posterior subhepatic space and right paracolic gutter. The collection surrounds the hepatic angle (H), explaining the loss of visualization by conventional radiologic techniques in these circumstances.

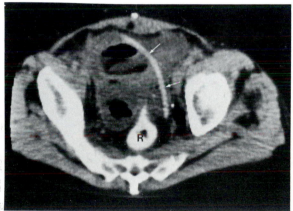

a

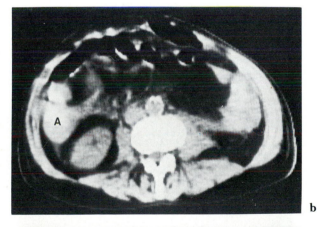

b

**Fig. 2–31. Extension of pelvic abscess to Morison's pouch.**
(a) CT scan of the pelvis, 10 days following sigmoid resection for carcinoma, demonstrates a large gas-containing abscess distending the pouch of Douglas and also compressing the contrast-filled rectum (R). A drainage catheter (arrows) is present.
(b) Scan at the level of the midabdomen reveals the abscess (A) progressing up the right paracolic gutter.
(c) CT of the upper abdomen documents extension of the abscess (A) into Morison's pouch, compressing the posterior contour of the liver.
(Courtesy of Leon Love, MD, Loyola University School of Medicine, Maywood, Ill.)

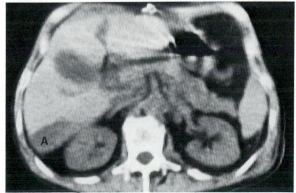

c

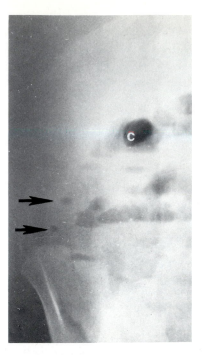

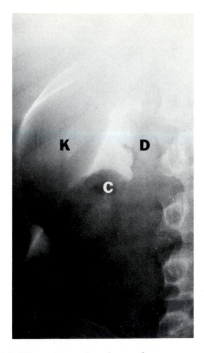

**Fig. 2–32. Right paracolic and anterior subhepatic abscesses,** postappendectomy.

Exudate containing a few gas bubbles (arrows) extends up the right paracolic gutter to a subhepatic abscess. This depresses the proximal transverse colon (C) and, by lifting the edge of the liver from its bed of extraperitoneal fat, results in loss of visualization of the hepatic angle. (From Meyers[6])

**Fig. 2–33. The triangular dependent recess of Morison's pouch** is opacified by a small amount of contrast agent.

This is bounded posteriorly by the kidney (K), medially by the descending duodenum (D), and inferiorly by the proximal transverse colon (C). (From Meyers[6])

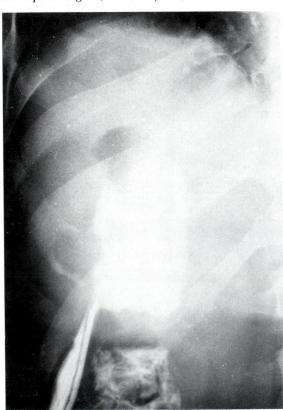

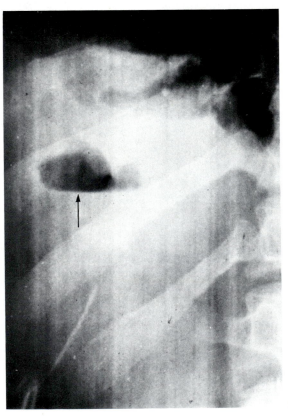

2-34

2-35

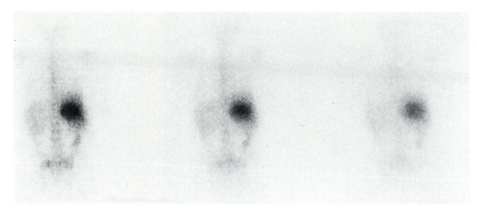

**Fig. 2–36. Morison's pouch abscess.**
Gallium-67 scan, three posterior images from tomoscan series, shows intensive activity in the posterior subhepatic area. (Courtesy of Paul B. Hoffer, MD, Yale University School of Medicine, New Haven, Conn.)

**Fig. 2–37. Fluid lateral to the liver.**
**(a)** Plain film visualization of the lateral margin of the right lobe (arrows) is highlighted by the differences in density between the intraperitoneal fluid and the displaced liver.
**(b)** These changes are confirmed by tomography following the effect of total body opacification.

▷

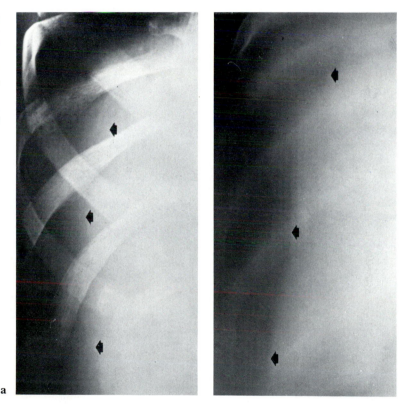

a                                                                                        b

◁————————————————————————————————————————————————————————————▷

**Fig. 2–34. Abscess of Morison's pouch.**
Injection into the localized abscess cavity through a drainage tube identifies its size and position. Note the relationship of the abscess to the 10th and 11th posterior ribs. Residual barium outlines the hepatic flexure of the colon, which serves as the inferior boundary of the abscess.
   The development of pyogenic membranes may prevent spread to other compartments. (From Meyers[6])

**Fig. 2–35. Abscess of Morison's pouch.**
Erect view identifies a conspicuous air–fluid level (arrow) characteristically in relation to the upper pole of the right kidney at the level of the 11th rib.

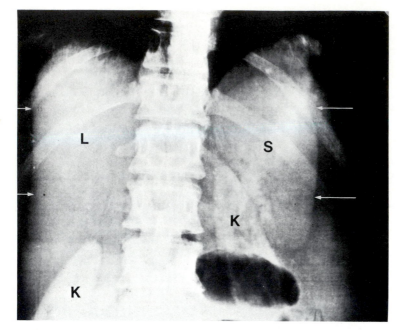

**Fig. 2–38. Fluid lateral to the liver and spleen.**
The enhancement of visualization of the liver (L) and spleen (S) during intravenous infusion of contrast medium clearly demonstrates their medial displacement in a case of ascites. Arrows point out their lateral borders. These changes help to explain the occasional plain-film observation of Hellmer's sign. K = kidneys.

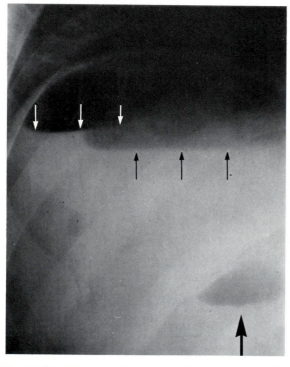

**Fig. 2–39. Right subhepatic and subphrenic abscesses.**
Upright film demonstrates an abscess within Morison's pouch (single arrow) and two air–fluid levels beneath the diaphragm (arrows), representing collections in the right subphrenic spaces over the dome of the liver.

ondary to the attenuation coefficients between ascitic fluid and the hepatic parenchyma.[29,32] Blood, however, does not possess any difference in attenuation from the liver to be seen in this manner.

It is important to recognize that only after Morison's pouch is contaminated does the infected material reach the right subphrenic space (Figs. 2–39 through 2–43). The fluid extends around the inferior edge of the liver or laterally from Morison's pouch along the inferior reflection of the right coronary ligament and then ascends in the flank to the space above the dome of the liver. Pyogenic membranes may compartmentalize an abscess solely to Morison's pouch (Figs. 2–34 and 2–35). Characteristically, this presents as a discrete air-fluid level posteriorly at the level of the 10th to 12th ribs. Whether further spread occurs is probably related to many factors, including particularly the rapidity with which the infection develops and the virulence of the infecting organisms. Fluid collections in the right posterior subphrenic space cannot extend medial to the coronary ligamentous attachments (Figs. 2–42 and 2–43). This is a useful landmark, then, in the distinction from other processes.[33,34] Direct passage from the right subphrenic space across the midline to the

**Fig. 2–40. Right posterior subhepatic and right subphrenic abscesses following a Billroth II procedure.** CT scan demonstrates progression of Morison's pouch abscess (A1) to subphrenic abscess (A2), with compression of the liver (L).

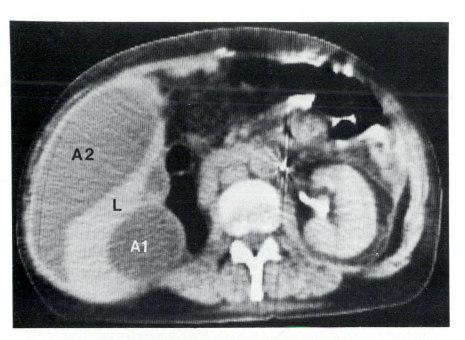

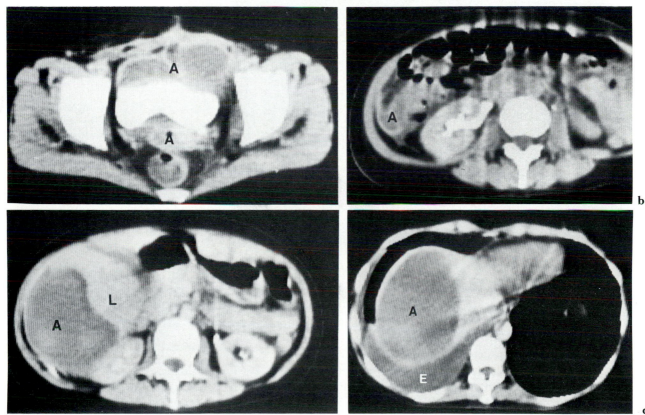

**Fig. 2–41. Extension of pelvic abscesses to right subhepatic and subphrenic spaces,** following hysterectomy. CT scans demonstrate extension of abscess (A) from **(a)** pouch of Douglas and anterior paravesical spaces, along **(b)** the right paracolic gutter, to **(c)** the right anterior and posterior subhepatic spaces, compressing the liver (L), and then **(d)** over the dome of the liver to the anterior and posterior subphrenic spaces, where the infection has elicited a pleural effusion (E). (Courtesy of Leon Love, MD, Loyola University School of Medicine, Maywood, Ill.)

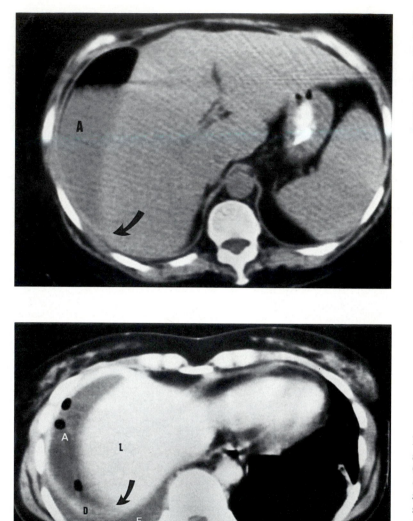

**Fig. 2–43. Right subphrenic abscess and pleural effusion.**
CT shows a gas-containing abscess (A) in the right subphrenic space and a pleural effusion (E). The abscess does not extend medial to the attachment of the superior coronary ligament (arrow) in contrast to the pleural effusion, which extends into the medial costophrenic angle. D = diaphragm, L = liver.

left subphrenic space is prevented by the falciform ligament.

These dynamics of flow explain the incidence and location of intraperitoneal abscesses reported empirically in large clinical series. The frequency of subphrenic and subhepatic abscesses is two to three times greater on the right than on the left,[3,9] and the most common site is Morison's pouch.[9] Abscesses localized solely to the right anterior subhepatic space are relatively uncommon. Abscesses of Morison's pouch and the right subphrenic space often coexist. Clinical evidence of abscesses limited to the right subphrenic space, however, is not uncommon, but it can be assumed that some contamination of

the right posterior subhepatic space had already occurred, perhaps manifested only by some residual inflammatory adhesions.

*Hydrostatic Considerations.* In addition to the anatomic pathways and action of gravity, variations in intraperitoneal pressure also determine the distribution of peritoneal fluid. Egress from the pelvis upward is not a function simply of overflow. Fluid surmounts the sacral promontory and flank muscles to extend upward, whether the patient is horizontal or erect. Autio[35] first documented the intraperitoneal extension of radiographic contrast medium into the upper abdominal recesses even in the erect position. Ten milliliters of oily contrast medium were introduced into the ileocecal, paracecal, and paraduodenal regions of 38 patients in connection with appendectomy or cholecystectomy. Although the oil derivative tended to fragment, it had an advantage in that it persisted in the peritoneal cavity for a least 3 days before being absorbed. It was therefore possible to see that its distribution on the first day, when the patient was supine, was the same as that on later days, when the patient was erect for lengthy periods of time, and achieved its final disposition within 3 hours of insertion. The contrast medium moved both down into the pelvis and up into the subphrenic space via the two-way avenue of the right paracolic gutter.

The hydrostatic pressure of the contents of the abdominal cavity together with the flexibility of a portion of the abdominal wall determine, for the most part, the pressure within the abdominal cavity. Overholt[36] demonstrated in animals that the hydrostatic pressure in the subdiaphragmatic region is lower than that elsewhere in the abdomen and that the pressure varies with respiration. The intraperitoneal pressure in the upper abdomen is subatmospheric and decreases further during inspiration. This negative subdiaphragmatic pressure and its relation to breathing are maintained in the horizontal or erect position. This is explained by the outward movement of the ribs during inspiration, which enlarges the space in the upper abdomen more than it is decreased by the descent of the diaphragm. Salkin[37] subsequently confirmed these observations in humans, noting in a series of 50 cases that most showed an intraperitoneal pressure of from 0 to $-30$ mm $H_2O$ and that pressure is less in the epigastrium than in the hypogastrium. Drye[38] recorded that in the supine position intraperitoneal pressure averages 8 cm $H_2O$ and in the upright position pressure in the lower abdomen is almost three times as great as in the supine position. These pressure differences with positional and respiratory variations have been confirmed by others. Hydrostatic pressure differences between the lower and upper abdomen are capable then, even in the upright position, of conveying infected material.

Fluid introduced into the right supramesocolic area follows similar pathways.[6] Preferential flow is directly into Morison's pouch, with pro-

gression to the right subphrenic space and, via the right paracolic gutter, to the pelvis. In 1940, Mitchell,[11] using sequential injections of barium emulsions in infant cadavers, concluded that exudates do not progress directly from beneath the liver to the subphrenic area but first follow a circuitous route over and ventral to the proximal transverse colon to contaminate the right infracolic space. Although many of his basic observations have been subsequently confirmed, he incorrectly concluded that the right paracolic gutter is not the major path of communication by which infection spreads to and from the upper and lower peritoneal compartments. It was not until the development of peritoneography that the effects of intraabdominal pressure gradients and body movements *in vivo* on the flow of fluid were accurately observed radiologically.[6,14]

## Lesser Sac Abscesses

Anatomically, Morison's pouch communicates with the lesser sac via the epiploic foramen. Noninfected intraperitoneal fluid originating within the greater peritoneal cavity may thus readily gain entrance to the lesser sac (Figs. 2–44 through 2–46). However, this slitlike connection is easily sealed off by adhesions, so the lesser sac is not usually contaminated in generalized peritonitis unless the primary infection arises in the walls of the lesser sac itself. Abscesses here are therefore encountered most often following perforated posterior ulcers of the stomach or duodenal bulb and pancreatitis (Figs. 2–47 through 2–52).

Lesser sac abscesses typically distend the space and displace the stomach anteriorly and the transverse colon inferiorly. I have noted that adhesions developing along the peritoneal fold raised by the left gastric artery often clearly partition an abscess to one of its two major compartments (Figs. 2–48, 2–49, and 2–52 through 2–55). Infection may occasionally follow acute rupture of the gallbladder, presumably since the bile is discharged into the lesser sac before the foramen can be sealed off (Fig. 2–56). Perforation of the posterior wall of the intraabdominal esophagus extends directly into the lesser sac.[39]

## Left Subphrenic Abscesses

Abscesses in the left subphrenic space may result from perforated anterior ulcers of the

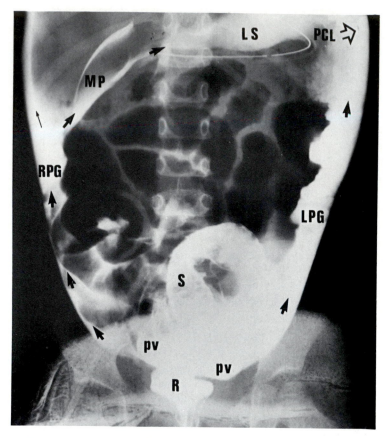

**Fig. 2–44. Extension of intraperitoneal fluid into the lesser sac.**
Contrast enema performed in a child following perforation of the rectosigmoid junction (R = rectum, S = sigmoid colon). Extravasation opacifies the paravesical fossae (pv) and the right paracolic gutter (RPG). Flow continues to Morison's pouch (MP), through the epiploic foramen to the lesser sac (LS). Extension up the left paracolic gutter (LPG) is impeded at the phrenicocolic ligament (PCL). (Courtesy of William Thompson, MD, University of Minnesota School of Medicine, Minneapolis, MN)

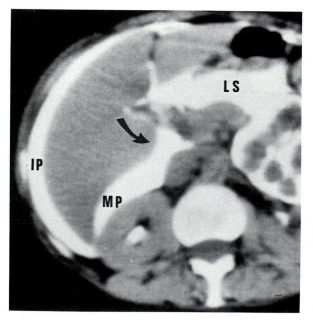

◁

**Fig. 2–45. Extension of intraperitoneal fluid into the lesser sac.**
Following intraperitoneal (IP) injection of water-soluble contrast medium, CT demonstrates direct communication of fluid from Morison's pouch (MP) through the epiploic foramen (arrow) to the lesser sac (LS).

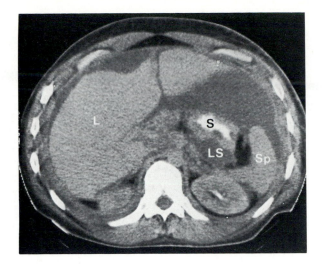

**Fig. 2–46. Entrance of noninfected intraperitoneal fluid into the lesser sac.**
CT scan in a patient with gastric linitis plastica demonstrates ascitic fluid within the lesser sac (LS) behind the contrast-filled thickened stomach (S), as well as within the greater peritoneal cavity around the liver (L) and spleen (Sp). The lesser sac fluid is bounded laterally by the gastrosplenic and splenorenal ligaments.

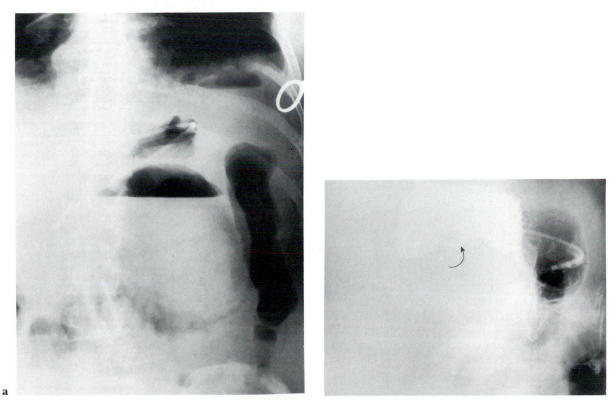

a
b

**Fig. 2–47. Lesser sac abscess** following perforation of a posterior gastric ulcer.
**(a)** Erect plain film at admission shows a large gas-containing abscess within the lesser sac displacing the transverse colon downward. (A smaller component extends beneath the left diaphragm.)
**(b)** After surgical drainage, cross-table lateral film of an upper GI series with water-soluble contrast medium demonstrates a posterior ulcer of the stomach (arrow) to be the underlying cause.

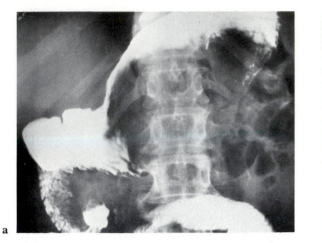
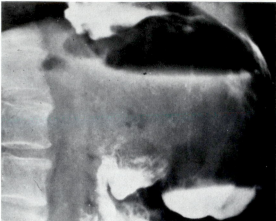

a                                                                                                          b

**Fig. 2–48. Lesser sac abscess** following perforation of a posterior gastric ulcer.
    Frontal **(a)** and erect lateral **(b)** views demonstrate a large gas-containing abscess behind the stomach. The collection is compartmentalized within the lateral compartment of the omental bursa by adhesions along the peritoneal fold of the left gastric artery.

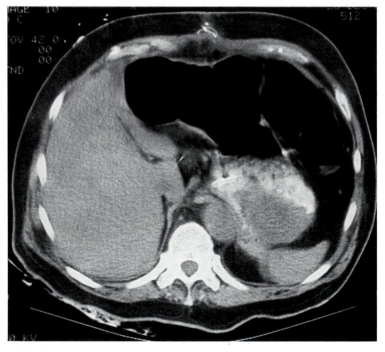

**Fig. 2–49. Lesser sac abscess.**
Following surgery for a perforated gastric ulcer, CT demonstrates communication of oral contrast medium to retrogastric abscess collection in the lateral compartment of the lesser sac. The abscess is bounded laterally by the gastrosplenic ligament.

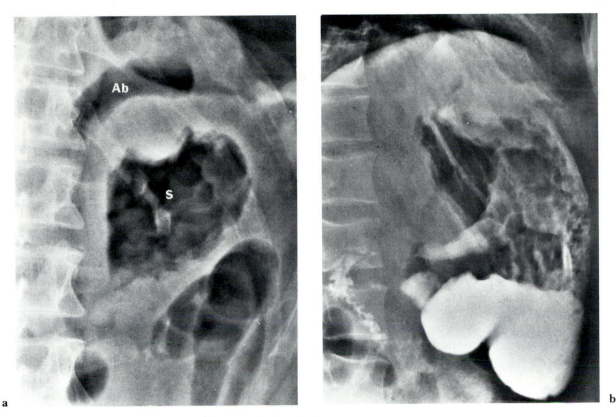

**Fig. 2–50. Lesser sac abscess** secondary to duodenal ulcer.
**(a)** Right lateral decubitus plain film. There is a loculated gas-containing abscess (Ab) compressing the top of the fundus of the stomach (S). On a frontal projection, this might suggest a subphrenic collection within the greater peritoneal cavity. There are associated changes at the base of the left lung.
**(b)** Upper GI series. Lateral view shows extravasation into the lesser sac behind the stomach from a posterior ulcer of the duodenal bulb.

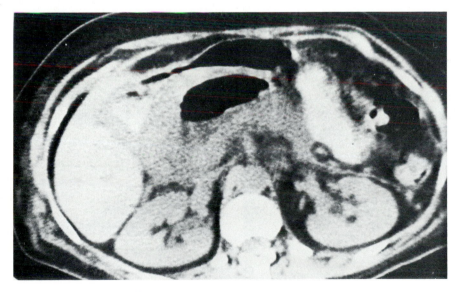

**Fig. 2–51. Lesser sac abscess** secondary to pancreatitis.
CT scan demonstrates a large gas-producing abscess of the pancreas distending the lesser sac and displacing the stomach anteriorly. (Courtesy of Daniel Wise, MD, Toronto Western Hospital, Toronto, Canada)

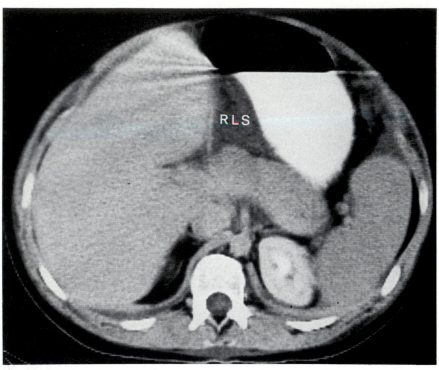

**Fig. 2–52. Pancreatic fluid within medial compartment of lesser sac.**
In this patient with acute pancreatitis, there is fluid loculation within the right (medial) compartment of the lesser sac (RLS).

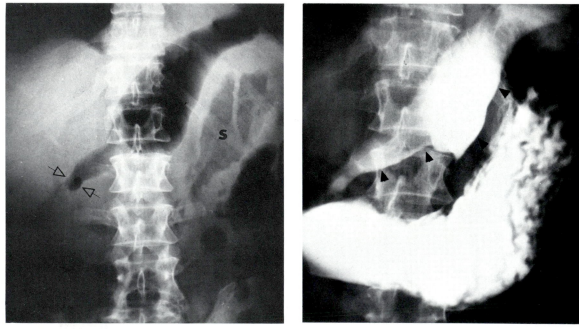

a                                                                                                                    b

**Fig. 2–53. Lesser sac abscess.**
(a) Well-defined loculated gas collection superior to the stomach (S), identified by its rugal outlines. The collection is continuous with a circular lucency at its base (arrows). There are associated changes at the left lung base.
(b) GI series demonstrates extravasation from a large duodenal ulcer accounting for the circular lucency on the plain film, into the medial compartment of the lesser sac, demarcated inferiorly by the fold (arrowheads) raised by the left gastric artery.

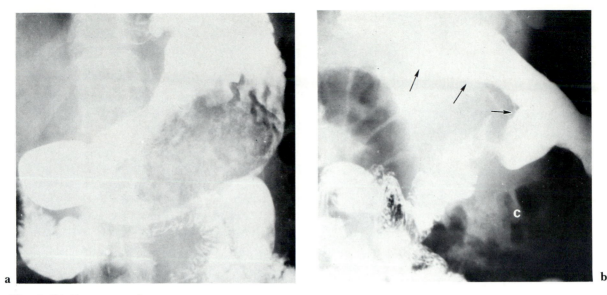

**Fig. 2–54. Lesser sac abscess.**
Frontal **(a)** and lateral **(b)** projections demonstrate a large retrogastric mass displacing the stomach anteriorly (arrows) and depressing the transverse colon (C). These changes localize the abscess behind the stomach and gastrocolic ligament and above the transverse mesocolon. The collection is compartmentalized within the lateral compartment of the omental bursa.

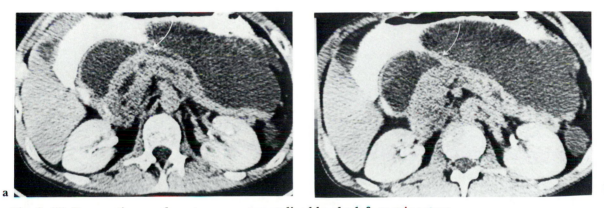

**Fig. 2–55. Pancreatic pseudocysts compartmentalized by the left gastric artery.**
CT scan at two different levels **(a** and **b)** demonstrates partition of pseudocysts obliterating the lesser sac by attachment (arrow) to the posterior wall of the contrast-filled stomach along the plane of the peritoneal fold of the left gastric artery.

stomach or duodenal bulb, but are seen particularly as complications of gastric or colonic surgery and of splenectomy.

The most consistent aspect of flow of fluid arising in the left upper quadrant is that it is preferentially directed upward to the subphrenic area, where an abscess typically coalesces.[6] This is a function of the negative intraabdominal pressure beneath the diaphragm related to respiration.

Figure 2–57 details the pathway from a perforation of the anterior wall of the stomach extending deep to the left lobe of the liver to abscess development in the immediate left subphrenic area. Coalescence of an abscess between the stomach and the left lobe of the liver is unusual. A similar direct cephalad extension is shown in an instance of colonic perforation in Figure 2–58, and other instances of post-splenectomy abscesses in Figures 2–59 and 2–60.

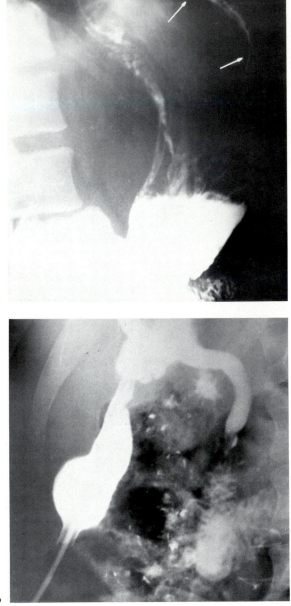

Anastomotic leaks are being increasingly recognized as a source of postoperative left subphrenic abscesses. These may be small and loculated (Fig. 2–61) or extensive (Figs. 2–62 and 2–63).

When the volume of infected material in the left subphrenic space is considerable, one of two routes becomes available:

1. Spread may occur across the midline, beneath the free edge of the falciform ligament, to the right subhepatic, right subphrenic, and then the right paracolic recesses. Figure 2–64 shows the pathways of infection across three quadrants of the abdomen, arising from a perforated ulcer of the stomach.

2. More often, the infected material simply overflows the strut of the phrenicocolic ligament. Ordinarily, inferior extension from the left subphrenic space tends to be arrested by this strong peritoneal reflection. However, large amounts simply proceed over it to the left paracolic gutter and then the pelvis (Figs. 2–65 and 2–66). From this site, contamination may rise up the paracolic gutter to the subhepatic and subphrenic spaces on the right.

Infection arising in the pelvis may extend upward to some degree within the shallow left paracolic gutter, where the relatively slow flow may permit the development of adhesions and thereby coalescence into an abscess (Figs. 2–67 and 2–68). Medial displacement of the descending colon may result and discrete gas shadows may be seen in the area of the infected fluid. Bulging of the posterolateral abdominal wall may be evident. The properitoneal fat line, radiologically referred to as the "flank stripe," is generally maintained. Loss of clear visualization of this implies extension of the infection across the peritoneal surface into the abdominal wall. Livingston's description[41] that "fluid may well upward out of the pelvis . . . to pass into the left paracolic groove, to extend farther upward into the perisplenic space" is generally not true. I have noted that an intact phrenicocolic ligament usually prevents spread to the left subphrenic area. This explains the repeatedly noted infrequency of left upper quadrant abscesses following generalized peritonitis. However, if the phrenicocolic ligament had been excised previously, as is done in splenectomy and in surgical mobilization of the splenic flexure of

**Fig. 2–56. Lesser sac abscess** secondary to perforated gallbladder.
**(a)** Initial upper GI series shows a large retrogastric mass and left pulmonary basilar changes.
**(b)** Contrast injection through a paracolic drainage tube demonstrates that the catheter has inadvertently entered a site of gallbladder rupture.

**Fig. 2–57. Left subphrenic abscess** from anterior gastric perforation.

**(a)** Extensive scirrhous carcinoma of the stomach.

**(b** and **c)** Following gastroscopy, with accidental perforation of the anterior gastric wall, repeat study shows contrast material extends from the stomach (S) anterior to the lesser omentum (LO). It tracks to a large abscess (arrow) beneath the diaphragm and above the colon (C), which is opacified by residual barium.

(From Meyers[6])

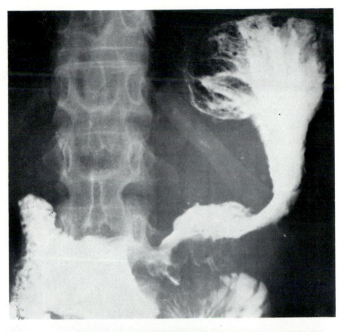

a

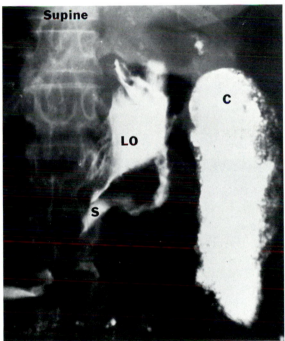

b

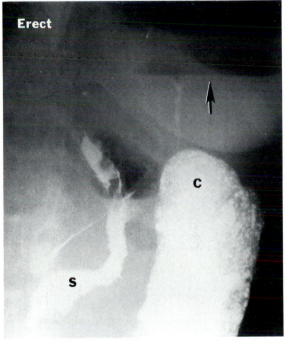

c

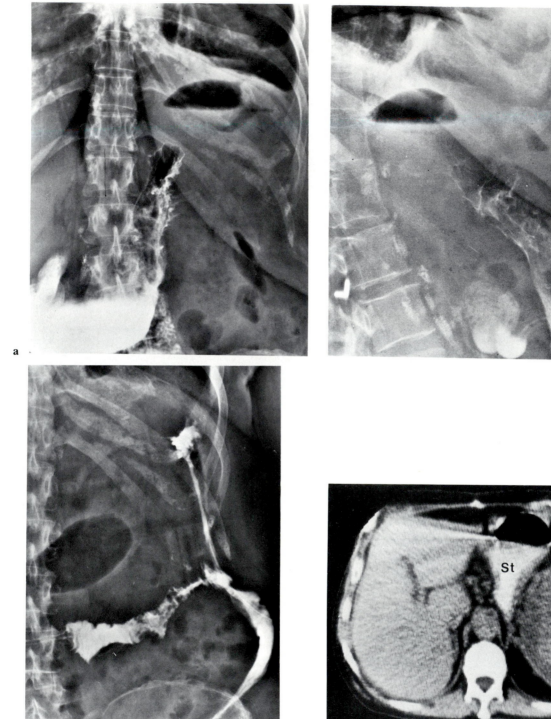

**Fig. 2–58. Left subphrenic abscess,** postsplenectomy.
**(a** and **b)** Erect frontal and lateral views demonstrate a large air–fluid collection extending lateral and superior to the stomach.
**(c)** Barium enema study shows a postsurgical perforation of the splenic flexure with a sinus tract leading to the subphrenic abscess.

**Fig. 2–59. Left subphrenic abscess,** postsplenectomy. CT scan demonstrates large gas-containing abscess (A) in the splenic bed behind and lateral to the contrast-filled stomach (St). (Courtesy of Leon Love, MD, Loyola University School of Medicine, Maywood, Ill.)

**Fig. 2–60. Left subphrenic abscess,** postsplenectomy. CT scan demonstrates a huge abscess (A) in the splenic bed, displacing the contrast-filled stomach (St) anteriorly and medially. (Courtesy of Leon Love, MD, Loyola University School of Medicine, Maywood, Ill.)                                   ▷

**Fig. 2–61. Chronic loculated left subphrenic abscess** secondary to anastomotic leak, following gastrectomy and esophagojejunostomy. Frontal (**a**) and lateral (**b**) views.

▽

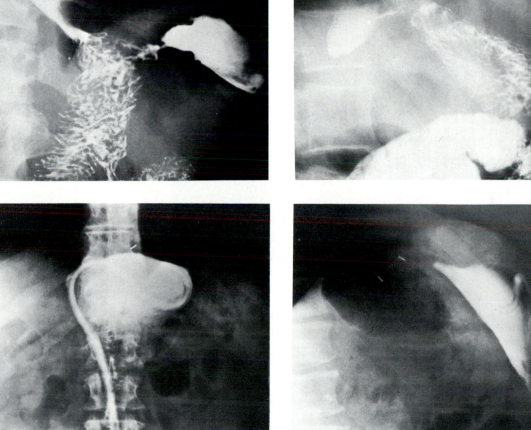

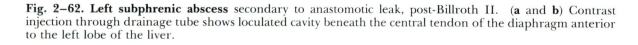

**Fig. 2–62. Left subphrenic abscess** secondary to anastomotic leak, post-Billroth II.   (**a** and **b**) Contrast injection through drainage tube shows loculated cavity beneath the central tendon of the diaphragm anterior to the left lobe of the liver.

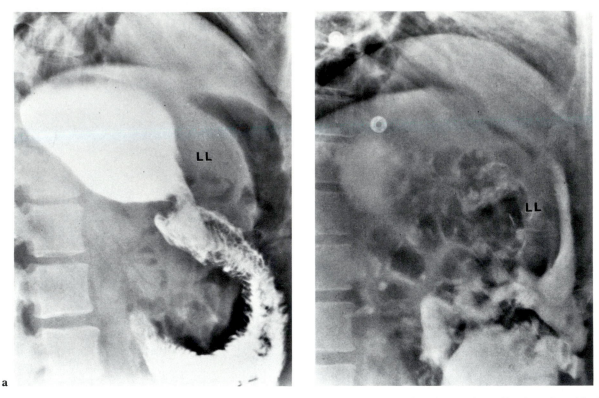

a                                                                              b

**Fig. 2–63. Left subphrenic abscess** secondary to anastomotic leak, post-Billroth II. The collection, first filled with gas and later opacified, seeks the subphrenic area anterior to the left lobe of the liver (LL).

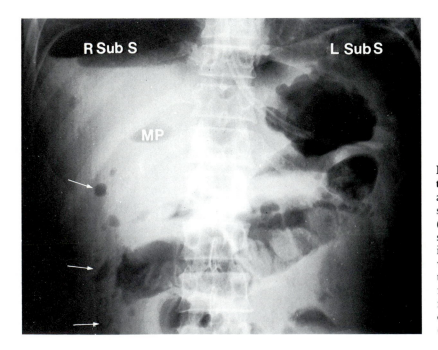

**Fig. 2–64. Perforation of an anterior wall gastric ulcer** leads to abscesses of the left subphrenic space (LSubS), Morison's pouch (MP), and the right subphrenic space (RSubS). The gas-containing exudate extends along the visceral surface of the liver to the right paracolic gutter (arrows). This case illustrates the flow of exudate across three quadrants of the abdomen. (From Meyers[6])

**Fig. 2–65. Extravasated contrast material in the left upper quadrant** (1) at the time of percutaneous splenoportography can be traced to overflow the phrenicocolic ligament (PL) and proceed down the left paracolic gutter (2) to the pelvis (3). From here it ascends the right paracolic gutter (4) to the subhepatic spaces (5). This illustrates the dynamic pathways of fluid across the four quadrants of the abdomen.

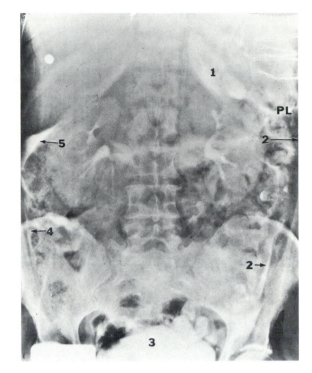

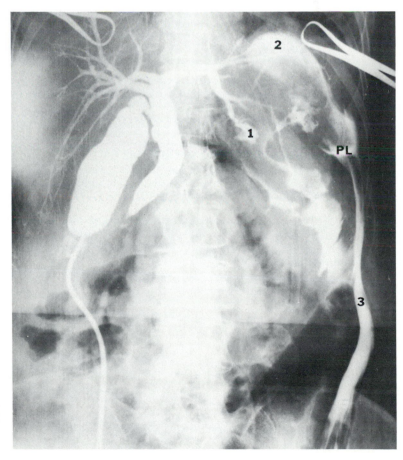

**Fig. 2–66. Stab wound of liver.**
Injection through cholecystotomy tube shows extravasation from left lobe of liver (1). This seeks the left subphrenic space (2), overflows the phrenicocolic ligament (PL), and progresses down the left paracolic gutter (3) to the pelvis.

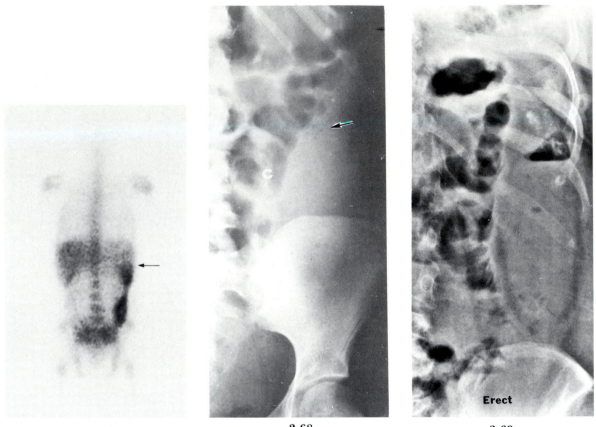

2-67                                    2-68                                    2-69

**Fig. 2–67. Phlegmon in left paracolic gutter,** postappendectomy.
Gallium-67 scan demonstrates activity extending up the left paracolic gutter with an abrupt cut-off at the level of the phrenicocolic ligament (arrow). This activity is not in the colon and did not clear following repeated enemas. Activity in the pelvis is associated with surgical drains in this area. (Courtesy of Paul B. Hoffer, MD, Yale University School of Medicine, New Haven, Conn.)

**Fig. 2–68. Localized abscess of the left paracolic gutter,** 2 weeks after a cesarean section.
The mass displaces the descending colon (C) medially and bulges the flank structures laterally. It is ill defined inferiorly and superiorly at which point several small discrete gas bubbles are present (arrow). Cephalad flow to the left subphrenic space is prevented by the phrenicocolic ligament in this case.

**Fig. 2–69. Abscess of left paracolic gutter extending into the perisplenic space.**
Following a resection of the sigmoid colon with mobilization of the splenic flexure and excision of the phrenicocolic ligament, the large gas-producing infected collection in the gutter is not restrained from progressing into the perisplenic area.

the colon, infection may readily spread from the left paracolic gutter to the subphrenic space (Figs. 2–69 and 2–70).

## Summary of Pathways

Figure 2–71 summarizes the major pathways of spread of intraperitoneal infections. Given the source of contamination, an understanding of

the dynamics of spread allows the anticipation of a remote abscess at a specific site.

Postoperative changes of normal anatomic barriers may cause subsequent development of abscesses in unusual or unexpected locations[42] (Fig. 2–72).

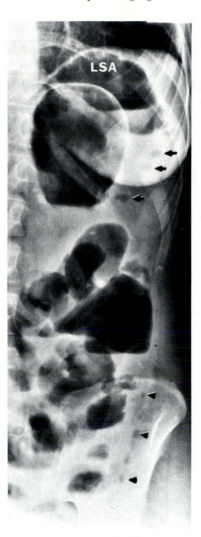

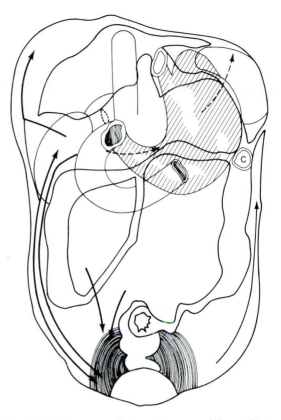

**Fig. 2–71. Diagram of the pathways of flow of intra-peritoneal exudates.**
(See Fig. 2–2.) Broken arrows indicate spread anterior to the stomach to the left subphrenic area. C = splenic flexure of colon. (Modified from Meyers[6])

**Fig. 2–70. Left paracolic and subphrenic abscesses.** Following splenectomy and excision of the phrenicocolic ligament, intestinal infarction within the pelvis leads to infected exudate in the left paracolic gutter (arrows). This progresses without interruption to the development of a left subphrenic abscess (LSA).

# The Sectional and Isotopic Imaging Modalities

The sectional imaging modalities have not only confirmed the pathways of extension but have provided a striking advance in the diagnosis and localization of intraperitoneal abscesses[27] (Table 2–2).

Ultrasonography has a sensitivity of almost 95% and a specificity approaching 100% if the study is not limited by bowel gas, obesity, and surgical wounds and bandages. The absence of ionizing radiation makes it particularly safe in evaluating children and young women. Abscesses present generally as irregular fluid collections with indistinct margins. Ultrasonography is too time consuming, however, to serve as a survey evaluation of the entire abdomen in suspected abscesses; it is best used when localizing features have been indicated.

Computed tomography may reveal an abscess as a mass with low attenuation value displacing surrounding structures, occasionally with a peripheral rim of higher density which may show contrast enhancement; there may be thickening or obliteration of neighboring fascial planes, and the frequent presence of gas bubbles or air–fluid levels usually allows definitive diagnosis. CT may diagnose and accurately define the extent of involvement in at least 90% of cases, depending on the size of the abscess. It provides

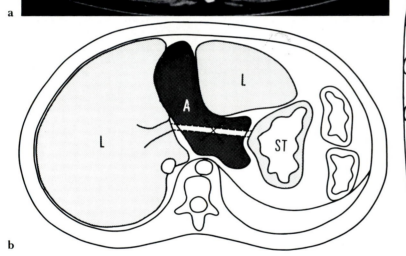

**Fig. 2–72. Spread of abscess following transection of gastrohepatic ligament.**

**(a)** The gastrohepatic ligament was operatively transected. This permits the spread of abscess (arrows) from the ventrally located gastrohepatic recess between the stomach (ST) and left lobe of liver (L) to the superior recess of the lesser sac.

**(b and c)** Cross-sectional and sagittal drawings showing spread of abscess (A) permitted by removal of the anatomic barrier of the gastrohepatic ligament. C = colon, LS = lesser sac. (Reproduced from Pokieser et al[42])

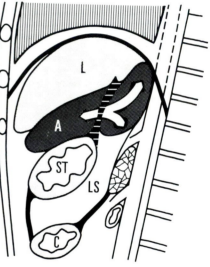

**Table 2–2.** Accuracy of sectional and isotopic imaging modalities in the diagnosis of intraabdominal abscess[a]

| Modality | Sensitivity (true-positive rate) (%) | Specificity (true-negative rate) (%) |
|---|---|---|
| Gallium Scanning | 50–100 (generally 75–85)[b] | 75–100 (generally 85–95)[c] |
| Ultrasonography | 75–95 (generally 90–95) | 95–100 |
| Computed tomography | 90–100 | 100 |

[a] Statistics derived from Forgacs,[46] Haaga,[47] Hopkins,[44] Knochel,[48] Kumar,[49] Taylor,[50] and Wolverson.[51]

[b] False positives: Healing incision, LUQ bowel postsplenectomy, tumors, nonabscess inflammation (pyelonephritis, inflammatory or ischemic bowel disease)

[c] False negatives: Large acute abscesses and secondarily infected hematomas, pseudocyst.

**Table 2–3.** Diagnostic algorithm for suspected abdominal abscess

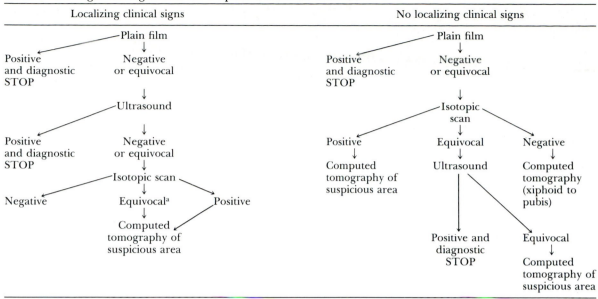

<sup>a</sup> If equivocal or positive in area not already examined by ultrasound, ultrasound should be repeated prior to CT.

precise differentiation with excellent anatomic detail. Radiation dosage is comparable to that from an average barium study. The characteristic signs on ultrasonography and CT usually permit clear distinction from other postoperative fluid collections such as seroma and lymphocysts.

Ultrasonography is superior to conventional radiography and probably to CT for detection of minor intraperitoneal fluid.[24,28] A study has shown that magnetic resonance imaging (MRI) provides equivalent information to CT concerning the presence and extent of intraabdominal fluid collections.[43]

The overall accuracy for gallium-67 examination is highly dependent on the type of patient studied; the presence of a surgical incision as well as nonspecific uptake in inflammatory but nonsuppurative lesions, bowel, and tumors may be mistaken for an abscess. Despite the use of cleansing enemas for repeated gallium scans, differentiation of an abscess from normal bowel may still occasionally be difficult. The technique provides relatively poor resolution and has a higher false-positive and false-negative rate than either ultrasonography or computed tomography. Although 6-hour delay scans have been advocated,[44] they are difficult to interpret because of high background radioactivity. A reliable diagnosis may be made from the 24-hour study, but 48- and sometimes 72-hour scans are necessary. This contrasts with the immediate results obtainable from ultrasonography and computed tomography.

[111]In-labeled leukocyte scanning, in contrast, results in superior image quality; moreover, no indium-111 normally appears in the gastrointestinal tract or its contents, or in the urinary collection system. However, intense uptake may occur in recent hematomas and less intense accumulations in any acute inflammatory lesion and in some noninflammatory states as well.[45]

Isotopic scans are particularly useful as an initial survey in suspected abscesses when there are no localizing clinical signs and plain-film findings are negative or equivocal.

Table 2-3 outlines a rational diagnostic algorithm in cases of suspected abdominal abscesses.[27]

# Management

Precise radiologic identification of an intraabdominal abscess permits the most appropriate route of drainage (see Fig. 2–8). Although antibiotics play an important role, drainage remains the cornerstone of therapy. Radiographic localization is particularly important in supramesocolic infections.

An abscess compartmentalized to the right posterior subhepatic space is best drained surgically by Ochsner's extrapleural approach through the bed of the resected 12th rib. The right posterior subphrenic space is drained via Trendelenburg's transpleural route; the 8th, 9th, 10th, or 11th ribs are resected subperiosteally, the pleural cavity is entered, the diaphragm tightly sutured around the pleural opening, and the subphrenic abscess drained after an incision is made through the diaphragm.

A transperitoneal approach is generally employed for surgical drainage of anterior subphrenic and subhepatic, left subphrenic, lesser sac, and multiple abscesses. It is especially advantageous since it permits a thorough evaluation of the extent of the purulent collection and drainage can be undertaken accordingly.

Ultrasound- and CT-guided aspiration and drainage of intraabdominal abscesses represent recent major advantages in management.[52-54]

# References

1. Connell TR, Stephens DH, Carlson HC, et al: Upper abdominal abscess: A continuing and deadly problem. AJR 134: 759–765, 1980
2. Wang SMS, Wilson SE: Subphrenic abscess: The new epidemiology. Arch Surg 112:934–936, 1977
3. Wetterfors J: Subphrenic abscess: A clinical study of 101 cases. Acta Chir Scand 117: 388–408, 1959
4. Samuel E, Duncan JG, Philip T, et al: Radiology of the postoperative abdomen. Clin Radiol 14: 133–148, 1963
5. Annotation: Subphrenic abscess: A changing pattern. Lancet 2: 301, 1970
6. Meyers MA: The spread and localization of acute intraperitoneal effusions. Radiology 95: 547–554, 1970
7. Morison R: The anatomy of the right hypochondrium relating especially to operations for gallstones. Br Med J 2: 968, 1894
8. Barnard HL: Surgical aspects of subphrenic spaces. Br Med J 1: 371–377, 1908
9. Ochsner A, DeBakey M: Subphrenic abscess: Collective review and an analysis of 3,608 collected and personal cases. Int Abstr Surg 66: 426–438, 1938
10. Harley HRS: Subphrenic abscess, with particular reference to the spread of infection. Hunterian Lecture. Ann R Coll Surg Engl 17: 201–224, 1955
11. Mitchell GAG: The spread of acute intraperitoneal effusions. Br J Surg 28: 291–313, 1940
12. Boyd DP: The anatomy and pathology of the subphrenic spaces. Surg Clin N Am 38: 619–626, 1958
13. Boyd DP: The subphrenic spaces and the emperor's new robes. N Engl J Med 275: 911–917, 1966
14. Meyers MA: Peritoneography: Normal and pathologic anatomy. AJR 117: 353–365, 1973
15. Whalen JP, Bierny JP: Classification of perihepatic abscesses. Radiology 92: 1427–1437, 1969
16. Wooler AH: Subphrenic abscess. Thorax 11: 211–222, 1956
17. Meyers MA: Roentgen significance of the phrenicocolic ligament. Radiology 95: 539–545, 1970
18. Vincent LM, Mauro MA, Mittelstaedt CA: The lesser sac and gastrohepatic recess: Sonographic appearance and differentiation of fluid collections. Radiology 150: 515–519, 1984
19. Weill FS, Perriguey G, Belloir A, et al: Ultrasonic anatomical study of the lesser omental sac: A pictorial essay. Europ J Radiol 3: 142–147, 1983
20. Dodds WJ, Foley DW, Lawson TL, et al: Anatomy and imaging of the lesser peritoneal sac. AJR 144: 567–575, 1985
21. Jeffrey RB, Federle MP, Goodman PC: Computed tomography of the lesser peritoneal sac. Radiology 141: 117–122, 1981
22. Meyers MA, Oliphant M, Berne AS, et al: The peritoneal ligaments and mesenteries: Pathways of intra-abdominal spread of disease. Annual oration. Radiology 163: 593–604, 1987
23. Meyers MA, Whalen JP: Radiologic aspects of intraabdominal abscesses. The Diagnosis and Treatment of Intraabdominal Abscesses. Edited by I Ariel, K Kazarian. Williams & Wilkins, Baltimore, 1971
24. Forsby J, Henriksson L: Detectability of intraperitoneal fluid by ultrasonography. Acta Radiol Diagn 25(Fasc. 5): 375–378, 1984
25. Yeh H-C, Wolf BS: Ultrasonography in ascites. Radiology 124: 783–790, 1977
26. Myerson PJ, Myerson D, Spencer RP: Anatomic patterns of Ga-67 distribution in localized and diffuse peritoneal inflammation: Case report. J Nucl Med 18: 977–980, 1977
27. Meyers MA: Abdominal abscesses. Pp 186–190. In Radiology Today. Edited by MW Donner, FHW Heuck. Springer-Verlag, Berlin, Heidelberg, 1981
28. Wojtowicz J, Rzymski K, Czarnecki R: A CT evaluation of the intraperitoneal fluid distribution. Fortschr Röntgenstr 137(1): 95–99, 1982
29. Jorulf H: Roentgen diagnosis of intraperitoneal fluid. A physical, anatomic, and clinical investigation. Acta Radiol Suppl 343, 1975
30. Auh YH, Rubenstein WA, Markisz JA, et al: In-

traperitoneal paravesical spaces: CT delineation with US correlation. Radiology 159: 311–317, 1986

31. Hellmer H: Die Konturen des rechten Leberlappens beim Ascites. Acta Radiol 23: 533–540, 1942

32. Love L, Demos TC, Reynes CJ, et al: Visualization of the lateral edge of the liver in ascites. Radiology 122: 619–622, 1977

33. Naidich DP, Megibow AJ, Hilton S, et al: Computed tomography of the diaphragm: Peridiaphragmatic fluid collection. J Comp Assist Tomogr 7: 641–649, 1983

34. Rubinstein WA, Auh YH, Whalen JP, et al: The perihepatic spaces: computed tomographic and ultrasound imaging. Radiology 149: 231–239, 1983

35. Autio V: The spread of intraperitoneal infection. Studies with roentgen contrast medium. Acta Chir Scand Suppl 321: 1–31, 1964

36. Overholt RH: Intraperitoneal pressure. Arch Surg 22: 691–703, 1931.

37. Salkin D: Intraabdominal pressure and its regulation. Am Rev Tubercu 30: 436–457, 1934

38. Drye JC: Intraperitoneal pressure in the human. Surg Gynecol Obstet 87: 472–475, 1948

39. Allen KS, Siskind BN, Burrell MI: Perforation of distal esophagus with lesser sac extension: CT demonstration. J Comp Assist Tomogr 10(4): 612–614, 1986

40. Halvorsen RA, Jones MA, Rice RP, Thompson WM: Anterior left subphrenic abscess: Characteristic plain film and CT appearance. AJR 139: 283–289, 1982

41. Livingston EM: A Clinical Study of the Abdominal Cavity and Peritoneum. Paul B Hoeber, New York, 1932

42. Pokieser H, Czembirek H, Frank W, et al: Septic lesions of the abdomen. In Radiology Today 3, edited by MW Donner, FHW Heuck. Springer-Verlag, New York, 1985

43. Cohen JM, Weinreb JC, Maravilla KR: Fluid collections in the intraperitoneal and extraperitoneal spaces: Comparison of MR and CT. Radiology 155: 705–708, 1985

44. Hopkins GB, Kan M, Mende CW: Early [67]Ga scintigraphy for the localization of abdominal abscesses. J Nucl Med 16: 990–992, 1975

45. McAfee JG, Samin A: In-111 labeled leukocytes: A review of problems in image interpretation. Radiology 155: 221–229, 1985

46. Forgacs P, Wahner HW, Keys TF, et al: Gallium scanning for the detection of abdominal abscesses. Am J Med 65: 949–954, 1978

47. Haaga JR, Weinstein AJ: CT-Guided percutaneous aspiration and drainage of abscesses. AJR 135: 1187–1194, 1980

48. Knochel JQ, Koehler PR, Lee TG, et al: Diagnosis of abdominal abscesses with computed tomography, ultrasound, and [111]In leukocyte scans. Radiology 137: 425–432, 1980

49. Kumar B, Alderson PO, Geisse G: The role of Ga-67 citrate imaging and diagnostic ultrasound in patients with suspected abdominal abscesses. J Nucl Med 18: 534–537, 1977

50. Taylor KJW, Sullivan DC, Wasson JF, et al: Ultrasound and gallium for the diagnosis of abdominal and pelvic abscesses. Gastrointest Radiol 3: 281–286, 1978

51. Wolverson MK, Jagannadharao B, Sundaram M, et al: CT as a primary diagnostic method in evaluating intraabdominal abscess. AJR 133: 1089–1095, 1979

52. Mueller PR, Simeone JF, Butch RJ, et al: Percutaneous drainage of subphrenic abscess: A review of 62 patients. AJR 147: 1237–1240, 1986

53. Mueller PR, van Sonnenberg E, Ferrucci JT Jr: Percutaneous drainage of 250 abdominal abscesses and fluid collections. II. Current procedural concepts. Radiology 151: 343–347, 1984

54. van Sonnenberg E, Mueller PR, Ferrucci JT Jr: Percutaneous drainage of 250 abdominal abscesses and fluid collections. I. Results, failures, and complications. Radiology 151: 337–341, 1984

55. Feldberg MAM: Computed Tomography of the Retroperitoneum: An Anatomical and Pathological Atlas with Emphasis on the Fascial Planes. Martinus Nijhoff, The Hague, 1983

# 3 Intraperitoneal Spread of Malignancies

## General Introduction

The spread of neoplasms within the peritoneal cavity occurs by direct invasion, intraperitoneal seeding, embolic metastases, and lymphatic extension.[1,2] Recent insights and basic correlation with the pathogenesis of the intraabdominal spread of malignancies have established that the *pattern* of involvement and the individual effects of secondary malignancies of the bowel often present characteristic radiologic features.[1,3–6] These reflect the mode of dissemination and thereby indicate the primary site. They are based on the application of certain gross anatomic relationships, the dynamic factors of the flow of ascites, and conditions of hematogenous dissemination.

Distinction between the major pathways of spread (Table 3–1) is of critical practical importance for several reasons: (a) It closely correlates the radiologic changes with the pathogenesis and provides a rational system for radiologic analysis. (b) Since it is not rare for a malignant neoplasm to be manifested initially by its gastrointestinal metastasis or extension,[7] recognition of the *type* of secondary involvement can aid in

the search for the primary lesion. Confronted with a lesion of the bowel that he can identify as secondary in nature, the clinical radiologist is then in a crucial position—by recognizing the particular mode of dissemination—to determine the further investigation required in the search for the primary lesion. (c) If there is a known primary tumor and gastrointestinal symptomatology develops, particular radiologic attention can be directed to the most likely sites in the abdomen for that type of lesion. In a patient with either a known or clinically occult primary malignancy, only nonspecific abdominal symptomatology may herald the development of intraperitoneal metastases. Not infrequently, these are attributed to other gastrointestinal disorders or perhaps to the side effects of chemotherapeutic drugs. (d) Identification of the type of secondary involvement of bowel can help in planning treatment. Awareness that involvement of a portion of the alimentary tract is secondary to invasion from an adjacent primary tumor allows for adequate preoperative preparation for wider surgical excision. Localized embolic metastases are subject to segmental resection.[7,8] Radiotherapy and chemotherapy may be reserved for disseminated metastases or implants.

Analysis of a large proved series[1] has demonstrated that each of the three major pathways of spread (direct invasion, seeding, and hematogenous metastases) accounts for roughly an equal number of cases of secondary neoplastic involvement of the bowel. Occasionally, more than one mechanism of spread may be encountered in any given patient. This is seen most frequently in intraperitoneal primary malignan-

**Table 3–1.** Classification of pathways of spread of secondary neoplasms to the bowel

Direct invasion
    From noncontiguous primary tumors
        Along mesenteric reflections
        By lymphatic permeation
    From contiguous primary tumors
Intraperitoneal seeding
Embolic metastases

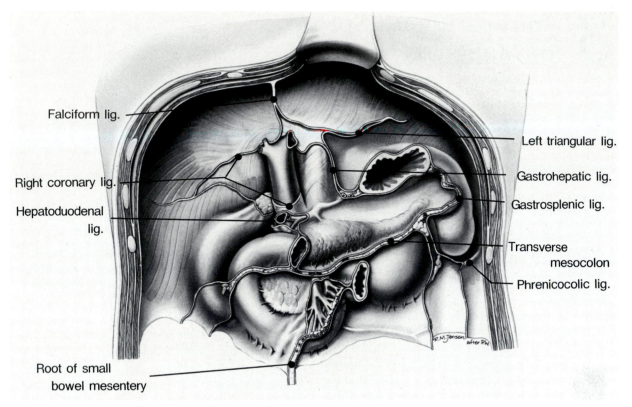

**Fig. 3–1. Peritoneal ligaments and mesenteries.**
Drawing of the posterior parietal wall of the upper abdomen showing the planes of peritoneal reflections constituting the major ligaments and mesenteries. Anatomic continuity is established along the "bare areas" at the roots of origin between intraperitoneal structures and between extraperitoneal and intraperitoneal sites. (From Meyers et al[9])

cies with both direct invasion and seeded metastases.

# Direct Invasion from Noncontiguous Primary Tumors

## Invasion along Mesenteric Reflections

The mesenteric reflections provide an important natural pathway for extension of primary neoplasms to other sites that may not be in actual contiguity.[1,9]

In the upper abdomen peritoneal reflections constitute nine major ligaments and mesenteries which provide continuity of anatomic planes for the spread of malignancies (Fig. 3–1; Table

3–2). These connect not only intraperitoneal sites, but also extend between intraperitoneal and extraperitoneal sites.[9–11] Neither the mesenteries nor the ligaments should be thought of as veillike membranes but rather as connective tissue–laden peritoneal reflections of often considerable substance. The areolar tissue within these planes contains lymphatics accompanying blood vessels so that this interconnecting abdominal network provides discrete pathways of

**Table 3–2.** Major upper abdominal peritoneal reflections

Gastrohepatic ligament
Hepatoduodenal ligament
Gastrocolic ligament
Transverse mesocolon
Duodenocolic ligament
Gastrosplenic ligament
Splenorenal ligament
Phrenicocolic ligament
Small bowel mesentery

**Fig. 3–2. The gastrohepatic and gastrosplenic ligaments.**
**(a)** The gastrohepatic ligament occupies the wedge-shaped area between the opacified stomach and the liver. The left gastric artery (large white arrows) as well as the coronary vein and accompanying lymphatics course through it. Posteriorly the ligament inserts in relationship to the bulbous enlargement of the right diaphragmatic crus. At this level it continues into the fissure for the ligamentum venosum (open arrow) between the tuber omentale (to) of the left lobe of the liver and the caudate lobe (cl).

The gastrosplenic ligament can also be identified by virtue of branches of the splenic vessels (small white arrows).
**(b)** At a slightly lower level, the gastrohepatic ligament is identified by the left gastric artery (black arrows) branching from the celiac artery (c). Here, the ligament continues into the porta hepatis, also known as the transverse fissure of the liver (open arrows). Ao = aorta. The gastrosplenic ligament is identified by its short gastric vessels and branches of the gastroepiploic vessels (white arrows).
(From Meyers et al[9])

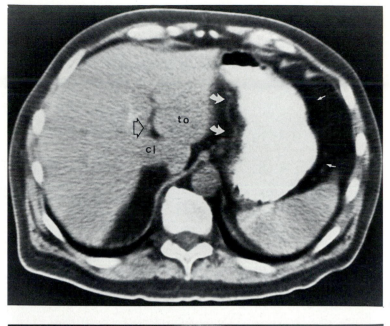

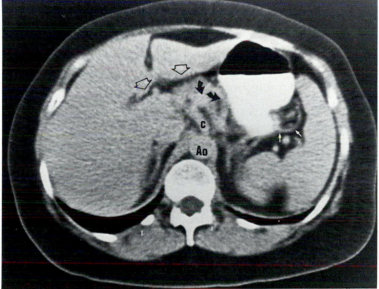

spread of disease. The ligaments and mesenteries are generally readily recognizable on CT by either their typical location and organ relationships or the landmarks provided by their major constituent vessels.

## Gastrohepatic Ligament and Hepatoduodenal Ligament

The gastrohepatic ligament (lesser omentum) extends between the lesser curvature of the stomach and the liver, attached in its upper portion deep within the fissure for the ligamentum venosum and more inferiorly with the porta hepatis. The subperitoneal areolar tissue of the gastrohepatic ligament continues into the liver as Glisson's capsule. The ligament is generally wedge-shaped and contains considerable adipose tissue, through which course the left gastric artery, coronary vein, and the left gastric nodal chain[12] (Fig. 3–2). Identification of the fissure for the ligamentum venosum immedi-

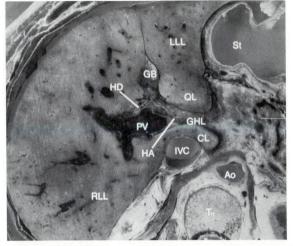

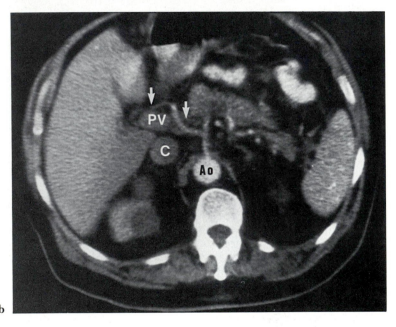

**Fig. 3–3. The hepatoduodenal ligament.**
(a) Anatomic cross-section demonstrates the relationships of the portal triad within the hepatoduodenal ligament at its insertion in the liver. HA = hepatic artery, PV = portal vein, HD = hepatic duct, RLL = right lobe of the liver, LLL = left lobe of the liver, QL = quadrate lobe, CL = caudate lobe, GHL = gastrohepatic ligament, GB = gallbladder, Ao = aorta, IVC = inferior vena cava.
(b) CT scan. The opacified hepatic artery (arrows) passes anteriorly to the portal vein (PV) as both structures, accompanied by the bile duct, course within the hepatoduodenal ligament. Immediately behind its free edge resides the epiploic foramen of Winslow, deep to which is the inferior vena cava (C). Right renal cysts are incidentally present. Ao = aorta.
(From Meyers et al[9])

ately inferior to the esophagogastric junction determines the CT sections in which the gastrohepatic ligament is readily evident.[12]

The free edge of the gastrohepatic ligament is known as the hepatoduodenal ligament, extending from the flexure between the first and second portions of the duodenum to the porta hepatis and transporting the portal triad. After the common hepatic artery gives off its gastroduodenal branch, the proper hepatic artery courses within the hepatoduodenal ligament anterior to the portal vein in most patients. The common bile duct also lies anterior to the portal vein, but is located lateral to the proper hepatic artery[13] (Fig. 3–3). It is thus evident that this "edge" is in truth a structure of considerable thickness. Immediately behind it is the epiploic foramen of Winslow leading into the lesser sac.

On CT, identification of the sites of the left gastric artery and the hepatic artery permits precise localization of disease spread to the gastrohepatic and hepatoduodenal ligaments, respectively (Fig. 3–4).

Although the lymphatics of the gastrohepatic ligament are frequent sites of metastases in cases of carcinoma of the stomach, distal esophagus, pancreas, breast, and lung, they also may give rise to lymphoma. Discrete nodal enlargement

**Fig. 3–4. CT identification of extension of mass lesions within discrete ligaments.**
In a case of lymphoma, following intravascular injection of contrast medium, nodal masses are readily identified within the upper abdominal ligaments accompanying their contained opacified visceral arteries arising from the aorta (Ao). c = celiac artery.

Masses are present within the gastrohepatic ligament (1) around the left gastric artery (g), within the hepatoduodenal ligament (2) around the hepatic artery (h), and in the splenorenal ligament (3) accompanying the splenic artery. Splenomegaly and retrocrural adenopathy are also present. (From Meyers et al[9])   ▷

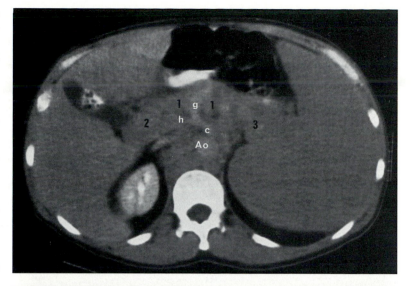

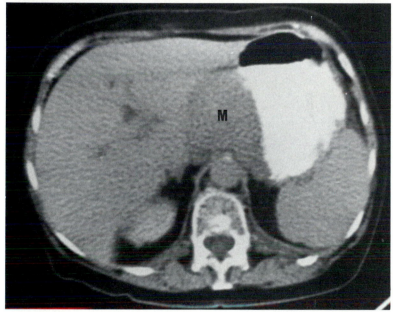

**Fig. 3–5. Nodal mass within the gastrohepatic ligament.**
Lymphomatous mass (M) occupies the wedge-shaped site of the gastrohepatic ligament, mildly separating the stomach and the liver.

may be identifiable or there may be gross mass involvement expanding the area, separating the stomach and liver, and resulting in organ distortion (Fig. 3–5).

The upper portion of the stomach and the left lobe of the liver bear an intimate relationship (Fig. 3–6a) connected by the gastrohepatic ligament, the areolar tissue of which is continuous with that constituting Glisson's capsule. This brief pathway permits invasion of the left hepatic lobe by carcinoma of the fundus and pars media of the stomach. The CT findings in such cases include loss of the fat plane and consequent lack of a definite boundary between the two organs[14] (Fig. 3–6b).

The hepatoduodenal ligament, when thickened, may be seen directly on CT coursing from its intraperitoneal relationships to its extraperitoneal insertion (Fig. 3–7). The portal structures pass into the retroperitoneum through the hepatoduodenal ligament. Lymphatic drainage from the gallbladder is initially to cystic and common bile duct nodes, then into the pancreaticoduodenal system (Fig. 3–8), with later

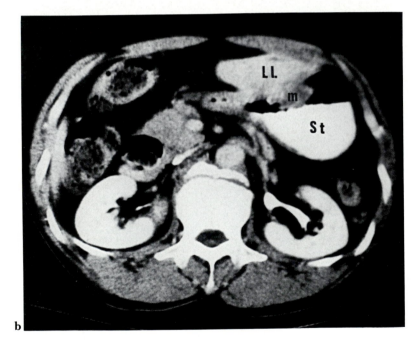

a

b

**Fig. 3–6. Hepatic invasion across the gastrohepatic ligament.**
(a) Anatomic cross-section demonstrates the intimate relationship of the stomach (St) and the left lobe of the liver (LL). The upper portion of the gastrohepatic ligament extends from the lesser curvature of the stomach to the fissure for the ligamentum venosum. Its areolar tissue is continuous with Glisson's capsule.
(b) CT scan in a patient with an infiltrating polypoid carcinoma of the stomach (St), shown as a soft-tissue mass (m) projecting into its lumen, demonstrates direct invasion of the overlying left lobe of the liver (LL). (From Meyers et al[9])

**Fig. 3–7. Inflammatory thickening of the hepatoduodenal ligament.**
Secondary to a penetrating post-bulbar duodenal ulcer with obstructive jaundice, there is mural thickening of the duodenum (D) and inflammatory thickening of the hepatoduodenal ligament (small arrows) which contains the dilated common bile duct (large arrow). (From Meyers et al[9])

▷

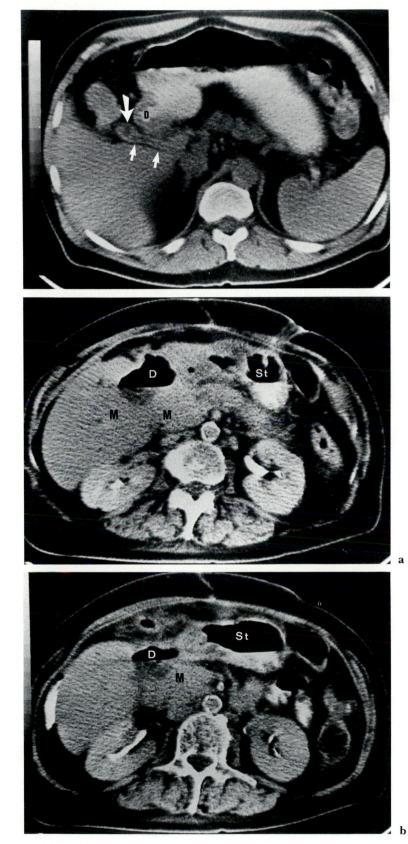

a

b

**Fig. 3–8. Inferior extension of gallbladder carcinoma along hepatoduodenal ligament.**
(**a** and **b**) A carcinomatous mass arising in the gallbladder extends along the hepatoduodenal ligament to paraduodenal and peripancreatic lymph node masses (M). The stomach (St) and duodenal bulb (D) are obstructed.

potential spread into the rest of the celiac axis or aortic nodes.[15]

## Gastrocolic Ligament

The gastrocolic ligament extends inferiorly from the greater curvature of the stomach to suspend the transverse colon and is traversed by the gastroepiploic vessels (Fig. 3–9). It inserts in relationship to the taenia omentalis, and injection studies and clinical observations have documented that spread of gastric lesions down the gastrocolic ligament involves first and predominantly the superior haustral row of the transverse colon[1,5,16,17] (Fig. 3–10), with highly characteristic changes on barium enema study. The wall becomes fixed and straightened, with selective loss of the contour of the haustral sacculations, and most characteristically, the mucosal folds are conspicuously tethered (Figs. 3–11 through 3–13). The term "tethering" is used to indicate that the mucosal folds lose their parallel orientation to each other and their axes, which are normally perpendicular to the lumen of the bowel, become randomly angulated. This change reflects the associated desmoplastic reaction within the gastrocolic ligament itself, acting in effect as a mass of adhesions. The uninvolved haustral contours of the inferior border of the transverse colon retain their pliability and are thrown into pseudosacculations (Figs. 3–12 and 3–13). Further distortion and fixed buckling of the mucosal pattern may occasionally produce the appearance of cobblestone linear and transverse ulcers (Fig. 3–13). The primary gastric carcinomas are usually scirrhous in nature and are frequently clinically occult. It is said that glandular adenocarcinomas spread mainly in the mucosa and submucosa with little serosal spread while scirrhous carcinomas spread in submucosa and muscle coats, probably via lymphatics.[8] The incidence of involvement of the gastrocolic ligament is over 90% once the cancer reaches the serosa.[18] Initially, the complex of these features on a barium enema examination may be mistaken for an intrinsic inflammatory process, such as granulomatous colitis,[19] since the processes share several pathologic and roentgenographic characteristics. These include unilateral mural involvement, nodular irregularities, pseudosaccular outpouchings, and the occasional appearance of ulcerations. However, the localization specifically to the superior bor-

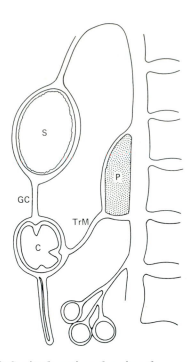

**Fig. 3–9. Sagittal section showing the mesenteric reflections to the transverse colon (C) from the stomach (S) and the pancreas (P).**
Note that the gastrocolic ligament (GC) inserts superiorly and the transverse mesocolon (TrM) posteroinferiorly. (From Meyers[1])

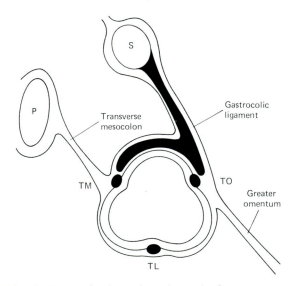

**Fig. 3–10. Sagittal section through the transverse colon, demarcated into its three constituent haustral rows by the taenia omentalis (TO), taenia mesocolica (TM), and taenia libera (TL).**
Extension of a malignancy from the stomach (S) through the gastrocolic ligament spreads preferentially to the TM–TO haustral row. This constitutes the superior border of the transverse colon. P = pancreas. (From Meyers et al[17])

**Fig. 3–11. Direct invasion of the transverse colon along the gastrocolic ligament from a scirrhous carcinoma of the stomach** (S). There is fixation and angulation of the mucosal folds along the superior contour (arrows) involving the TM–TO haustral row. The fixation results in pseudosaccular outpouchings from the uninvolved haustral row on the inferior border. (From Meyers and McSweeney[1])

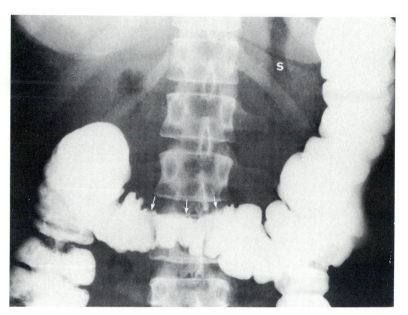

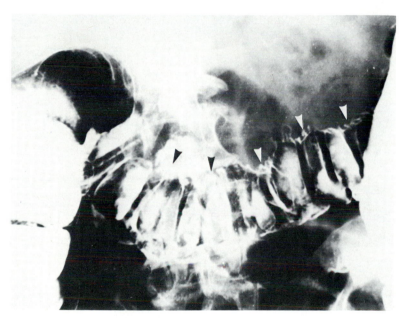

**Fig. 3–12. Carcinoma of the stomach extending down the gastrocolic ligament** involves first the TM–TO row on the superior contour of the transverse colon (arrowheads). Nodular irregularities are associated with tethering of the mucosal folds. (From Meyers[17])

der of the transverse colon and the identification of the tethered mucosal folds, a change not seen in granulomatous colitis, readily lead to the correct diagnosis.

A similar appearance may uncommonly be the result of seeded metastases on the gastrocolic ligaments,[20] but this is almost invariably accompanied by contiguous changes upon the greater curvature of the stomach and characteristic changes at other seeded sites.[21]

Even with extensive circumferential invasion, the greater degree of involvement with fixation and angulation of mucosal folds and mass effects tends to be maintained on the superior contour (Fig. 3–14).

Computed tomography documents that gastric carcinoma may extend into the ligament only partially, although certainly a sign of extramural spread, to perhaps only indent the underlying colon (Fig. 3–15) or may spread down

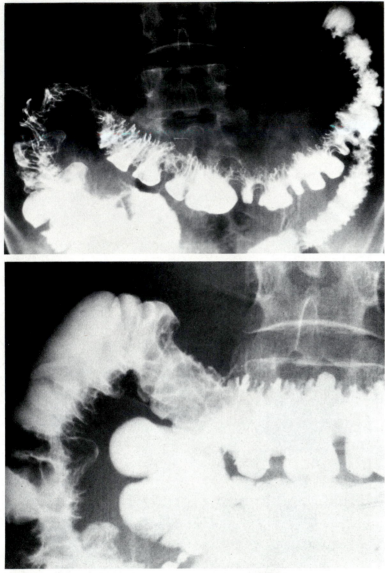

a

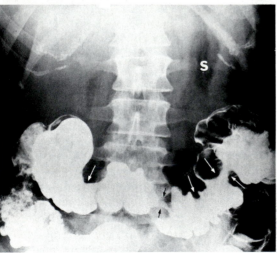

b

**Fig. 3–13. Gastric carcinoma spreading down the gastrocolic ligament.**
(a) Fixation and mucosal tethering along the entire superior border of the transverse colon. Prominent haustral pseudosacculations project from the uninvolved inferior contour.
(b) Spot film of hepatic flexure shows the appearance of cobblestone linear and transverse ulcers.

**Fig. 3–14. Circumferential invasion of the transverse colon from a scirrhous carcinoma of the stomach** (S).
The nodular masses (arrows) remain predominant on the superior contour.

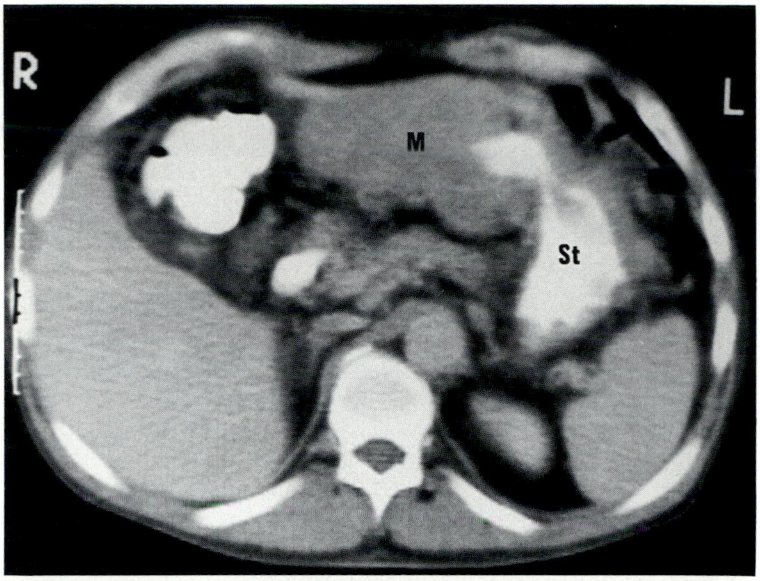

**Fig. 3–15. Extension of gastric carcinoma along gastrocolic ligament.**
**(a)** A large mass (M) representing carcinoma extends from the stomach (St).
**(b)** The mass extends inferiorly within the gastrocolic ligament to displace and compress the transverse colon (TC).
(From Meyers et al[9])

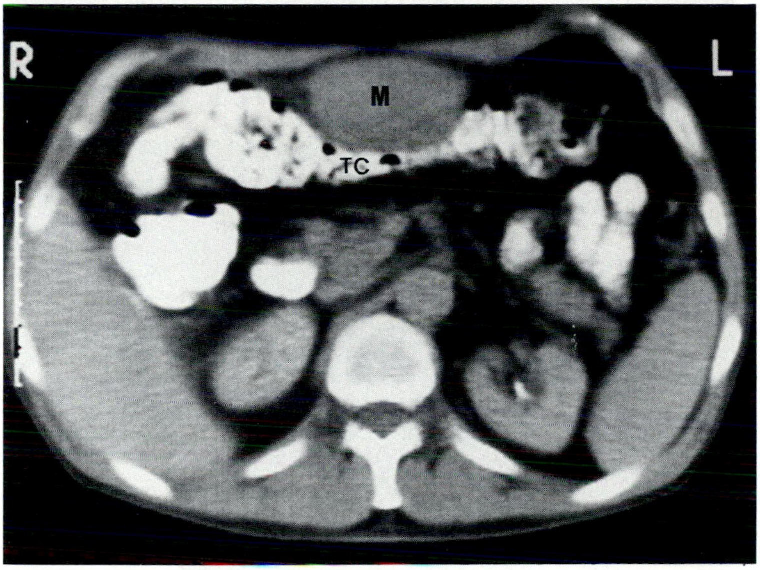

its length to clearly invade the upper haustral contour (Fig. 3–16), or progress to annular involvement of the transverse colon (Fig. 3–17).

The limit of anatomic continuity of the mesenteric reflections toward the left is at the level of the phrenicocolic ligament,[22] which extends from the anatomic splenic flexure to the diaphragm. At this point, the mesenteric transverse colon continues as the extraperitoneal descending colon. Spread of the process thus typically ends abruptly at the anatomic splenic flexure of the colon, just below the tip of the spleen (Figs. 3–18 through 3–20). A mass may further de-

velop within the phrenicocolic ligament itself (Fig. 3–21).

As evidence of the two-way street provided by the ligament, carcinoma of the transverse colon can extend superiorly to involve the greater curvature of the stomach[23] (Fig. 3–22). Further invasion may result in a malignant gastrocolic fistula (Fig. 3–23).

Ultrasonography and computed tomography may show not only abnormal mural thickening but also the intraabdominal tumor extension.[24–28] These modalities further refine capabilities in staging tumors, assessing surgical re-

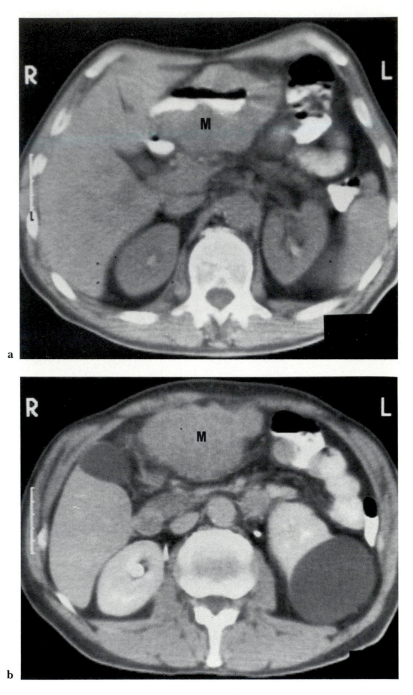

**Fig. 3–16. Extension of gastric carcinoma along gastrocolic ligament to the transverse colon with involvement of the upper haustral row.**
(a) A prominent mass (M) representing an annular carcinoma compresses the gastric lumen.
(b) The mass extends inferiorly into the gastrocolic ligament. An incidental left renal cyst is noted.
(c) At a level through the superior haustral row of the mid-transverse colon (TC), early infiltration by the mass is seen.
(d) At a level through lower haustral sacculations of the transverse colon, no further involvement by the malignant extension is present.

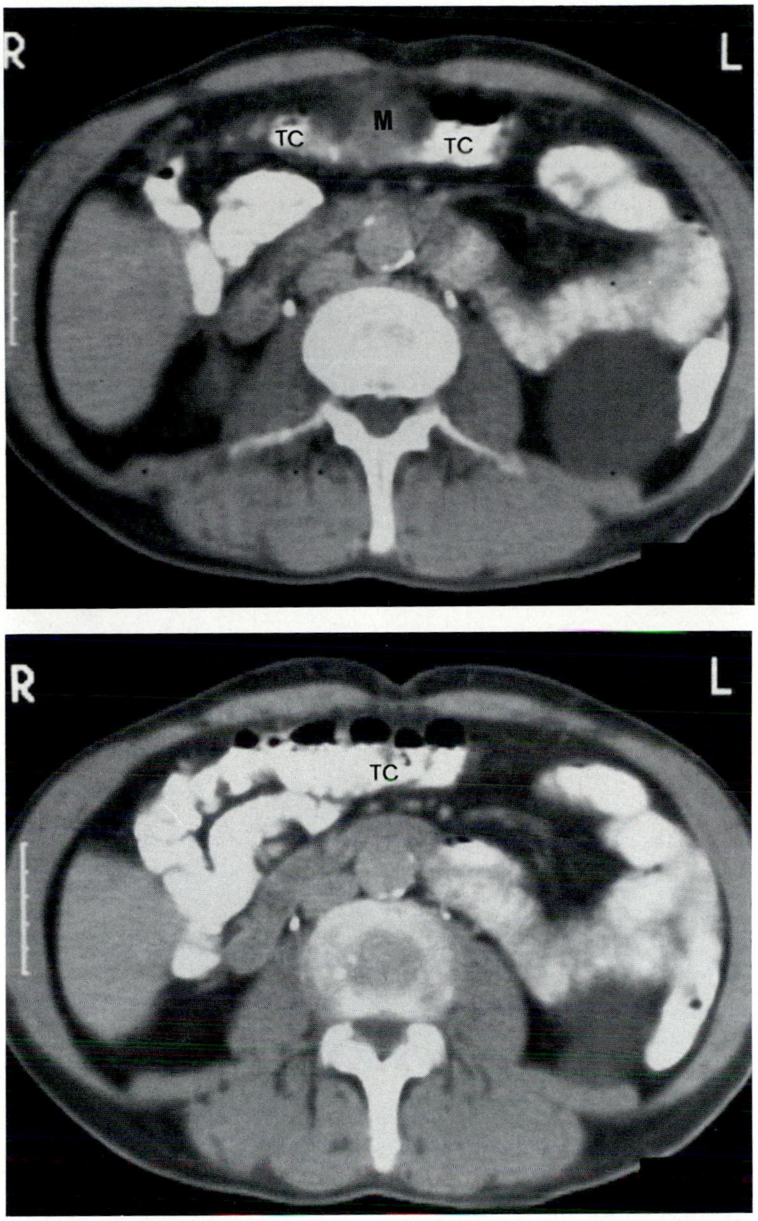

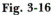

**Fig. 3-16**

sectability, evaluating tumor response, and detecting postoperative recurrence.

## Transverse Mesocolon and Duodenocolic Ligament

The root of the transverse mesocolon extends across the infraampullary segment of the descending duodenum, the head of the pancreas, and continues along the lower edge of the body and tail of the pancreas anteriorly to bear continuity with the splenorenal and phrenicocolic ligaments[6,29] (Fig. 3–24). Near the uncinate process of the pancreas it becomes confluent as well with the root of the small bowel mesentery. These bare areas thus establish anatomic planes of continuity between (1) the pancreas and (2) the transverse colon up to the anatomic splenic flexure, the spleen, and small bowel loops. The very beginning of the peritoneal reflections on the right, known as the duodenocolic ligament, further establishes continuity to the descending duodenum and posterior hepatic flexure.[6,30]

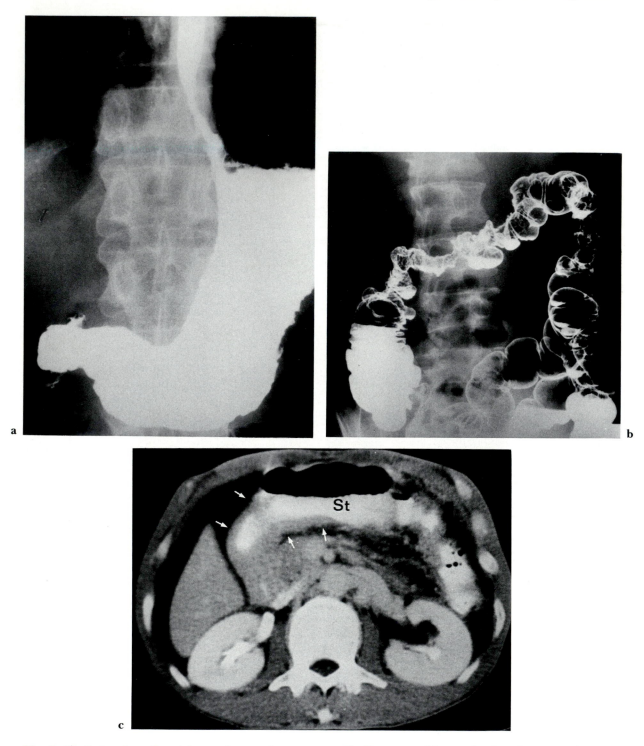

**Fig. 3–17. Extension of gastric carcinoma along gastrocolic ligament with annular involvement of transverse colon.**
(a) Upper GI series reveals a linitis plastica carcinoma of the stomach.
(b) Barium enema shows narrowing, rigidity, and angulation of the transverse colon.
(c) CT documents annular mural thickening (arrows) of the stomach (St) secondary to a scirrhous carcinoma.
(d) A lower CT scan through the opacified transverse colon (TC) confirms inferior extension along the gastrocolic ligament with annular infiltration (arrows), see p. 105.
(From Komaki[27]).

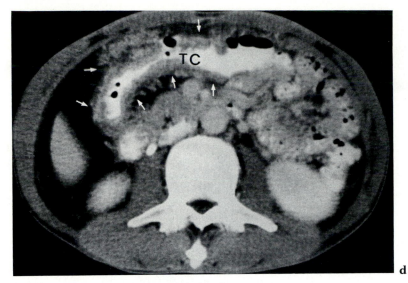

**Fig. 3-17**

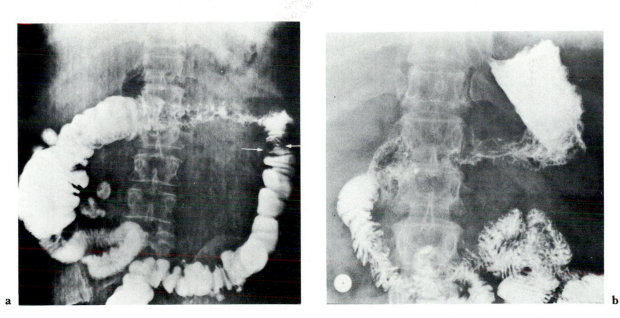

**Fig. 3–18. Direct invasion of the transverse colon from gastric carcinoma along the gastrocolic ligament.**
**(a)** Invasive desmoplastic changes involve the distal transverse colon, stopping abruptly at the anatomic splenic flexure (arrows).
**(b)** Upper GI series documents a primary scirrhous carcinoma of the stomach.

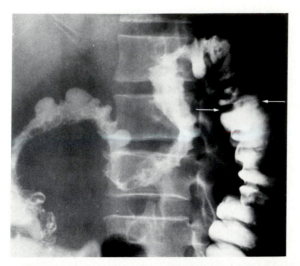

**Fig. 3–19. Annular strangulation of the transverse colon by spread from gastric carcinoma down the gastrocolic ligament.**
The severe extension involves the entire length and typically stops abruptly at the anatomic splenic flexure (arrows).

◁

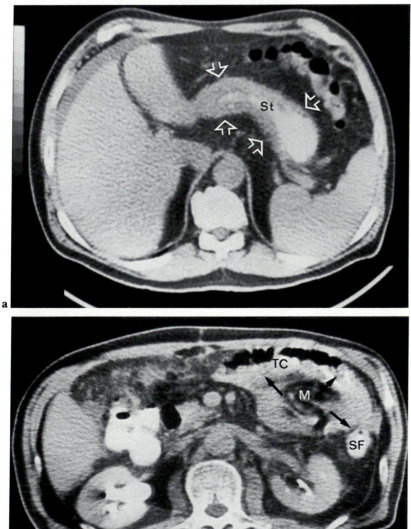

**Fig. 3–20. Extension of gastric carcinoma along gastrocolic ligament to anatomic splenic flexure of colon.**
**(a)** Mural thickening (arrows) of stomach (St) secondary to carcinoma.
**(b)** Mass extension (M) into the gastrocolic ligament to the transverse colon (TC) ending on the left at the anatomic splenic flexure of the colon (SF).

**Fig. 3–21. Extensive annular invasion along the length of the transverse colon from gastric carcinoma.**

The changes end abruptly at the level of the phrenicocolic ligament. At this point along the lateral aspect of the anatomic splenic flexure of the colon, a prominent serosal mass has developed (arrow). (From Meyers and McSweeney[1])  ▷

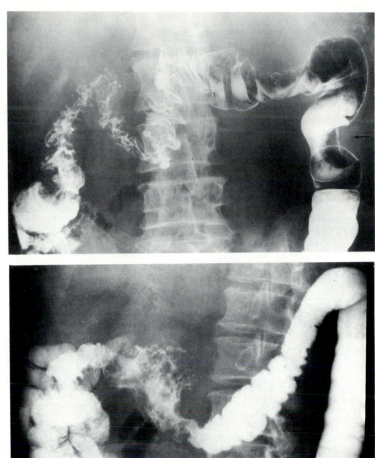

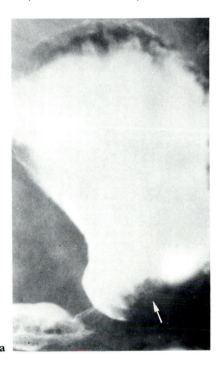

a

b

△

**Fig. 3–22. Transmural invasion of the stomach from colonic carcinoma.**

**(a)** There is nodular infiltration along the greater curvature (arrow).

**(b)** Spread has occurred along the gastrocolic ligament from a large primary carcinoma of the transverse colon.

▷

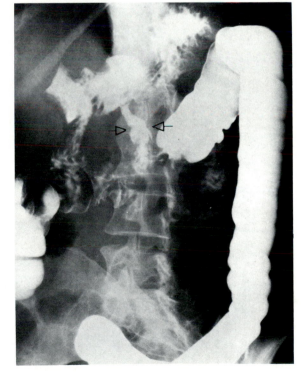

**Fig. 3–23. Gastrocolic fistula secondary to carcinoma of the transverse colon.**

Barium enema demonstrates that the small primary lesion has established a malignant fistulous tract along the gastrocolic ligament (arrows). (From Meyers and McSweeney[1])

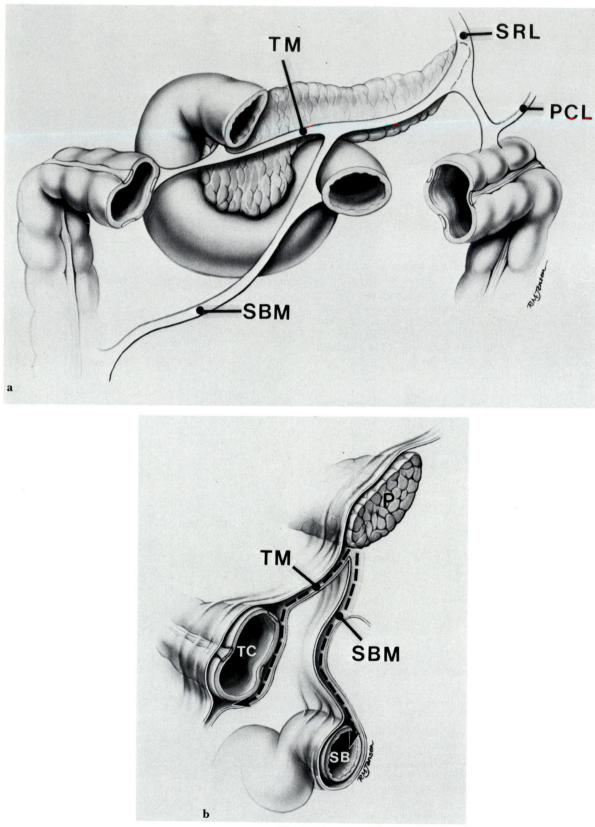

**Fig. 3-24**

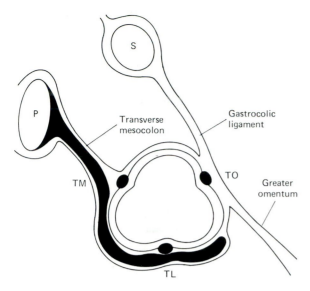

Fig. 3–25. Sagittal section through the transverse colon.
Extension of a malignancy from the pancreas (P) through the transverse mesocolon spreads preferentially downward along the TM–TL haustra toward the TO–TL row. This constitutes the inferior border of the transverse colon. S = stomach, TM = taenia mesocolica, TO = taenia omentalis, TL = taenia libera. (From Meyers et al[17])

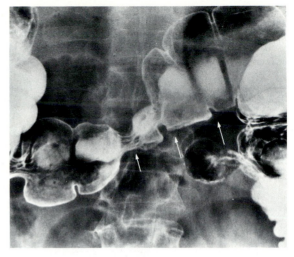

Fig. 3–26. Extension of carcinoma of the pancreas along the transverse mesocolon.
Barium enema documents flattening and fixation along the inferior border of the transverse colon (arrows).

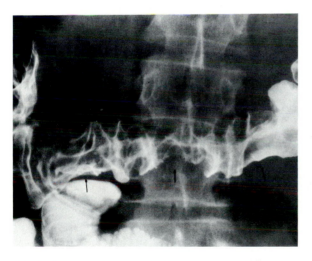

Fig. 3–27. Carcinoma of the pancreas with direct invasion of the transverse colon along the mesocolon.
The major extension is typically along the inferior contour (arrows), where multiple nodules are present.

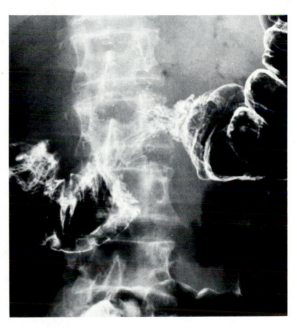

Fig. 3–28. Carcinoma of the pancreas extending along the transverse mesocolon.
This results in fixation and large mass along the inferior border of the transverse colon. (From Meyers and McSweeney[1])

Fig. 3–24. The transverse mesocolon: anatomic relationships and planes of spread.
(a) Frontal drawing showing the relationships of the transverse mesocolon (TM) and its continuity with the small bowel mesentery (SBM), the splenorenal ligament (SRL), and the phrenicocolic ligament (PCL).
(b) Lateral diagram. The arrowed-dashed lines show the planes of spread from the pancreas (P) to the transverse colon (TC) and small bowel (SB).
(From Meyers et al[9])

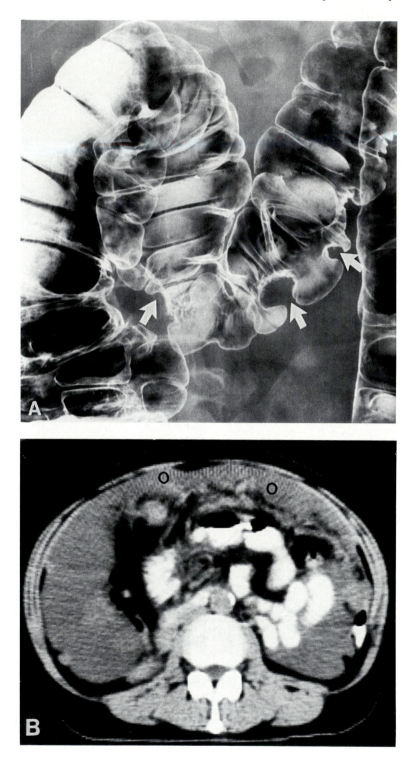

**Fig. 3–29. Seeded metastatic ovarian carcinoma on the greater omentum.**
(a) Barium enema shows multinodular infiltration of the inferior border of the transverse colon (arrows).
(b) CT demonstrates metastatic cakelike thickening of the greater omentum (O).
(Reproduced from Krestin et al[31])

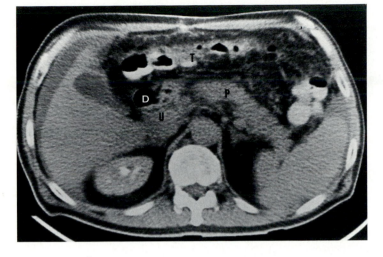

**Fig. 3–30. The transverse mesocolon.**
CT scan shows middle colic vessels branching in the fatty space between the uncinate process (U) and body of the pancreas (P) and the transverse colon (T). D = duodenum. Some ascites is present adjacent to the liver and spleen. (From Meyers et al[9])

The transverse mesocolon inserts in relation to the taenia mesocolica, and correlative studies have established that the preferential spread of pancreatic lesions along this mesentery is to the inferior border of the transverse colon[16,17] (Figs. 3–25 through 3–28). The haustral pattern on the uninvolved, pliable superior border may be thrown into a pseudosaccular appearance. Circumferential growth may develop, although usually the degree of invasion and fixation is not as extensive as may occur from indurated carcinoma of the stomach. Nevertheless, the greater involvement of the posteroinferior margin of the transverse colon on a barium enema study generally indicates the pancreas as the primary site. Rarely, similar changes may be encountered from seeded metastases on the greater omentum[31] (Fig. 3–29).

On CT, the transverse mesocolon is identified as the fatty plane extending from the pancreas, particularly at the level of the uncinate process, to the ventrally situated transverse colon with the middle colic vessels coursing through it (Fig. 3–30). In cases of pancreatic carcinoma, masslike or dendritic spread through the mesocolon can be precisely localized (Fig. 3–31).

These same ligaments provide mesenteric planes for direct extension to and from other sites. As the hepatic flexure of the colon crosses anterior to the descending duodenum, the two structures are in very close anatomic relationship, separated only by the duodenocolic ligament, constituting the short beginning of the transverse mesocolon[6] (Fig. 3–32). In this way, the paraduodenal area may be involved by direct spread from an infiltrating carcinoma of the hepatic flexure across the beginning reflection of the transverse mesocolon[6,30,32,33] (Figs. 3–33 and 3–34). Carcinomas of the right colon are notoriously clinically occult and the palpation of an epigastric or right upper quadrant mass in such a patient may lead to radiologic investigation being initiated with an upper GI series (Fig. 3–34a). This may be very misleading unless the underlying anatomic relationships are kept in mind and a barium enema study undertaken.

Direct lymphatic extension along the draining chain of lymph nodes may be identified occasionally by barium studies.[6,34] By its relationship to the central lymph nodes draining the colon, the duodenum may reflect changes of lymph node spread from a remote carcinoma of the colon. The lymphatic vessels draining the colon parallel the arterial supply. Those draining the right side of the colon are located near the origin of the superior mesenteric artery, in close relationship to the superior border of the horizontal (third) portion of the duodenum (Fig. 3–32). Those draining the distal transverse and descending colon are partially located in the

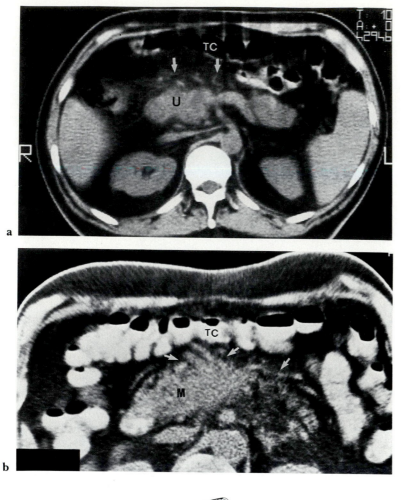

a

b

Fig. 3–31. Spread of pancreatic carcinoma into transverse mesocolon.
(a and b) In two different patients, arrows show extension of carcinoma of the uncinate process (U) and the body of the pancreas (M) as stellate and dendritic infiltrations of the transverse mesocolon toward the transverse colon (TC). (a, courtesy of Nancy O. Whitley, MD, University of Maryland, School of Medicine, Baltimore, MD)

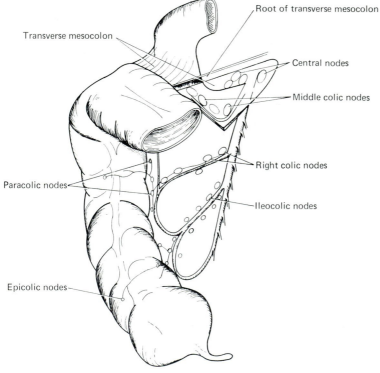

Transverse mesocolon

Root of transverse mesocolon

Central nodes

Middle colic nodes

Right colic nodes

Paracolic nodes

Ileocolic nodes

Epicolic nodes

Fig. 3–32. Duodenocolic relationships:
(1) The hepatic flexure of the colon and the descending duodenum are bridged by the transverse mesocolon.
(2) The central lymph nodes draining the right colon are in relationship to the duodenum.

**Fig. 3–33. Spread of carcinoma of right colon across duodenocolic ligament.**
**(a)** Barium enema shows an annular carcinoma of the distal ascending colon (arrow).
**(b** and **c)** CT scans demonstrate the mass (M) of the primary carcinoma and its spread across the duodenocolic ligament to paraduodenal-peripancreatic nodal masses (DC). D = duodenum.
(From Meyers et al[9])

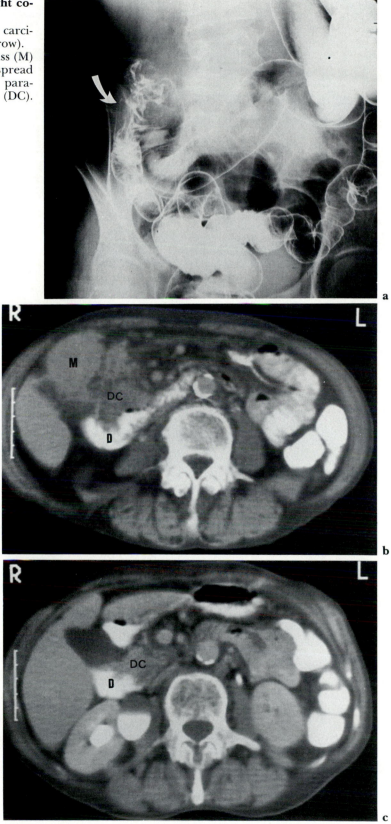

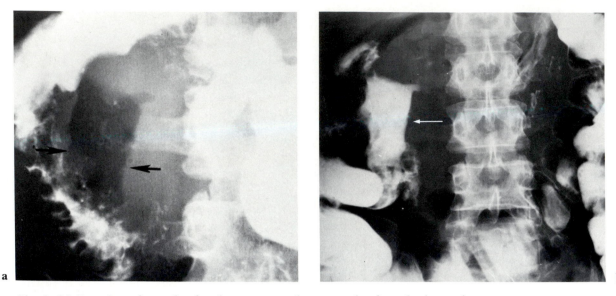

**Fig. 3–34. Invasion of paraduodenal area across the mesocolon by colonic carcinoma.**
(a) Upper gastrointestinal series demonstrates well-defined gas-containing abscess cavity (arrows) within a mass in the area of the head of the pancreas. Mucosal edema of the descending duodenum is present.
(b) A subsequent barium enema reveals a primary infiltrating carcinoma of the anterior hepatic flexure with opacification of a pericolonic–paraduodenal abscess (arrow).
(From Treitel et al[30])

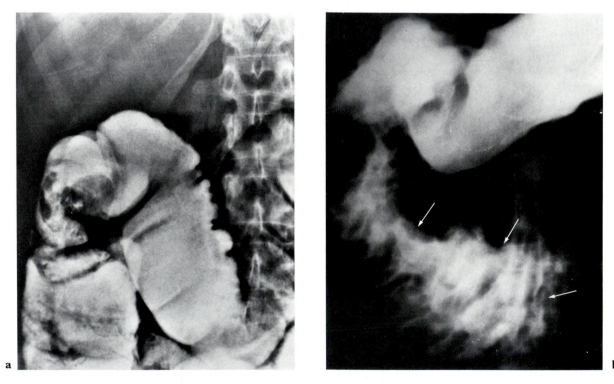

**Fig. 3–35. Nodal spread from colonic carcinoma.**
(a) Barium enema shows a polypoid carcinoma within the distal ascending colon.
(b) Upper gastrointestinal series documents metastases within the enlarged, draining lymph nodes by virtue of their extrinsic impressions upon the duodenum (arrows).

**Fig. 3–36. Metastases within the draining central inferior mesenteric lymph nodes from a carcinoma of the left colon.** These are shown by the extrinsic pressure effect on the lateral aspect of the duodenojejunal junction (arrows).

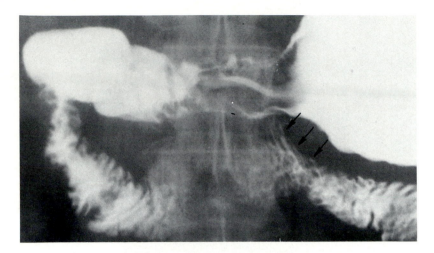

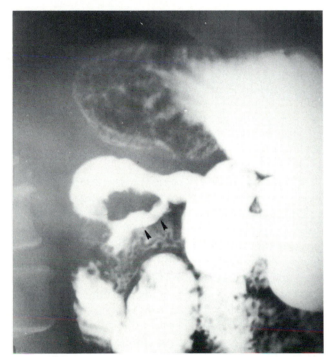

**Fig. 3–37. Duodeno-duodenal fistula.** Fifteen months following a right hemicolectomy for carcinoma of the hepatic flexure, upper GI series demonstrates the fistula (arrowheads), proved to be secondary to duodenal invasion by paraduodenal lymph node metastases. (Reproduced from Schabel SI, et al[35])

transverse mesocolon and near the ascending left colic branch of the inferior mesenteric artery, which courses lateral to the ascending (fourth) portion of the duodenum. By radiologically recognizing these changes of nodal impressions upon the superior contour of the third portion of the duodenum (Fig. 3–35) or upon the lateral aspect of the duodenojejunal junction (Fig. 3–36), it is possible to determine the extent of a colonic carcinoma preoperatively or the development of lymph node metastases

postoperatively.[6,34] Rarely, postoperative lymph node metastases may undergo necrosis and become manifest as duodeno-duodenal fistulas[35] (Figs. 3–37 and 3–38).

## Gastrosplenic Ligament; Splenorenal Ligament; Phrenicocolic Ligament

The peritoneal reflections in the left upper quadrant of the abdomen are shorter but are certainly no less important in providing avenues

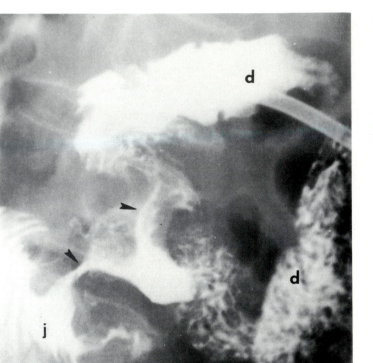

**Fig. 3–38. Duodeno-duodenal fistula.** Eight years following a right hemicolectomy for carcinoma of the ascending colon, upper GI series shows multiple fistulous tracts (arrowheads) between the second and third portions of the duodenum (d) and jejunum (j) secondary to a large mass of necrotic paraduodenal tumor. (Reproduced from Schabel SI, et al[35])

of spread of disease. Anatomic continuity between multiple sites is readily established.

The gastrosplenic ligament is continuous with the gastrocolic ligament and extends from the greater curvature of the stomach to the spleen (Fig. 3–39). It contains the left gastroepiploic and short gastric vessels. The splenorenal ligament (Fig. 3–39) invests the extremity of the pancreatic tail as it inserts toward or within the splenic hilus and also contains the distal splenic artery. Both ligaments form the boundaries of the lesser sac on the left.

The gastrosplenic ligament is identified on CT by its fat and vascular content at the site between the stomach and spleen (Figs. 3–2 and 3–40). It may be arranged into longitudinal pleats or a series of ruffles.[36,37] Radiologic localization of disease spread here can be very precise (Fig. 3–41) and is particularly helpful in the evaluation of extramural spread of gastric malignancies (Fig. 3–42). A tract may be formed in the gastrosplenic ligament to enable spread from the stomach to the development of a splenic abscess (Figs. 3–43 and 3–44). Although neoplasm in a contiguous organ has been considered a rare cause of splenic abscess in the past,[38] this pathogenesis is being increasingly recognized by computed tomography. Continuity with the splenorenal ligament allows spread of disease between the stomach, spleen, and tail of the pancreas (Figs. 3–45 through 3–47). This short ligament is identified less frequently by CT, but is generally indicated after intravenous contrast injection by the distal splenic artery or the proximal splenic vein.

The phrenicocolic ligament (Fig. 3–48a) extends from the anatomic splenic flexure of the colon to the diaphragm at the level of the 11th rib[22] and serves to support the spleen in the left upper quadrant. It is in most direct continuity with the splenorenal ligament and the transverse mesocolon. It can be identified occasionally on plain films[22] and clearly by peritoneography,[39] and on CT in cases of ascites it may be outlined in its characteristic position (Fig. 3–48b). The avenue of spread facilitated by the ligament's relationships explains the predisposition of carcinoma of the tail of the pancreas to involve the anatomic splenic flexure of the colon (Fig. 3–49).

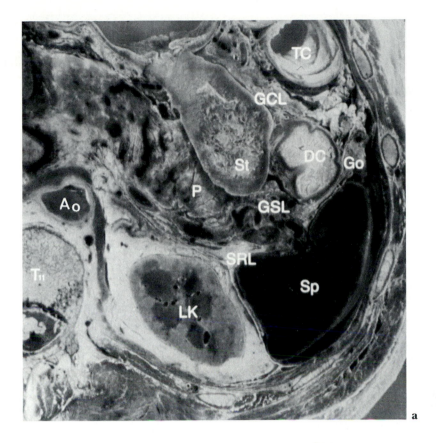

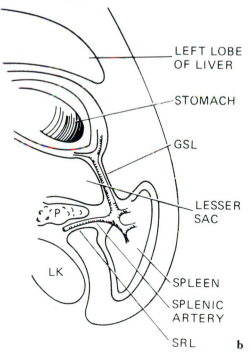

**Fig. 3–39. The gastrosplenic and splenorenal ligaments.**
**(a)** Anatomic cross-section at the level of T11 demonstrates the relationships of the gastrosplenic (GSL), splenorenal (SRL), and gastrocolic (GCL) ligaments. TC = transverse colon, DC = descending colon, St = stomach, P = pancreas, Go = greater omentum, Sp = spleen, LK = left kidney, Ao = aorta.
**(b)** Transverse diagram of the left upper quadrant shows the relationships of the gastrosplenic ligament (GSL) and splenorenal ligament (SRL).

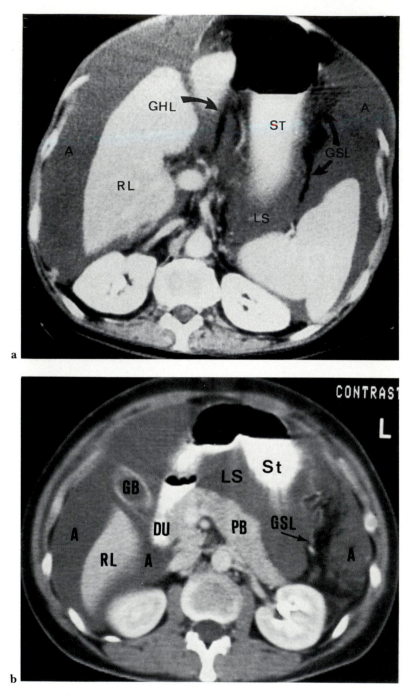

**Fig. 3–40. The gastrosplenic ligament.**
CT scans on two different patients with ascites (A) demonstrate the gastrosplenic ligament (GSL) by virtue of its fatty elements and contained blood vessels. RL = right lobe of the liver, GHL = gastrohepatic ligament, GB = gallbladder, St = stomach, DU = duodenum, PB = pancreatic body, LS = lesser sac.

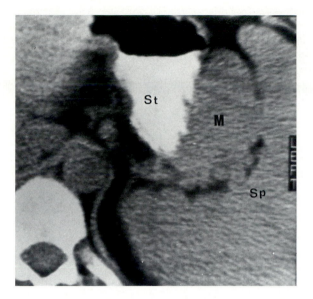

**Fig. 3–41. Lymphoma with the gastrosplenic ligament.**
Nodal mass (M) in the gastrosplenic ligament separates the stomach (St) from the enlarged spleen (Sp).

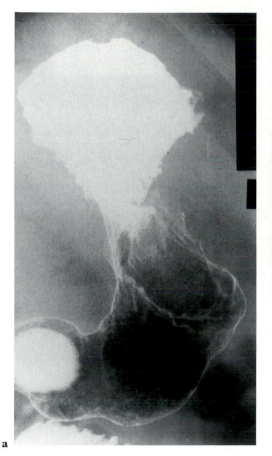

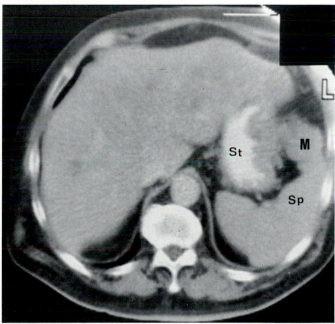

**Fig. 3–42. Extension of gastric carcinoma into gastrosplenic ligament.**
(a) Upper GI series demonstrates an infiltrating carcinoma of the greater curvature of the stomach. Extramural spread cannot be determined.
(b) CT scan documents nodal metastases (M) within the gastrosplenic ligament between the thickened irregular wall of the stomach (St) and the spleen (Sp).
(From Meyers et al[9])

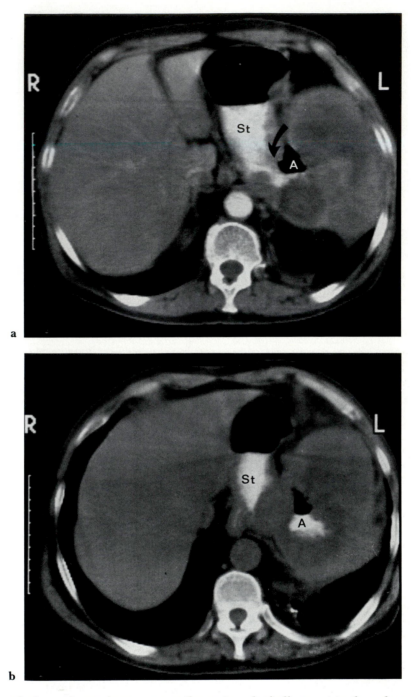

**Fig. 3–43. Spread of gastric carcinoma across the gastrosplenic ligament to the spleen.**
(a and b) Tract across the gastrosplenic ligament (arrow) establishes continuity between infiltrating carcinoma of stomach (St) and abscess cavity (A) within spleen.

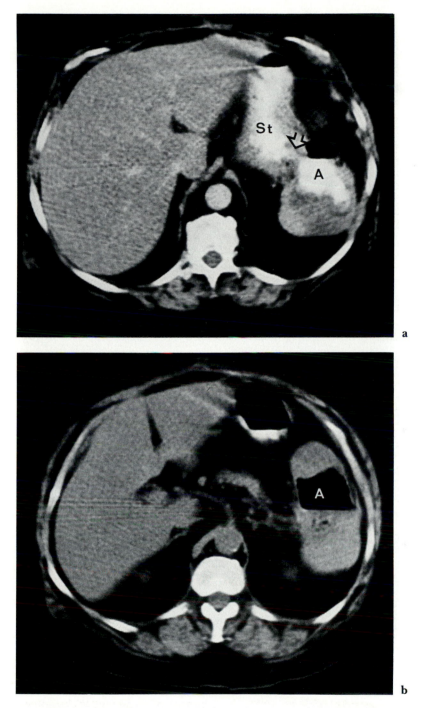

**Fig. 3–44. Spread of gastric lymphoma across the gastrosplenic ligament to the spleen.**
(**a** and **b**) Lymphomatous thickening of wall of stomach (St) directly continues across gastrosplenic ligament (arrow) to the development of a large communicating abscess cavity (A) within the spleen.

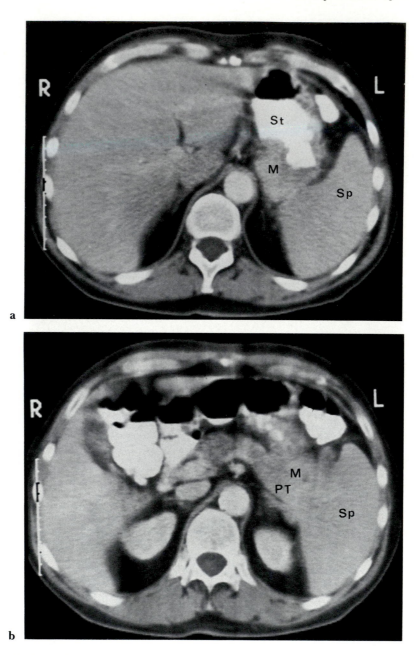

**Fig. 3–45. Spread of gastric carcinoma to gastrosplenic and splenorenal ligaments.**
**(a)** An ulcerated carcinoma of the stomach (St) extends as a mass (M) within the gastrosplenic ligament.
**(b)** At a lower level, the mass continues into the splenorenal ligament to displace the pancreatic tail (PT) posteriorly away from the spleen (Sp).

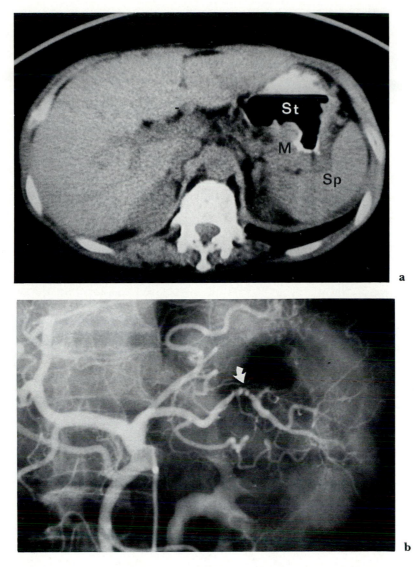

**Fig. 3–46. Continuity of gastric carcinoma into gastrosplenic and splenorenal ligaments.**
**(a)** The mass (M) of an ulcerated carcinoma of the stomach (St) extends into the gastrosplenic ligament in relation to the spleen (Sp).
**(b)** Celiac arteriogram documents extension into the splenorenal ligament by virtue of neoplastic beading of the splenic artery (arrow).

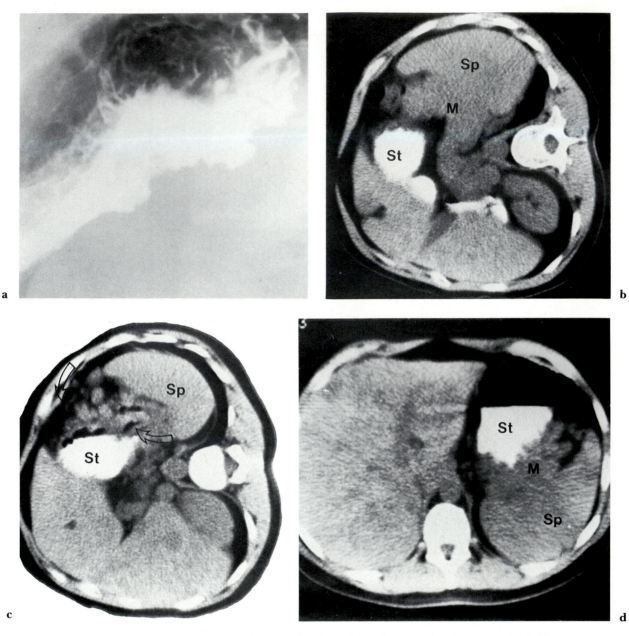

**Fig. 3–47. Carcinoma of the pancreas with extension into the splenorenal and gastrosplenic ligaments.**
**(a)** Lateral film of upper GI series shows fixed extrinsic defects involving posterior wall of gastric fundus.
**(b)** Computed tomography, right lateral decubitus projection, demonstrates carcinomatous mass (M) arising from tail of pancreas extending into the hilum of the spleen (Sp) and anteriorly toward the stomach (St).
**(c)** Decubitus scan at slightly higher level shows numerous serpentine venous collaterals (curved arrows). This is secondary to obstruction of the splenic vein, indicating invasion into the splenorenal ligament by the carcinoma.
**(d)** Supine scan at a more cephalad level shows the carcinomatous mass infiltrating the posterior wall of the stomach across the gastrosplenic ligament.

    These changes correspond to the finding on the upper GI series.

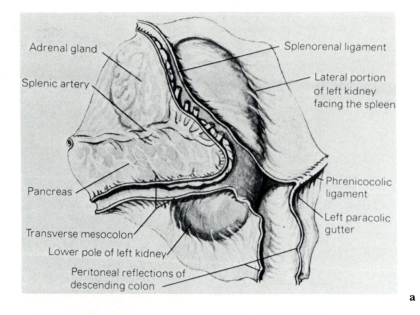

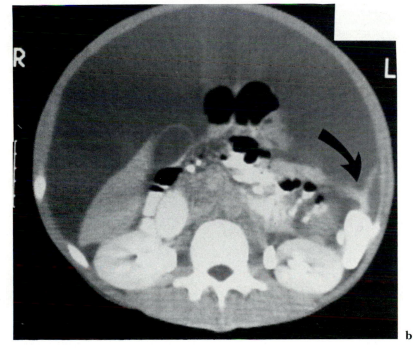

**Fig. 3–48. The phrenicocolic ligament.**
**(a)** Frontal drawing of the sites of the major posterior ligaments of the left upper quadrant shows that all have continuity with the phrenicocolic ligament.
**(b)** In a patient with ascites, CT scan demonstrates the phrenicocolic ligament (arrow) extending laterally from the region of the anatomic splenic flexure of the colon.
(From Meyers et al[9])

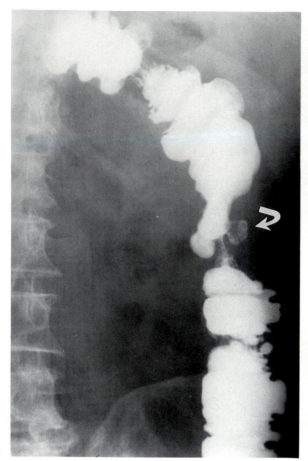

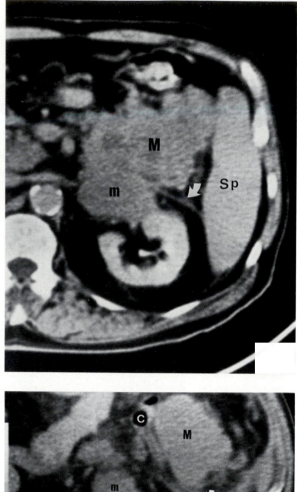

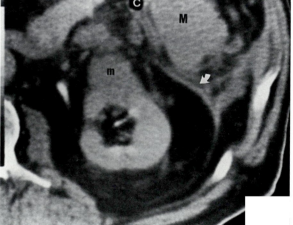

**Fig. 3–49. Spread of pancreatic carcinoma into phrenicocolic ligament.**
**(a)** Barium enema demonstrates lateral mass impression upon the anatomic splenic flexure of the colon (arrow). Incidental diverticula are present.
**(b)** CT scan shows a carcinomatous mass (M) arising from the tail of the pancreas anterior to the thickened anterior renal fascia (arrow) within the splenorenal ligament approaching the spleen (Sp). A component of the mass (m) has invaded the perirenal space.
**(c)** At a lower level, there is spread of the mass (M) into the phrenicocolic ligament anterior to the renal fascia (arrow) pressing upon the lateral aspect of the anatomic splenic flexure of the colon (C), as indicated initially by the barium enema. A component of the mass (m) has invaded the left kidney.

## Small Bowel Mesentery

The small bowel mesentery is a voluminous fat-laden peritoneal reflection. Whereas its root (Fig. 3–24) is only 15 cm long as it extends obliquely from the region of the pancreas to the right lower quadrant, the mesentery itself suspends 20–25 feet of jejunal and ileal loops.[40] This is achieved by its characteristic ruffled na-

ture which markedly lengthens its intestinal border. The mesenteric ruffles thereby provide routes of spread to one or multiple small bowel loops[41] (Fig. 3–50).

The normal small bowel mesentery is best appreciated on CT when its structural components are positioned to be imaged transaxially (Fig. 3–51). Its root is a bare area in continuity with the extraperitoneal anterior pararenal space.

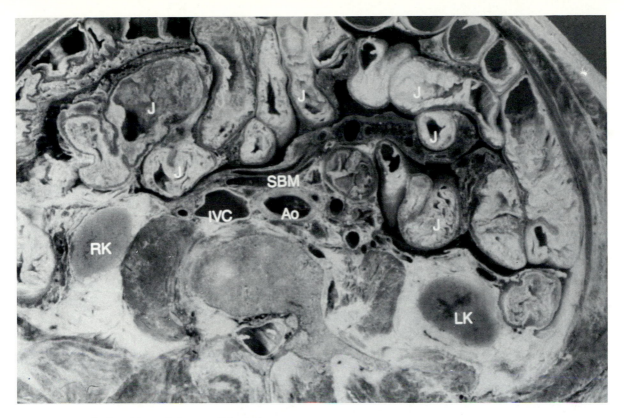

**Fig. 3–50. Relationships of the small bowel mesentery.**
Anatomic cross-section illustrates an extension of the small bowel mesentery (SBM) suspending jejunal loops (J). Anatomic continuity is established between the extraperitoneal anterior pararenal space and the intraperitoneal small bowel mesentery. RK = right kidney, LK = left kidney, Ao = aorta, IVC = inferior vena cava. (From Meyers et al[9])

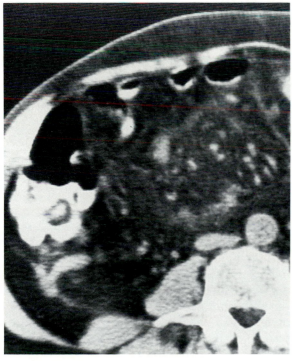

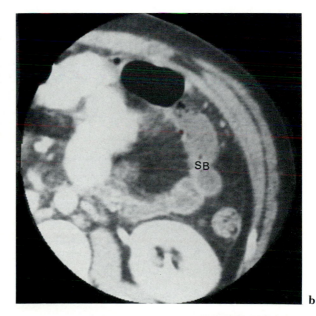

**Fig. 3–51. CT identification of the small bowel mesentery.**
(a and b) Branching vessels course through the fatty mesenteric tissue. In (b) discrete vasa recta penetrate the mesenteric border of a small bowel loop (SB).

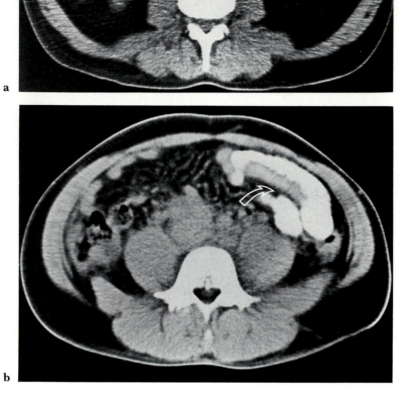

a

b

**Fig. 3–52. Spread of lymphoma within the mesentery.**
**(a)** A lymph node mass (M) expands within the lower portion of the root of the small bowel mesentery.
**(b)** In another patient, Hodgkin's lymphoma produces stellate infiltration of the small bowel mesentery and mural thickening of the mesenteric side of an opacified loop (arrow).
(From Meyers et al[9])

These features also explain many of the characteristic growth patterns of mesenteric lymphoma. This may present or originate within the mesenteric root (Fig. 3–52a), and extension may be seen as multiple or conglomerate densities or a stellate infiltration[42,43] of the mesentery. Lymphomatous mural involvement of a small bowel loop specifically on its mesenteric border may then be noted[41] (Fig. 3–52b).

When mesenteric lymphoma coexists with paraortic/paracaval adenopathy, a helpful differential feature on CT relies upon the integrity of the anterior pararenal fat. Even in the presence of a "sandwich sign" of a confluent lymphomatous mass infiltrating the mesenteric leaves and encasing the mesenteric vessels,[44] there remains a visible plane of demarcation from commonly accompanying retroperitoneal adenopathy[9] (Fig. 3–53).

## Invasion by Lymphatic Permeation

Lymphatic permeation plays an apparently minor role in the dissemination of secondary neoplasms of the bowel. The process refers to lymphatic-borne tumor emboli from a primary neoplasm of the bowel, which may not be arrested in the nearest lymph nodes along the chain of drainage. Rather, complete blockage of

**Fig. 3–53. Distinction of mesenteric and retroperitoneal masses.**
**(a)** In a patient with lymphoma, enlarged retroperitoneal nodes (N) can be distinguished from extensive mesenteric nodal masses (M) by virtue of an intact fat plane (arrows) of the anterior pararenal space. The mesenteric masses themselves exhibit the "sandwich" sign.
**(b)** The distinction between anatomically distinct compartments is further confirmed at a lower level by the partial interposition of opacified small bowel loops (arrows) approaching the root of the mesentery between the extraperitoneal tissues and the mesenteric mass (M).
(From Meyers et al[9])

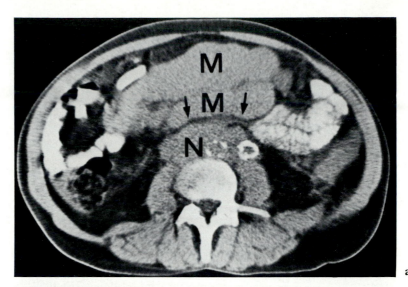

a

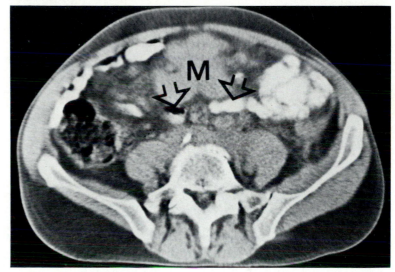

b

a more remote node can occur from cellular impaction, with retrograde passage along other afferent channels to involve a segment of bowel adjacent to, or at some distance from, the primary carcinoma (Fig. 3–54). It has been documented that metastatic tumor cells may be carried for considerable distances beyond the usual route by this altered lymph flow.[45] This process may play a role in anastomotic recurrence following resection of the colon for carcinoma (Fig. 3–55). It appears to be a major factor in some cases of local bowel metastases.[46,47]

The deranged lymph flow in the initial stages may be radiologically demonstrated as edema in the wall of the bowel with mucosal thickening,

luminal narrowing, and loss of colonic haustration. As the metastatic lymphatic edema increases, nodular tumor deposits occur which may be evident as "thumbprinting" in the colon and "cobblestoning" of the small intestine (Fig. 3–56), changes mimicking inflammatory bowel disease.[46,47] Radiologic demonstration of these findings indicates that extensive lymphatic permeation has occurred and that resection will not be curative.[45] The process can also result in diversion of lymph flow into veins through direct lymphaticovenous communications[48] or through shared channels intrinsic to lymph nodes.[49]

Lymphatic permeation also explains the rare

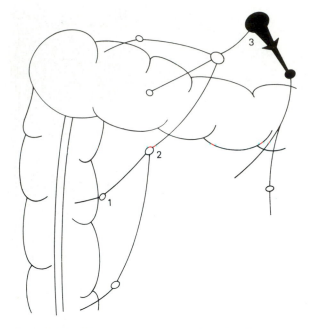

**Fig. 3–54. The mechanism of lymphatic permeation.**
Tumor cells may be transported through the draining chain of lymph nodes (1,2) to impact a more central node (3), with retrograde permeation then occurring.

form of insidious widespread linitis plastica of the intestines which can follow carcinoma of the stomach.[50]

# Direct Invasion from Contiguous Primary Tumors

Intrinsic involvement of the alimentary tract by an immediately contiguous neoplasm indicates that a locally aggressive tumor has usually broken through fascial planes.[1,51,52] The most common primaries arise in the ovary, uterus, prostate, and kidney.

With pelvic tumors, the cardinal roentgen signs include an identifiable mass and invasion of the wall of adjacent bowel, often over a considerable length, usually without overhanging margins (Fig. 3–57). Tethering of mucosal folds is often a conspicuous feature. In a female, the most common primary that directly invades the large intestine is *carcinoma of the ovary*. On the left, the *inferior* border of the sigmoid colon is characteristically involved first. Stages of in-

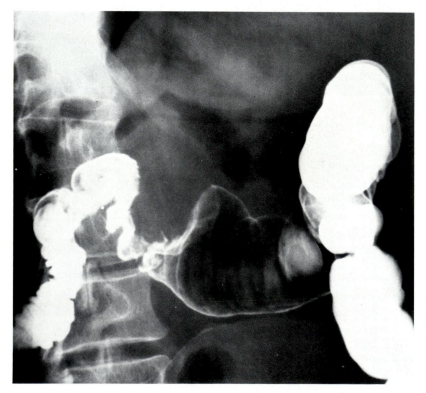

**Fig. 3–55. Anastomotic recurrence.**
This occurred following right hemicolectomy for carcinoma and ileotransverse colostomy. Lymphatic permeation may be a contributing factor.

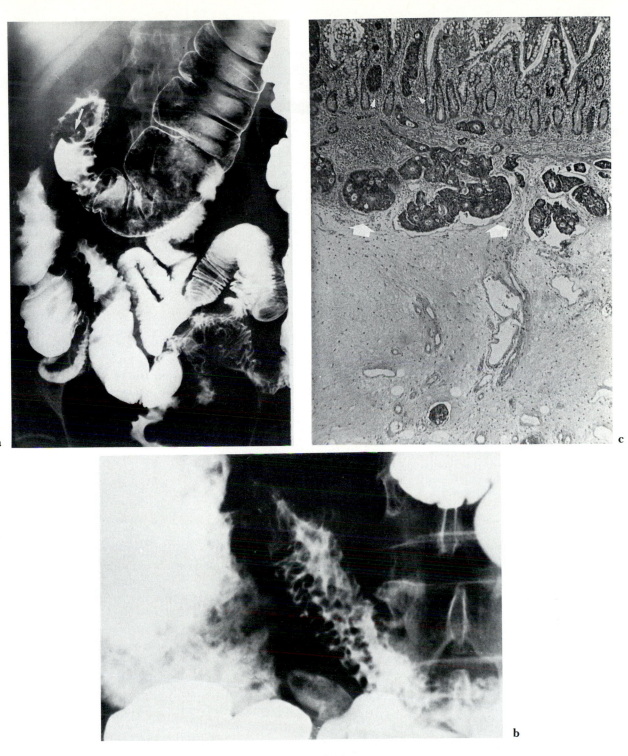

**Fig. 3–56. Carcinoma of the hepatic flexure with lymphatic permeation simulating Crohn's disease.**
**(a)** Barium enema shows a severe long stenosis in the hepatic flexure secondary to a primary adenocarcinoma with colocolonic fistulization (arrow). "Thumbprinting" is present in the ascending colon and terminal ileum, and the appendix shows spiculation and nodularity.
**(b)** Small bowel examination demonstrates a "cobblestone" appearance in the terminal ileum and thickening of the ileocecal valve.
**(c)** Histologic findings include submucous lymphatic infiltration by carcinoma cells (arrows). Some metastatic cell groups are invading the normal intestinal mucosa in retrograde fashion (arrowheads).
(Reproduced from Perez C, et al[47])

131

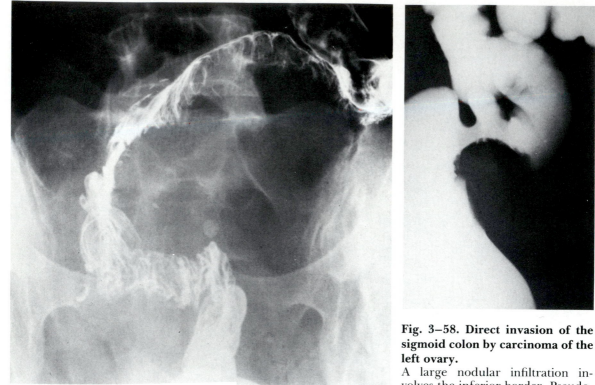

**Fig. 3–58. Direct invasion of the sigmoid colon by carcinoma of the left ovary.**
A large nodular infiltration involves the inferior border. Pseudosacculations result on the pliable superior border. (From Meyers MA[5])

**Fig. 3–57. Direct invasion of the sigmoid colon by a leiomyosarcoma (malignant fibroid) of the uterus.**
Large pelvic mass displaces and fixes the colon, with gross distortion and tethering of the mucosal folds from the associated desmoplastic reaction. (From Meyers and McSweeney[1])

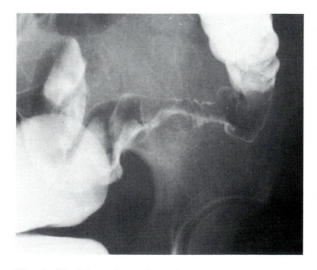

**Fig. 3–59. Direct invasion of the sigmoid colon by carcinoma of the left ovary.**
Nodular infiltrations involve the inferior border.

volvement range from fixation with nodular irregularities (Figs. 3–58 through 3–60) or gross desmoplastic angulation of mucosal folds (Fig. 3–61) to annular involvement (Fig. 3–62).

Advanced *prostatic carcinoma* can spread across Denonvillier's fascia to invade the rectum anteriorly or circumferentially[1,53] (Figs. 3–63 and 3–64). Winter[54] reported that 26 of 225 (11%) patients with carcinoma of the prostate had rectal involvement. Young[55] found 12 instances of rectal mucosal involvement at autopsy in 800 patients with prostatic carcinoma, an incidence of 1.5%. Annular type constriction of the rectum may cause partial to complete obstruction.

*Renal neoplasms* may invade adjacent segments of bowel directly, possibly as recurrences many years after resection of the primary tumor. The late manifestations of renal metastasis

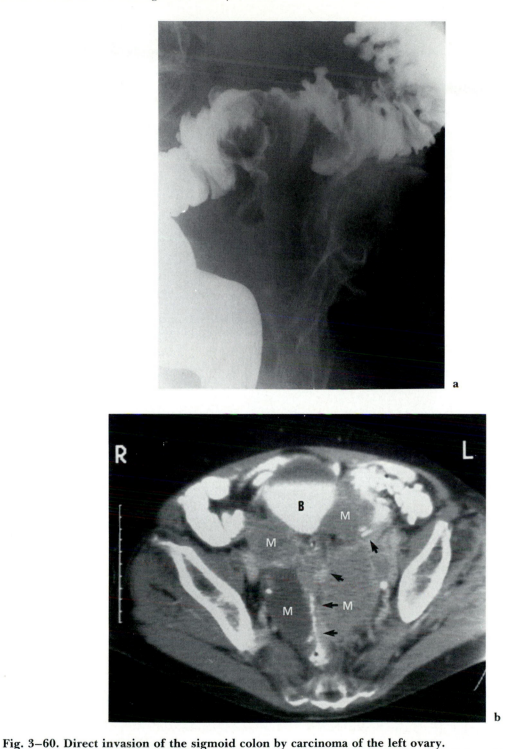

**Fig. 3–60. Direct invasion of the sigmoid colon by carcinoma of the left ovary.**
(a) Barium enema shows gross nodular invasion extending from inferior border of sigmoid colon.
(b) CT demonstrates the presence of bilateral ovarian carcinomatous masses (M), with those on the left straightening and displacing the markedly narrowed sigmoid colon (arrows). B = urinary bladder.
(Courtesy of Michiel Feldberg, MD, University of Utrecht, The Netherlands)

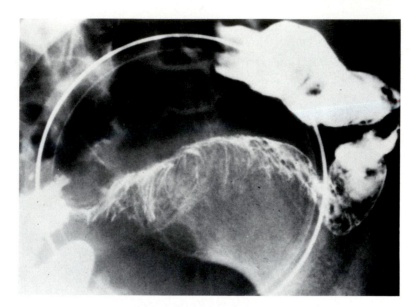

**Fig. 3–61. Direct invasion of the sigmoid colon by carcinoma of the left ovary.**
Mass displacement and fixation of the inferior border are accompanied by striking mucosal tethering.

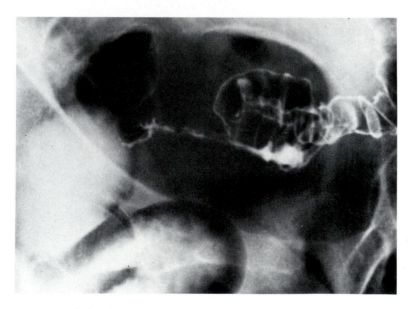

**Fig. 3–62. Direct invasion of the sigmoid colon by carcinoma of the left ovary.**
Extension has progressed to annular involvement.

may occur as long as 30 years after diagnosis. The delay in extension from the nephrectomy site may be due to the poor blood supply of the scar.[56] With growth, they tend to produce bulky intraluminal masses without significant obstruction, since they generally do not elicit a desmoplastic response.[1,57,58] Occasionally, they may produce luminal narrowing with mucosal destruction, simulating a primary carcinoma of the bowel (Fig. 3–65). Recognition of the usual sites of involvement and identification of any extraluminal soft-tissue mass lead to the correct diagnosis. On the right, the descending duodenum (Figs. 3–65 and 3–66) and, on the left, the distal transverse colon or proximal descending colon (Figs. 3–67 through 3–69) are most often involved. At times, jejunal loops may be affected (Figs. 3–70 through 3–72).

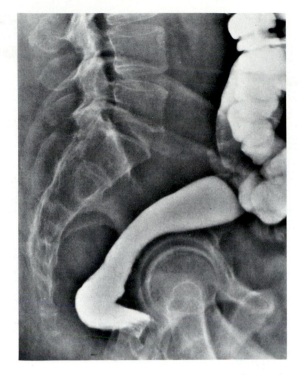

**Fig. 3–63. Annular rectal invasion by prostatic carcinoma.**
The surrounding extrinsic mass narrows the rectal lumen.

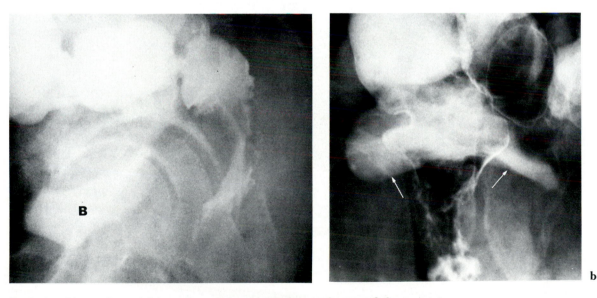

a                                                                                                      b

**Fig. 3–64. Circumferential invasion of the rectum by carcinoma of the prostate.**
(a) Lateral view. Note the widened retrorectal and rectovesical spaces, as well as the mucosal alterations in the rectum. Urinary bladder (B) opacified by simultaneous intravenous urography. (From Meyers and McSweeney[1])
(b) Frontal view. The superior border of the annular involvement of the rectum corresponds to the base of the urinary bladder (arrows), which is elevated by the enlarged prostate gland.

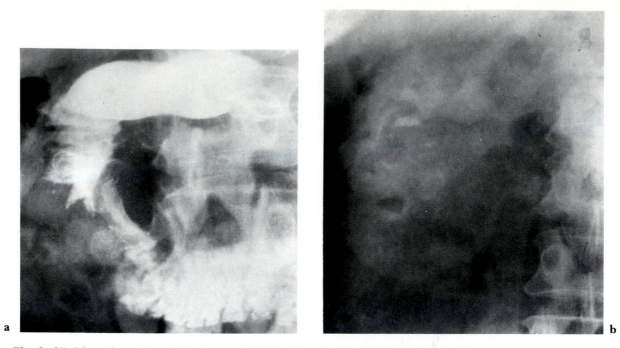

a                                           b

**Fig. 3–65. Direct invasion of the descending duodenum by right renal hypernephroma.**
**(a)** Mucosal destruction simulates a primary neoplasm of the duodenum. (From Meyers and McSweeney[1])
**(b)** Intravenous urogram shows large mass with a few faint calcifications within the lower pole of the right kidney, displacing the collecting system.

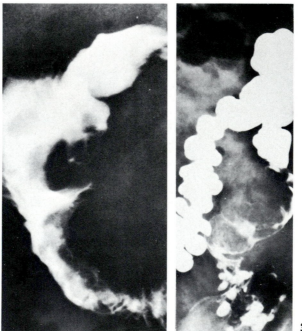

3-66                                           3-67

**Fig. 3–66. Direct invasion of the descending duodenum by right renal hypernephroma.**
This results in multiple polypoid intramural masses of varying sizes, without angulation.

**Fig. 3–67. Direct invasion of the colon by left renal hypernephroma.**
Large polypoid masses extend intraluminally and widen the caliber of the colon, without angulation or obstruction.

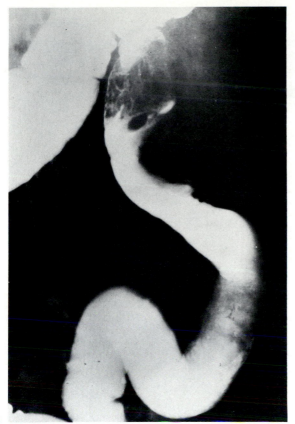

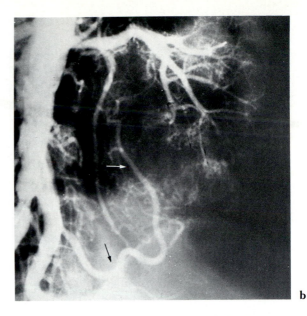

**Fig. 3–68. Direct invasion of the colon by left renal carcinoma.**

**(a)** Extrinsic and intramural masses of the distal transverse and proximal descending colon with bulky polypoid intraluminal extensions. There is no obstruction or acute angulation. (From Meyers and McSweeney[1])

**(b)** Abdominal aortogram shows neovascularity from the renal artery. In addition, a hugely dilated inferior mesenteric artery (arrows) contributes blood supply to the tumor invasion of the colon.

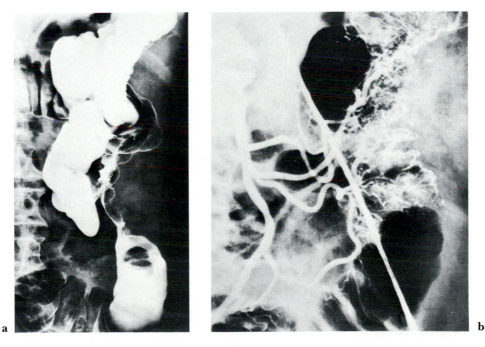

**Fig. 3–69. Direct invasion of the colon by left renal hypernephroma.**

**(a)** Extrinsic masses deform and narrow the descending colon and grow into its lumen.

**(b)** Selective inferior mesenteric arteriogram demonstrates a plethora of neovascularity within the invaded colon.

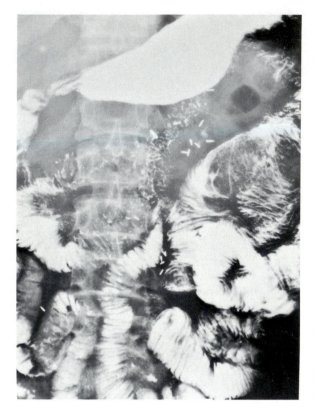

**Fig. 3–70. Direct invasion of the jejunum by left renal hypernephroma.**
Following a nephrectomy, recurrent tumor invades overlying jejunal loops as bulky intramural and intraluminal growths.

◁

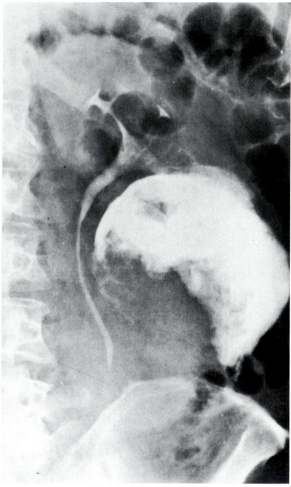

a                                                                                                                              b

**Fig. 3–71. Direct invasion of the jejunum by left renal hypernephroma.**
(a) Compression spot film demonstrates infiltration of the mesentery and jejunal loops.
(b) Percutaneous puncture of neoplastic mass arising from lower pole of left kidney shows its polypoid components.

**Fig. 3–72. Direct invasion of the jejunum by recurrence of hypernephroma, post–right nephrectomy.**

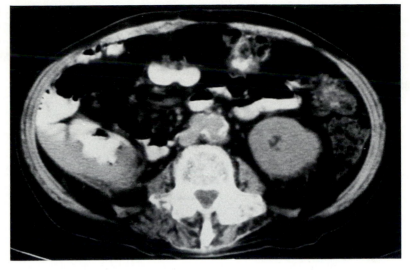

# Intraperitoneal Seeding

It has been classically assumed that transcoelomic spread is a random event or, at least, a function of serosal implantation in the immediate area of a primary neoplasm. However, I have shown that the deposition and growth of secondarily seeded neoplasms in the abdomen depend on the natural flow of ascites within the peritoneal recesses.[3] A primary neoplasm or even its intraabdominal lymph node metastases, in breaking through into the peritoneal cavity, can shed cells into the ascitic fluid induced. The degree of ascites need not be great for the transportation and deposition of malignant cells. I have documented that intraperitoneal fluid, rather than being static, continually follows a circulation through the abdomen.[3,39,59] These dynamic pathways of distribution and sequential spread depend particularly on mesenteric reflections and peritoneal recesses, as well as on the forces of gravity and negative subdiaphragmatic pressure.

## Anatomic Features

The peritoneal cavity is subdivided by peritoneal reflections and mesenteric attachments into several compartments and recesses (Fig. 3–73a). These are anatomically continuous, either directly or indirectly.

The major barrier dividing the abdominal cavity is the *transverse mesocolon*. Below this, the obliquely oriented *small bowel mesentery* divides the inframesocolic space into two compartments of unequal size—the *right* and *left infracolic spaces*. Its main axis, nevertheless, is directed toward the right lower quadrant in relation to the terminal ileum and cecum. The right infracolic space terminates at their junction. The left infracolic space is open anatomically to the pelvis to the right of the midline; toward the left, it is restricted from continuity with the pelvic cavity by the sigmoid mesocolon.

The *right* and *left paracolic gutters* are lateral to the attachments of the peritoneal reflections of the ascending and descending colon. They represent potential communications between the lower abdomen and pelvis below with the supramesocolic area above. On the left, however, the phrenicocolic ligament[22] partially separates the paracolic gutter from the perisplenic (left subphrenic) space. This ligament extends from the splenic flexure of the colon to the diaphragm at the level of the 11th rib.

The *pelvis* is the most dependent portion of the peritoneal cavity in either the supine or erect position. Its compartments include the midline cul-de-sac or *pouch of Douglas* (rectovaginal pouch in the female and rectovesical pouch in the male) and the *lateral paravesical recesses*.

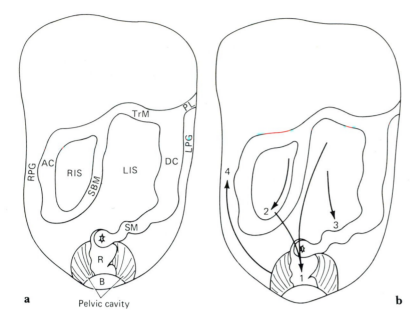

a

**Fig. 3–73. (a) Posterior peritoneal reflections and intraabdominal spaces.**
TrM = transverse mesocolon, PL = phrenicocolic ligament, SBM = small bowel mesentery, AC = attachment of ascending colon, DC = attachment of descending colon, SM = sigmoid mesocolon, R = rectum, B = urinary bladder, RIS = right infracolic space, LIS = left infracolic space, RPG = right paracolic gutter, LPG = left paracolic gutter.
**(b) Diagram of the pathways of flow of intraperitoneal fluid and the four predominant sites in the lower abdomen.**

b

## Pathways of Ascitic Flow

The transverse mesocolon, small bowel mesentery, sigmoid mesocolon, and the peritoneal attachments of the ascending and descending colon clearly serve as watersheds directing the flow of ascites (Fig. 3–73b). The force of gravity operates to pool peritoneal fluid in dependent peritoneal recesses. Fluid in the inframesocolic compartments preferentially seeks the pelvic cavity. From the left infracolic space, some fluid is temporarily arrested along the superior plane of the sigmoid mesocolon but gradually channels into the pelvis. From the right infracolic space, spread occurs along the small bowel mesentery. It is not until a pool is formed at the apex, at the termination of the ileum with the cecum, that some fluid begins to overflow into the pelvis. The pouch of Douglas is first filled and then, symmetrically, the lateral paravesical recesses (Fig. 3–74). From this point, the fluid ascends both paracolic gutters. Passage up the shallower left one is slow and weak, and cephalad extension is limited by the phrenicocolic gutter. The major flow from the pelvis is up the right paracolic gutter. It continues to the right subhepatic and right subphrenic spaces. The right paracolic gutter serves also as the main communication from the upper to the lower abdominal compartments. Freely movable fluid collecting in the right upper quadrant also continues to be redirected downward along this channel to the pelvis.

Four predominant sites in the lower abdomen are therefore identified clearly as the preferential, repeated, or arrested flow of ascitic fluid: (a) the pelvic cavity, particularly the pouch of Douglas, (b) the right lower quadrant at the termination of the small bowel mesentery, (c) the superior aspect of the sigmoid mesocolon, and (d) the right paracolic gutter. These pathways are illustrated in Figure 3–73b.

## Seeded Sites

Stasis or pooling of ascitic fluid favors the processes of deposition, fixation, and growth of seeded malignant cells. The seeded deposits coalesce and are then fixed to the serosal surfaces by fibrinous adhesions that quickly become organized.[60]

Analysis of a series of proved cases has shown that the sites of lodgment and growth of intraperitoneal seeded metastases clearly follow the pathways of flow of ascitic fluid.[3] The pouch of Douglas is involved in over 50%, the lower small bowel mesentery in about 40%, the sigmoid mesocolon in about 20%, and the right paracolic gutter in about 20% of cases. In males, the primary carcinoma most often arises in the gastro-

**Fig. 3–74. Pelvic drainage of intra-peritoneal fluid.**
Intraperitoneal opaque contrast material first gravitates to the pelvic cavity, filling the midline pouch of Douglas (PD) and then the two paravesical recesses (PV). B = urinary bladder.

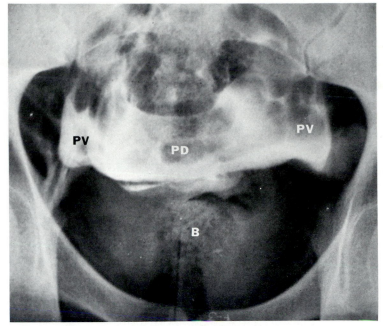

intestinal tract (stomach, colon, pancreas), and in females, in the genital system (ovary).[61–63]

## Pouch of Douglas (Rectosigmoid Junction): Radiologic Features

Intraperitoneal fluid consistently seeks the pouch of Douglas, the most caudal and posterior part of the peritoneal cavity, and then the lateral paravesical recesses (Fig. 3–74). The lower extension of the peritoneal reflections, comprising the pouch of Douglas, projects generally at the level of the lower second to upper fourth sacral segment (Fig. 3–75). This variability is determined by the developmental fixation of the peritoneum to Denonvillier's fascia (rectovaginal or rectovesical septum) and the degree to which the urinary bladder and rectum are distended.[64] It is a particularly useful landmark, demarcating the junction between the rectum and sigmoid colon. Thus, it is apparent that the ventral surface of the rectosigmoid junction faces the pouch of Douglas.

Seeding at this site is most common. On barium enema study, this results in a characteristic pattern of fixed parallel folds or a nodular indentation on the anterior aspect of the rectosigmoid junction[3,65] (Figs. 3–76 and 3–77). These changes reflect the coalescence of deposits with a dense fibrous reaction. This may be clinically

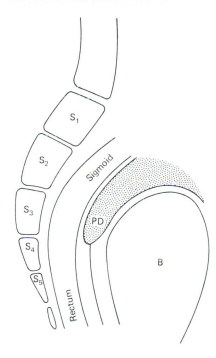

**Fig. 3–75. Sagittal view of relationships of pouch of Douglas** (PD).
This is the lower continuation of the peritoneal cavity between the rectosigmoid and the urinary bladder (B). (From Meyers[3])

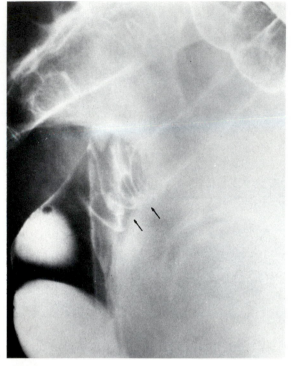

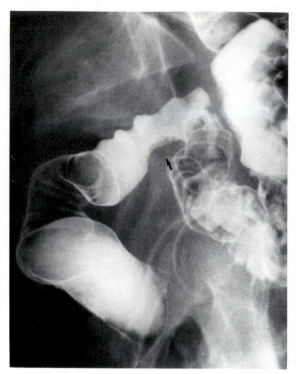

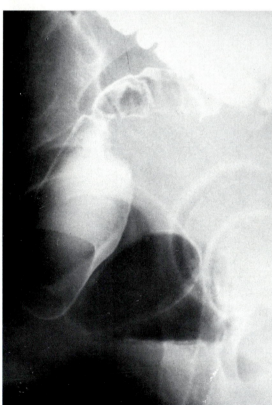

**Fig. 3–76. Different cases of metastatic seeding in the pouch of Douglas.**
Associated desmoplastic response characteristically results in (a) fixed transverse parallel folds, (b) nodular mass, or (c) mass with mucosal tethering along the ventral aspect of the rectosigmoid junction.

The primary tumors were (a) carcinoma of the ovary, (b) carcinoma of the pancreas, and (c) carcinoma of the stomach.
(From Meyers and McSweeney[1])

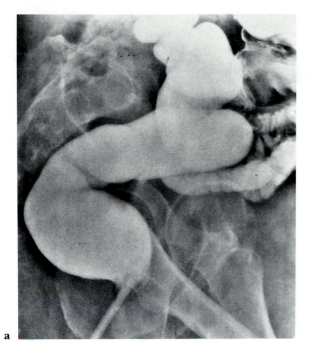

a

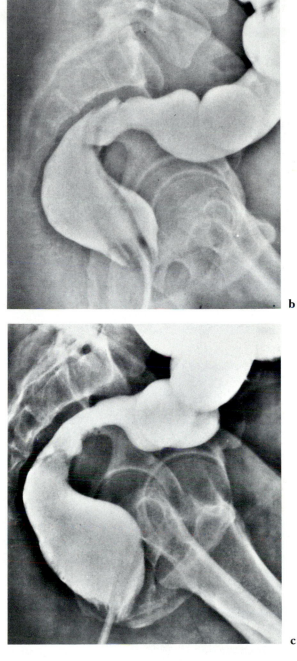

b

c

**Fig. 3–77. Progressive changes of metastatic seeding in the pouch of Douglas.**
Deposits from a primary carcinoma of the splenic flexure of the colon result in increasing mass impression on the rectosigmoid.
**(b)** and **(c)** 5 months and 1 year, respectively, after **(a)**.

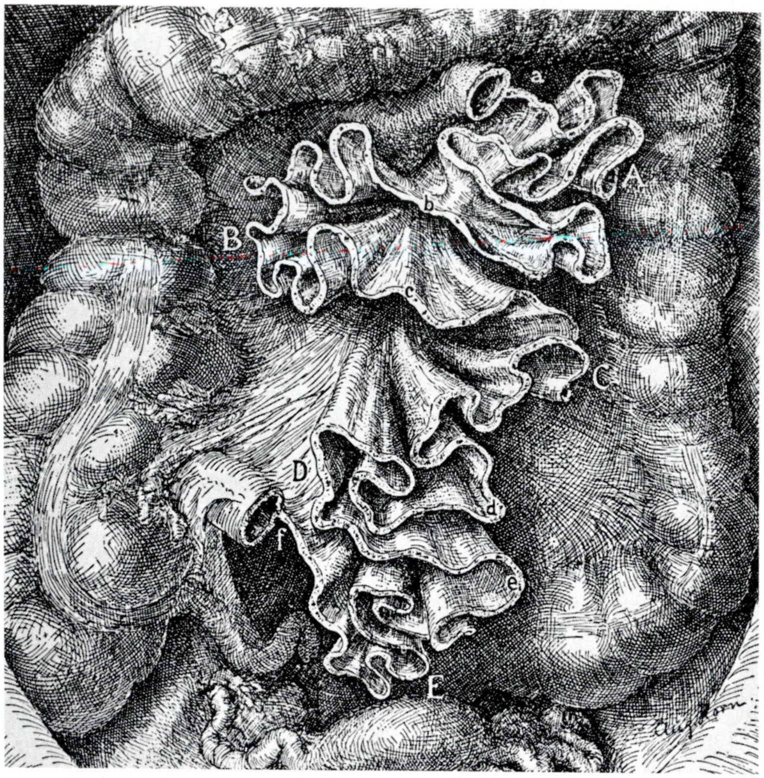

**Fig. 3–78. The small bowel mesentery, illustrating its ruffled nature.** A series of peritoneal recesses is formed along its right side. (Reprinted with permission from Kelly HA: Appendicitis and Other Diseases of the Vermiform Appendix. JB Lippincott Co, Philadelphia, 1909)

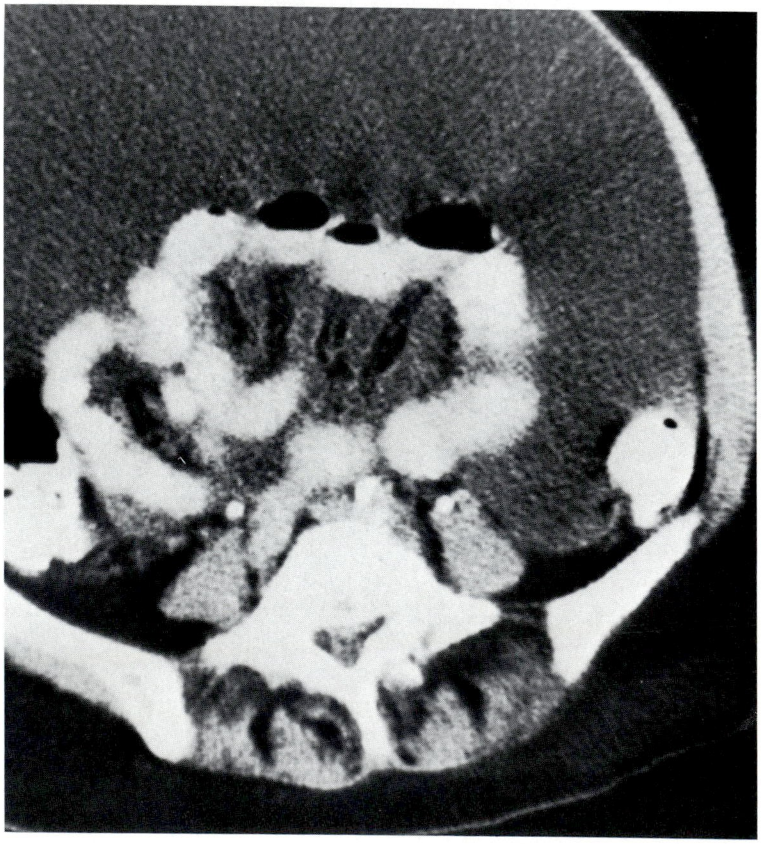

**Fig. 3–79. Ascitic fluid collecting between mesenteric folds.** Computed tomography documents ascitic fluid pooling between the folds of the small bowel mesentery. The latter are seen as lucent bands, reflecting their adipose nature, radiating from the root to opacified small bowel loops.

palpable as the classic Blumer's shelf.[64,66] It is thought that the factor essential to the development of a rectal shelf tumor is pathologic fixation of the uppermost part of Denonvillier's fascia.[64] The nodular impression on the ventral aspect of the rectosigmoid junction from seeding in the pouch of Douglas may be duplicated by endometriosis, periproctitis, tumors, inflammation of the seminal vesicles,[64,65] or postirradiation changes. The presence of ascites, however, indicates these findings as part of peritoneal carcinomatosis.

## Lower Small Bowel Mesentery (Terminal Ileum and Cecum): Radiologic Features

The root of the small bowel mesentery extends from the left side of the second lumbar vertebra downward to the right, across the aorta and inferior vena cava, to the right sacroiliac joint, a distance of only about 15 cm. From the root, a series of mesenteric ruffles support the small bowel loops (Fig. 3–78). These fanlike mesenteric extensions contribute to the characteristic undulating nature and position of the coils of small bowel, which averages 15 to 20 ft in length. Distally, the mesentery inserts most often at the cecocolic junction. A series of peritoneal recesses is thus formed extending along the right side of the ruffled small bowel mesentery obliquely toward the right lower quadrant of the abdomen. I have shown that these also serve to pool collections of ascitic fluid[1,3,4] (Fig. 3–79). Spread here occurs in a series of cascades or rivulets from one mesenteric ruffle to the next, directed along the axis of the small bowel mesentery toward the right lower quadrant in relation to distal ileal loops and the cecum (Fig. 3–80). It is here, within the lower recesses of the small bowel mesentery, that the most consistent pool of fluid forms before overflow into the pelvis occurs.

Seeded deposits lodging within the lower recesses of the small bowel mesentery in the right infracolic space are clinically identifiable in over 40% of cases by their displacement of distal ileal loops, perhaps with pressure effects also upon the medial contour of the cecum and ascending colon.

Symmetric growth within multiple adjacent mesenteric recesses results in discrete separation of ileal loops in the right lower quadrant.

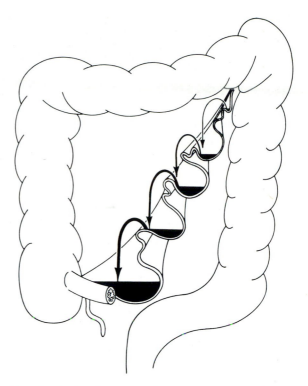

**Fig. 3–80. The flow of ascites forms a series of pools within the recesses of the small bowel mesentery.** The most consistent drainage is to its lower end, in relation to distal ileal loops and the cecum. (From Meyers[4])

Angulated tethering of mucosal folds indicates associated fibrous response. Significantly, these and any serosal masses are therefore identifiable on the concave borders, which are suspended by the mesenteric ruffles.[4] The narrowed loops may be aligned in a parallel configuration which I describe as "palisading" (Fig. 3–81). The axis of the serosal masses as well as of the affected intestinal loops conforms to the axis of the small bowel mesentery. As the seeded growths become somewhat larger, they may displace the bowel loops in a gently arcuate manner (Fig. 3–82). The striking symmetry of size, mass displacement from the mesenteric border of the loops, and orientation to the mesenteric ruffles in the right lower quadrant characterize the process. The seeded metastases on the serosal aspect of ileal loops in the right lower quadrant are typically localized to the concave mesenteric borders.

If the desmoplastic response to the seeded metastases is severe, marked fixation and angulation of ileal loops in the right lower quadrant

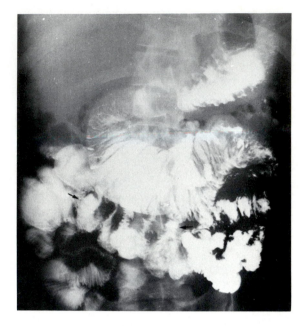

**Fig. 3–81. Seeded gastric carcinoma along lower small bowel mesentery.**
There is palisaded separation of ileal loops in the right lower quadrant (arrows). Mucosal folds are mildly tethered. (Sites of obstruction are also present proximally.) (From Meyers[4])

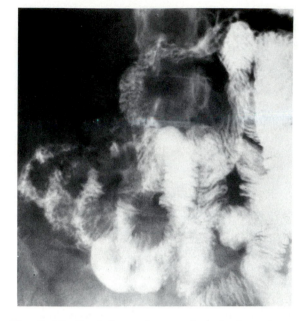

**Fig. 3–82. Seeded ovarian carcinoma along lower small bowel mesentery.**
There is striking scalloped displacement of multiple ileal loops in the lower right quadrant, following the axis of the mesenteric recesses. The mucosal folds are mildly tethered. (From Meyers and McSweeney[1])

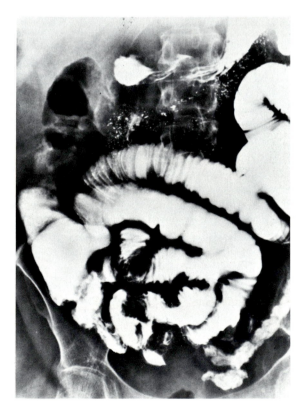

result (Figs. 3–83 and 3–84). The most extreme fibrous reaction has been encountered in metastatic seeding from pancreatic carcinoma and mucin-producing gastric carcinoma. Serosal mass displacement may remain evident. The points of acute angulation tend to conform to the axis of the mesentery. Despite the narrowing and sharp course, obstruction may not be conspicuous.

If no significant fibrous reaction is elicited as the metastases increase in size, gross extrinsic mass displacement may be shown (Fig. 3–85). The mesenteric masses, however, tend to be multiple, and they maintain their relationship to the lower small bowel mesentery (Fig. 3–86). They displace ileal loops predominantly inferiorly and medially and may exert pressure on the

◁——————————————————————

**Fig. 3–83. Seeded ovarian carcinoma along lower small bowel mesentery.**
Nodular serosal masses on the mesenteric borders of distal ileal loops are associated with fibrotic narrowing and angulation. These produce some proximal obstruction.

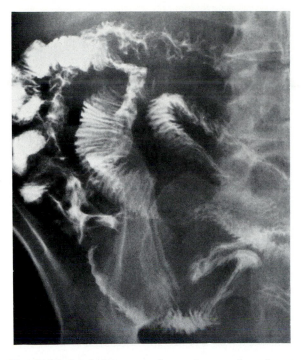

**Fig. 3–84. Seeded pancreatic carcinoma along lower small bowel mesentery.**
Mass separation and striking angulation of fixed ileal loops in right lower quadrant from extensive desmoplastic reaction. (From Meyers[4])

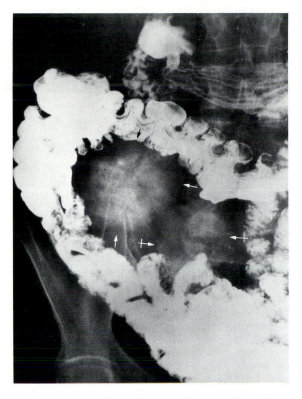

**Fig. 3–85. Seeded ovarian carcinoma along lower small bowel mesentery.**
Two masses with psammomatous calcifications in the right lower quadrant displace ileal loops and press on the ascending and transverse colon. (From Meyers and McSweeney[1])

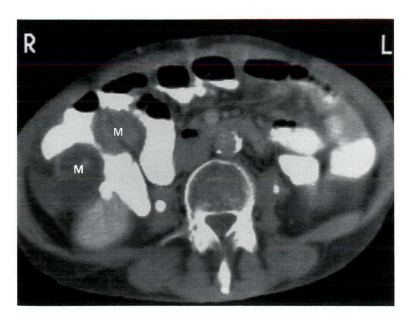

**Fig. 3–86. Seeded ovarian carcinoma along lower small bowel mesentery.**
Metastatic masses (M) compress the ileocecal region and an adjacent ileal loop. There is early tethering of mucosal folds. Ascites is present.

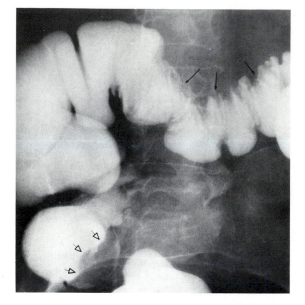

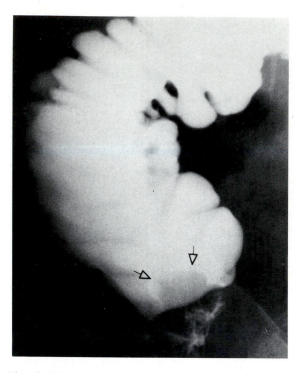

**Fig. 3–87. Seeded carcinoma of the gallbladder along lower small bowel mesentery.**
This results in a mass eccentrically indenting the medial contour of the cecum (open arrows). There is also direct invasion of the transverse colon (black arrows). (From Meyers[4])

**Fig. 3–88. Seeded gastric carcinoma along lower small bowel mesentery.**
Lobulated mass indents the inferior contour of the cecum (arrows). The distal ileum is angulated and deformed by mass impressions. (From Meyers[4])

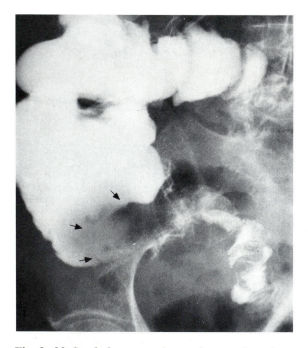

**Fig. 3–89. Seeded pancreatic carcinoma along lower small bowel mesentery.**
Large lobulated mass with nodular excrescences grossly indents the inferior contour of the cecum (arrows). There is also mass pressure on the terminal ileum with fibrous angulation. (From Meyers[4])

ascending colon medially and the proximal transverse colon inferiorly.

Since the small bowel mesentery most commonly inserts at the cecocolic junction, the effects of seeded metastases on the cecum are shown typically on its medial and inferior contours.[4] The level of involvement is thus usually below the ileocecal valve in the caput of the cecum. The extrinsic mass indenting the cecum may be smooth or lobulated (Figs. 3–87 and 3–88), of variable size (Fig. 3–89), and at times, may encircle the cecum (Fig. 3–90). The mass changes on the cecum are not, in themselves, specific for seeded metastases and may simulate appendiceal abnormalities, other mesenteric masses, or even primary lesions of the cecum. However, they are almost invariably accompanied by the more characteristic changes involving distal small bowel loops. If first appreciated on a barium enema study, these can be identified by reflux into the terminal ileum (Figs. 3–88 and 3–89) or in a subsequent small bowel series. The association of findings may occasionally closely simulate granulomatous enterocoli-

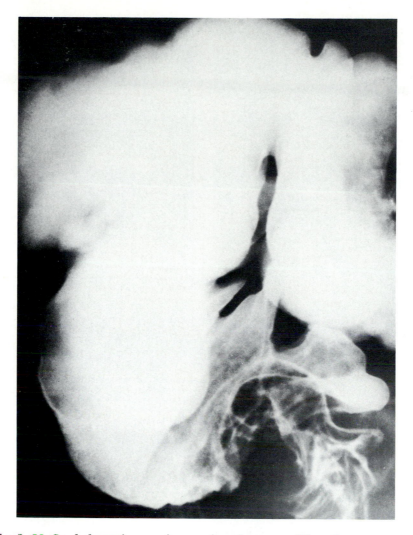

**Fig. 3–90. Seeded ovarian carcinoma along lower small bowel mesentery.**
Annular mass narrowing of apex of cecum. (From Meyers[4])

tis[19] (Fig. 3–91). The small bowel alterations are usually not difficult to distinguish from other common disease states. The lack of inflammatory features, such as spasm, ulcerations, and sinus tracts, and the characteristic spectrum of changes help in the differential diagnosis from regional enteritis, tuberculosis, amebiasis, and peritoneal adhesions. When the seeded metastases are diffuse throughout the small bowel (Fig. 3–92), the changes secondary to the desmoplastic process may resemble carcinoid or radiation enteritis. Fixed angulation and alternating areas of narrowing and dilatation are accompanied by serosal masses identifiable on the mesenteric borders and conspicuous tethering of mucosal folds.

## Sigmoid Colon: Radiologic Features

Lodgment and growth of deposits arrested along the barrier of the sigmoid mesocolon in the left lower quadrant result in changes characteristically localized to the superior border of the sigmoid colon (Figs. 3–93 and 3–94). The associated desmoplastic reaction causes tethering of the mucosal folds. These lose their axis normally perpendicular to the lumen of the bowel and become angulated, often toward a common point in the mesentery at the site of the secondary lesion (Figs. 3–95 through 3–97). Even when annular invasion from the seeded metastases has occurred, the sigmoid colon tends to show preponderant changes on its su-

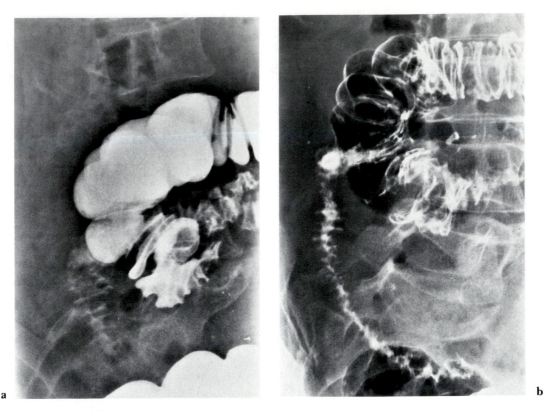

a                                                                                                   b

**Fig. 3–91. Seeded pancreatic carcinoma along lower small bowel.**
(a) Barium enema with (b) air-contrast studies demonstrate changes involving the cecum and terminal ileum closely simulating granulomatous enterocolitis. (From Meyers[4])

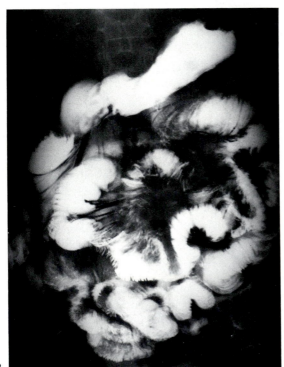

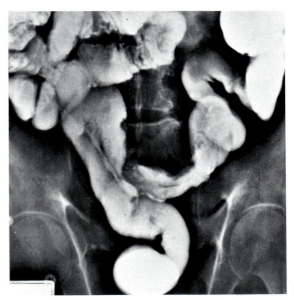

3-92                                                                                                3-93

**Fig. 3–94. Seeding in the sigmoid mesocolon
from ovarian mucinous carcinoma.**
Computed tomography shows the metastases
involving the superior aspect of the sigmoid
colon (SC).                                   ▷

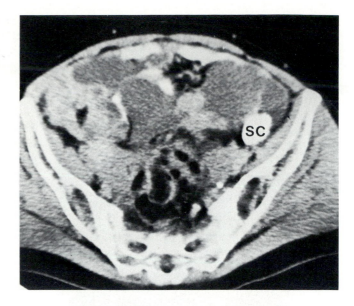

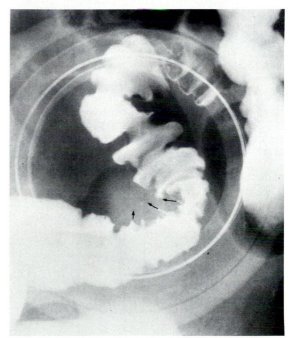

▷

**Fig. 3–95. Intraperitoneal seeding in the sigmoid
mesocolon from pancreatic carcinoma.**
The desmoplastic reaction accompanying the deposits causes tethering of the mucosal folds along the
superior border of the sigmoid colon, angulated toward a common site in the mesentery (arrows). (From
Meyers[3])

**Fig. 3–92. Diffuse seeded metastases from gastric carcinoma along small bowel mesentery.**
Serosal masses are present predominantly on the mesenteric borders of small bowel loops, including the ileum
in the right lower quadrant. The mucosal folds are tethered, and there are angulations and alternating
constrictions of loops. These changes are consequent to the fibrotic reaction.

**Fig. 3–93. Seeding in the sigmoid mesocolon from colonic carcinoma.**
Metastatic mass impresses the superior contour of the sigmoid colon.

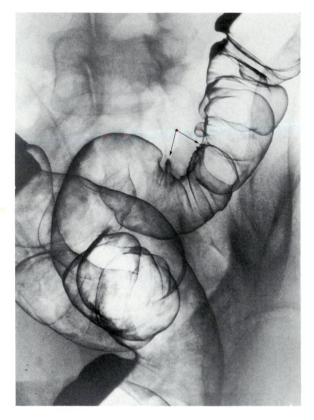

**Fig. 3–96. Intraperitoneal seeding in the sigmoid mesocolon from gastric carcinoma.**
The desmoplastic response tethers mucosal folds along the superior border of the sigmoid colon (arrows). (Reproduced from Maruyama M: Radiologic Diagnosis of Polyps and Carcinoma of the Large Bowel. Igaku-Shoin Ltd, Tokyo, New York, 1977)

perior border (Fig. 3–98). This localization occurs in more than 20% of cases of metastatic seeding.

## Right Paracolic Gutter (Cecum and Ascending Colon): Radiologic Features

Following the flow of ascitic fluid from the pelvis preferentially upward within the right paracolic gutter, deposition and growth in this peritoneal recess are shown by mass changes lateral and posterior to the cecum and proximal ascending colon (Fig. 3–99). Tethering of mucosal folds or angulated fixation of a small bowel loop in this area may occur as a consequence of an associated fibrous reaction (Fig. 3–100). This localization occurs in 18% of cases.

## Seeded Perihepatic and Subdiaphragmatic Metastases

Conventional radiologic studies have disclosed the intraperitoneal spread of seeded metastases to the supramesocolic compartment only on occasion. This pathway of spread is illustrated graphically in Fig. 3–101 in an instance of a spilled ovarian dermoid cyst.[67]

Transcoelomic migration of fluid, particles, and cells cephalad toward the undersurface of the diaphragm is caused by changes in intraperitoneal pressure during breathing and the topographic arrangement of the peritoneal re-

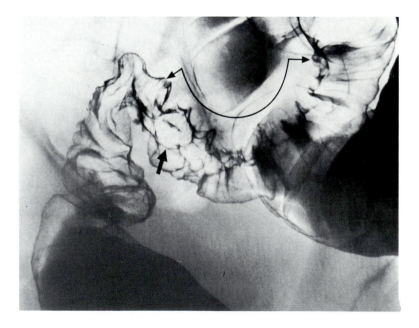

**Fig. 3–97. Metastatic seeding in sigmoid mesocolon.**
The superior margin of the sigmoid colon is involved over a considerable length with infiltrative and desmoplastic mucosal changes (arrow line). Mucosal elevation seen *en face* suggests submucosal tumor (arrow). (Reproduced from Marayuma M: Radiologic Diagnosis of Polyps and Carinoma of the Large Bowel. Igaku-Shoin Ltd, Tokyo, New York, 1977)

**Fig. 3–98. Metastatic seeding in the sigmoid meso-colon from gastric carcinoma.**
Circumferential invasion has occurred but the predominant effect can be identified on the superior contour of the sigmoid colon. (From Meyers et al[19])

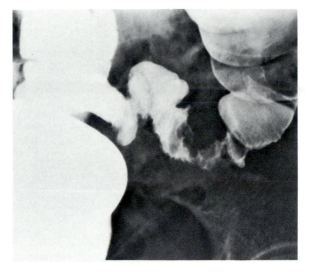

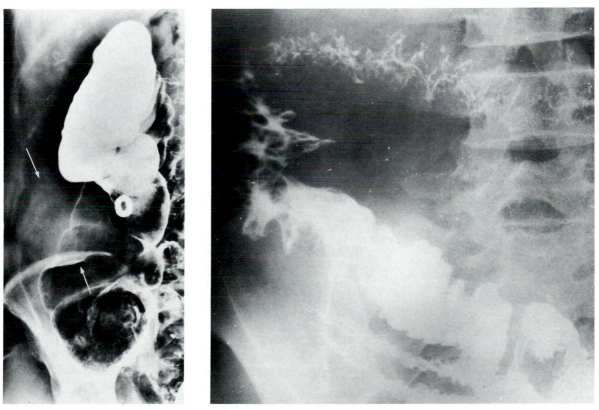

-99

3-100

**Fig. 3–99. Seeding in right paracolic gutter from ovarian carcinoma.**
Metastatic mass displaces the lateral aspect of the ascending colon (arrows).

**Fig. 3–100. Intraperitoneal seeding in the right paracolic gutter from gastric carcinoma.**
Nodular masses displace the ascending colon anteriorly and medially, and cause angulated fixation of a small bowel loop. (From Meyers and McSweeney[1])

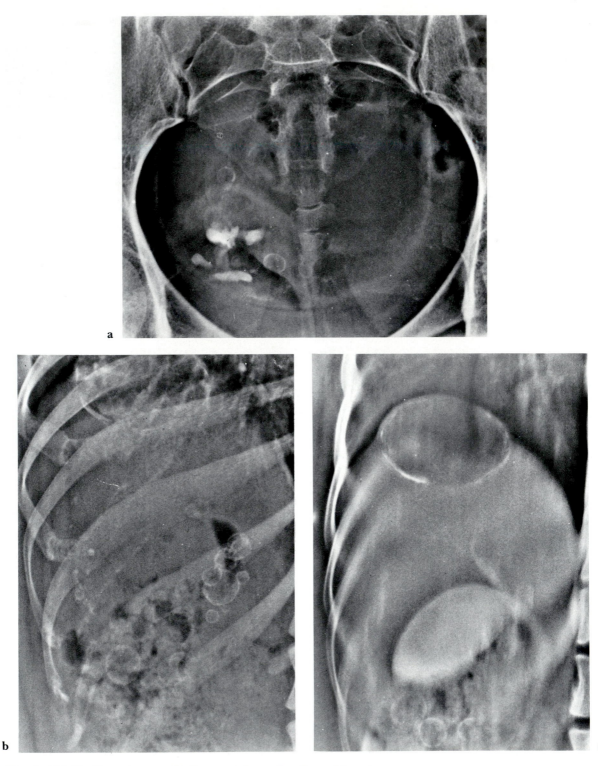

**Fig. 3–101. Perihepatic spread of ruptured ovarian dermoid cyst.**
(a) Plain film of the pelvis identifies the fatty radiolucency of a large dermoid cyst of the ovary. It contains toothlike and multiple small cystic calcifications.
(b) Plain film. Multiple cystlike calcifications in the right subphrenic and subhepatic areas.
(c) Intravenous cholangiogram with tomography verifies the location of the calcified structures. These represent perihepatic satellite cysts implanted from the ruptured dermoid of the ovary.

cesses.[3,59] In ovarian carcinoma, free tumor cells are shed from gross or microscopic tumor excrescences on the capsule of the primary tumor. These free-floating cells have been shown to be removed from the peritoneal cavity through lymphatic channels located in the diaphragm.[68,69] However, absorption does not take place evenly over the whole diaphragmatic surface, but is more extensive on the right side, overlying the liver.[70,71] Drainage occurs into submesothelial lymphatic capillaries of the diaphragm, which penetrate through the muscle to intercommunicate with a comparable plexus arising on the pleural surface. From the diaphragm, lymphatic drainage primarily occurs to the anterior mediastinal lymph nodes.[70,72–74] This pathway is quantitatively the most significant, accounting for 80% of the clearance from the peritoneal cavity. Partial or complete obstruction of the diaphragmatic lymph channels by ovarian carcinoma tumor cells facilitates the accumulation of malignant ascites and creates favorable conditions for the implantation of tumor cells at other sites in the peritoneal cavity.[68] Nearly 90% of patients with ovarian carcinoma have peritoneal implants at autopsy, and 60–70% have ascites.[75]

It is being increasingly recognized that metastatic ovarian implants along the right hemidiaphragm and liver capsule are frequent. Peritoneoscopic studies have shown metastatic diaphragmatic involvement in 61% of patients with ovarian carcinoma,[76] and more significantly, that in 21 to 34% of patients otherwise diagnosed as having stage I or stage II disease there is seeding on the undersurface of the diaphragm, particularly on the right.[77–80] These implants are generally only 2–3 mm in diameter (Fig. 3–102), but may reach a size of several centimeters.[81]

The perihepatic dissemination of ovarian carcinoma is now being increasingly detected by computed tomography. Peritoneal implants may be seen as nodular, plaquelike, or sheetlike masses[82] (Figs. 3–103 and 3–104), and deposits as small as 1 cm from ovarian carcinoma may be detected, often outlined by ascites.[81,83]

In mucinous cystadenocarcinoma of the ovary, the gelatinous material produced by seeded metastases may be first seen as a mantle over the right lobe of the liver (Fig. 3–105). With progression to the condition known as

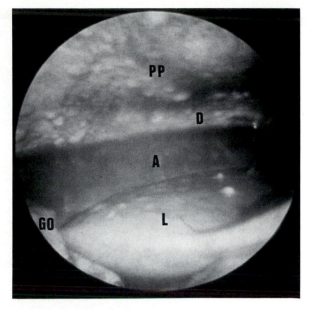
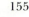

**Fig. 3–102. Perihepatic seeded ovarian carcinoma shown by peritoneoscopy.**
Multiple small nodules are present on the liver (L) and the parietal peritoneum (PP) of the abdominal wall and diaphragm (D). A = ascites, GO = greater omentum. (Courtesy of Charles Lightdale, MD, Memorial Sloan-Kettering Cancer Center, New York, NY)

pseudomyxoma peritonei, the characteristic findings of scalloping of the liver edge by the cystic collections and septated ascites may be evident[84] (Fig. 3–106). Delineation by the falciform ligament is a characteristic landmark of the process of intraperitoneal seeding.[39,59] Dense, punctate perihepatic calcifications in a case of pseudomyxoma peritonei from mucinous adenocarcinoma of the appendix following intraperitoneal chemotherapy has been reported.[85]

In serous cystadenocarcinoma of the ovary, calcified perihepatic metastatic implants may be detected.[86–88] This is the most common type of ovarian carcinoma and contains histologic calcification, psammoma bodies, in approximately 30% of cases.[89] The perihepatic calcifications are seen related to the right hemidiaphragm (Fig. 3–107) and liver surface (Figs. 3–108 and 3–109), even up to the immediate subphrenic region (Fig. 3–110), as well as on the falciform ligament (Figs. 3–108 and 3–109). Calcified implants have also been noted in the right paracolic gutter, in Morison's pouch, and adjacent to the spleen.[86,88]

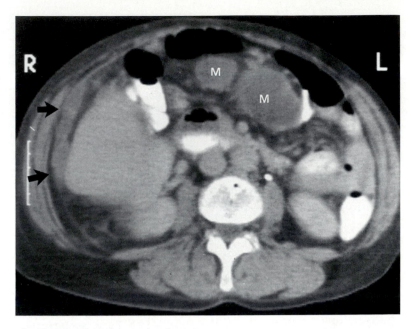

**Fig. 3–103. Metastatic "caking" of the parietal peritoneum.**
Seeded metastases from ovarian carcinoma have resulted in plaquelike thickening of the parietal peritoneum lateral to the right lobe of the liver (arrows). Mesenteric masses (M) are also present. (Courtesy of Michiel Feldberg, MD, University of Utrecht, The Netherlands)

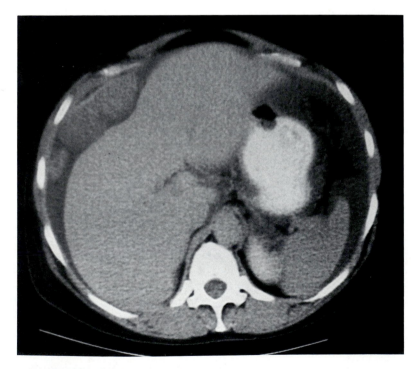

**Fig. 3–104. Perihepatic diaphragmatic metastatic nodules.**
Seeded implants from ovarian carcinoma are seen as prominent nodular masses on the parietal peritoneum overlying the diaphragm impressing upon the liver. Ascites is present.

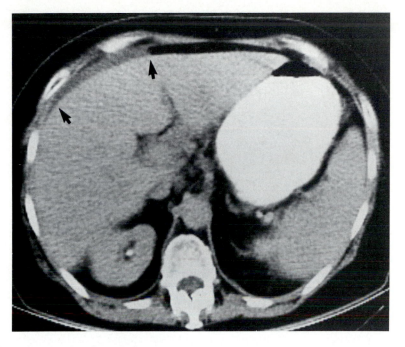

**Fig. 3–105. Perihepatic mantle of seeded metastases.**
A thin mantle of low density material representing early seeding from a mucinous ovarian carcinoma is adjacent to the liver (arrows). It extends anteriorly to the level of the falciform ligament. There is no appreciable ascites.

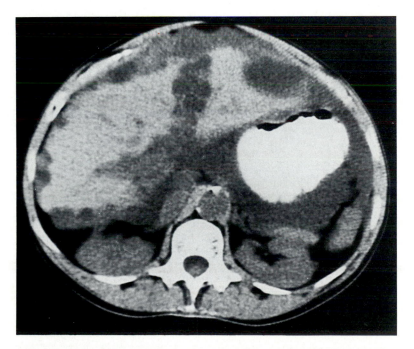

**Fig. 3–106. Pseudomyxoma peritonei secondary to mucinous cystadenocarcinoma of the ovary.**
Gelatinous cysts of varying densities produce scalloped indentations upon the liver. Discrete cysts bound the falciform ligament. Fluid collections in both the greater peritoneal cavity and lesser sac are inhomogeneous.

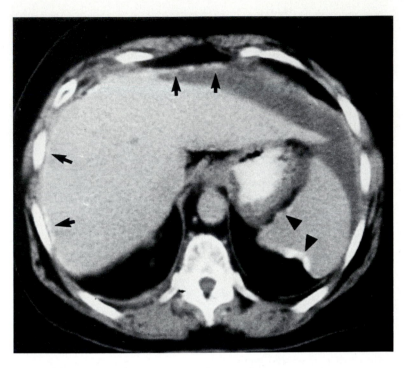

**Fig. 3–107. Calcified perihepatic implants from ovarian carcinoma.**
CT shows calcification along the right border of the liver that extends anteriorly along the diaphragm (arrows), where it is separated from the liver by ascites. Perisplenic calcification is also present (arrowheads). (Reproduced from Mitchell D, et al[86])

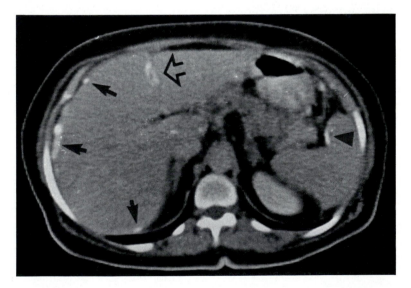

**Fig. 3–108. Calcified perihepatic implants from ovarian carcinoma.**
Calcified metastatic deposits are present on the surface of the liver (arrows) and on the falciform ligament (open arrow). Perisplenic calcification is also evident (arrowhead). (Reproduced from Pandolfo I, et al[87])

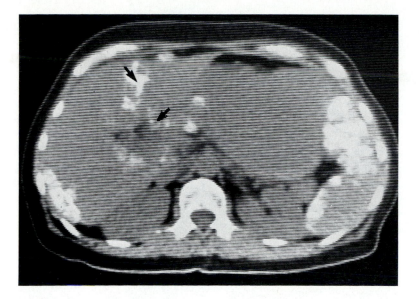

**Fig. 3–109. Calcified perihepatic implants from ovarian carcinoma.**
Calcified metastatic deposits are seen along the liver surface, the ligamentum teres and falciform ligament (arrows), and spleen. (Reproduced from Solomon A, Rubinstein Z[88])

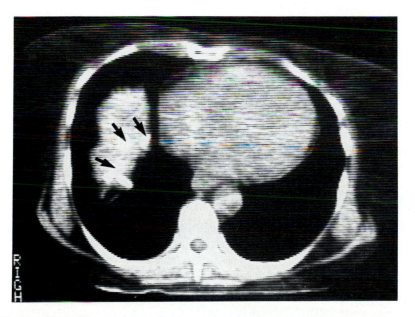

**Fig. 3–110. Calcified perihepatic metastases from ovarian carcinoma.**
The secondary malignancies have been transported and implanted in the immediate subdiaphragmatic region (arrows). (Reproduced from Solomon A, Rubinstein Z[88])

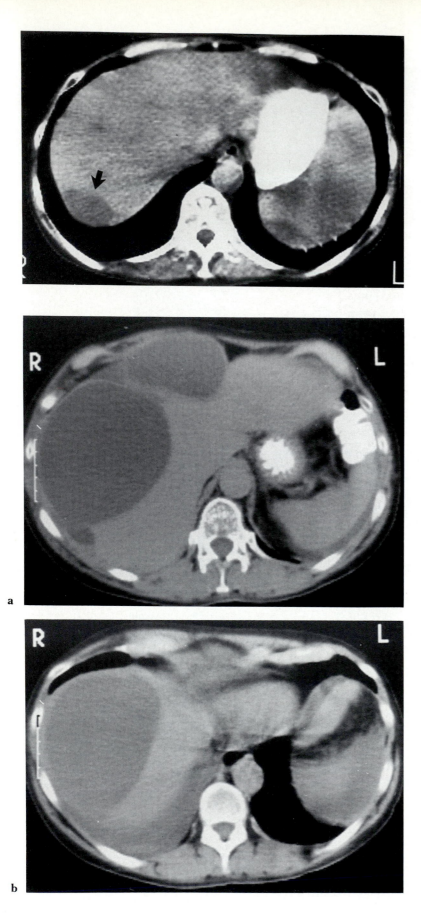

**Fig. 3–111. Subcapsular liver metastasis from ovarian carcinoma** on the posterior contour of the right lobe of the liver (arrow). ◁

a

b

**Fig. 3–112. Subcapsular liver metastases from ovarian carcinoma.** (a and b) Bilobed or confluent lesions involve the liver. Ascites and a right pleural effusion are present. (Courtesy of Michiel Feldberg, MD, University of Utrecht, The Netherlands)

**Fig. 3–113. Omental caking from seeded metastases** is seen as a solid mass between the anterior abdominal wall and bowel. It extends anteriorly to form an umbilical mass.

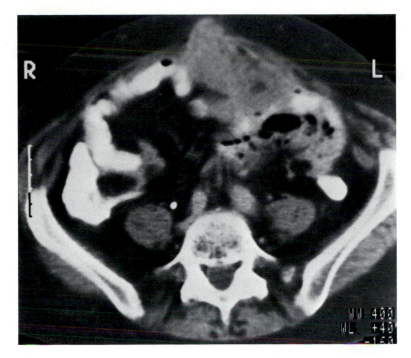

Subcapsular liver metastases have been observed by computed tomography in 13 cases of ovarian carcinoma by Triller and colleagues.[81] These are seen as rounded or oval low-density lesions between the liver capsule and the liver parenchyma, generally of 0.5–1 cm diameter and infrequently approaching 8 cm (Figs. 3–111 and 3–112). They are characteristically located in the dorsomedial and dorsolateral parts of the right liver lobe and may be associated with peritoneal metastases in Morison's pouch. Presumably cancer cells implanted on the liver surface infiltrate the capsule as well as the liver parenchyma and develop at these sites as subcapsular metastates.[60,81] The lesion may regress after chemotherapy.

## Seeded Metastases on the Greater Omentum

In disseminated carcinomatosis, most commonly from ovarian carcinoma, seeded metastases on the greater omentum may be readily evident by computed tomography. The lesions range from discrete linear and nodular densities to thick, solid omental masses described as "caking"[90,91] (Fig. 3–113). A densely calcified omental cake secondary to a metastatic serous cystadenocarcinoma of the ovary rich in psammoma bodies has been reported.[87]

## Multiple Sites

Multiple sites of seeded deposition are somewhat more common than a solitary focus. They may be appreciated on a barium enema study with reflux into the terminal ileum or in a subsequent small bowel series. Seeding in other disparate sites may be related to adhesions from previous inflammation or abdominal operations.

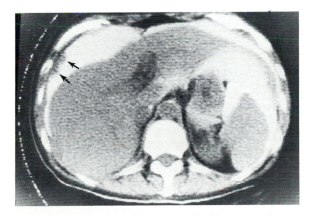

**Fig. 3–114. Peritoneal seeded metastases.** Computed tomography after intraperitoneal infusion of contrast medium demonstrates filling defects in right upper quadrant (arrows) representing studding of peritoneal surface from metastases. (Reproduced from Dunnick NR, et al[93])

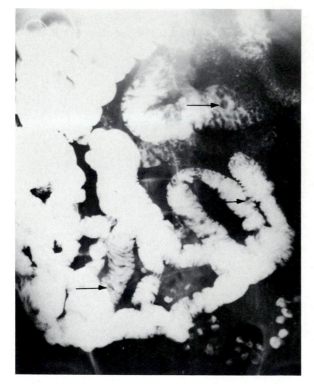

**Fig. 3–115. Metastatic melanoma to small bowel.** Multiple, small, almost uniform submucosal nodular masses are scattered throughout the entire small bowel. Some lesions are indicated by arrows. (Reproduced from Oddson TA, et al[98])

Computed tomography may clearly demonstrate localized or diffuse involvement of the peritoneum and its reflections and recesses.[5,82,91,92] Supplementing computed tomography with positive-contrast peritoneography[39,93–95] may further enhance the demonstration of small peritoneal implants (Fig. 3–114).

## Embolic Metastases

The most common primary neoplasms that embolize to bowel include melanoma and tumors

of the breast and lung. The presenting picture is usually one of incomplete obstruction or bleeding, often occurring several years after treatment of the original neoplasm. At times, the symptoms of the bowel metastases may be the first clinical manifestation of an occult primary malignancy.[7,8,96,97] Partial or complete obstruction is the result of the bulk of the metastatic mass, accompanied by either angulation of the bowel from a fibrotic response or intussusception. The appearance of a hematogenous metastasis to bowel depends on the characteristics of the lesions.[1] These include both the degree of vascularity relative to the rate of growth and the desmoplastic capabilities.

## Metastatic Melanoma

Metastatic melanoma is by far the most common of these tumors to be encountered clinically, and it may be taken as a particular prototype. The hematogenous deposition is usually in the submucosal layer where they may be seen early as small mural nodules (Fig. 3–115), and growth typically results in polypoid masses with a bulky extension into the lumen.[7,8,98] There is no significant desmoplastic response. Central ulceration is especially common as the metastasis outgrows its blood supply. In smaller lesions, this may be identified as a "bull's eye" or "target" lesion (Fig. 3–116), in which characteristically the borders of the filling defect are well defined and the ulcer is quite large in proportion to the metastatic mass (Fig. 3–117). Linear fissures over the surface of the mass, radiating distinctly to the central collection, produce a "spokewheel" pattern[1,98] (Fig. 3–118). In the larger lesions, necrosis may be reflected as a large excavating lesion yielding an appearance of aneurysmal dilatation[98–100] (Figs. 3–119 through 3–122). Intussusception may be associated with the larger polypoid masses[98] (Fig. 3–121).

Dissemination may be single (Fig. 3–123) but is more often multiple. Although metastatic

⟶

**Fig. 3–117. Metastatic melanoma to duodenal bulb.**
**(a)** A filling defect with sharply demarcated borders contains a proportionately large ulcer crater. These features are helpful in identifying this lesion as a submucosal nodule with secondary central ulceration, in contrast to a benign peptic ulcer with surrounding edema, the borders of which usually fade away gradually.
**(b)** Gross specimen demonstrates prominent submucosal mass (arrows) with central ulceration (arrowheads). Pathologically, this type of hematogenous metastasis is described as a "buttercup" lesion.
(From Meyers and McSweeney[1])

**Fig. 3–116. Metastatic melanoma to stomach.**
The multiple, centrally ulcerated submucosal lesions are seen en face and tangentially along the curvatures as *bull's-eye* lesions. (From Meyers and McSweeney[1])

▷

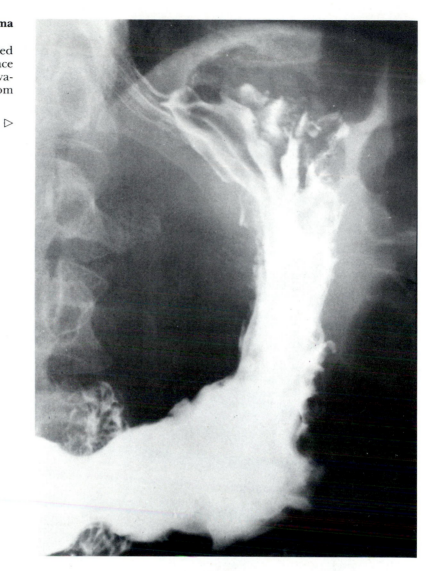

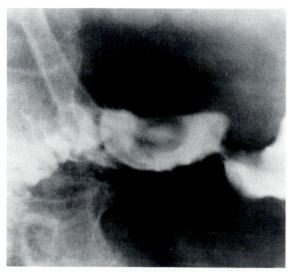

a

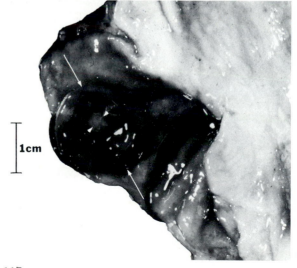

1cm

b

Fig. 3-117

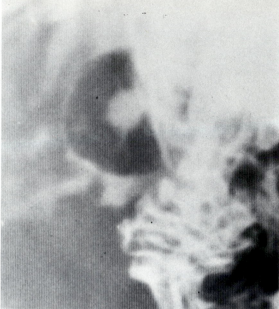

a

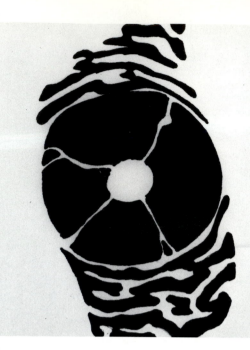

b

△

**Fig. 3–118. Metastatic melanoma to stomach.**
**(a)** On the greater curvature, there is a centrally ulcerated submucosal mass. Radiating linear fissure ulcerations result in a distinctive "spokewheel" configuration.
**(b)** Diagramatic representation of **(a)**.
(From Meyers and McSweeney[1])

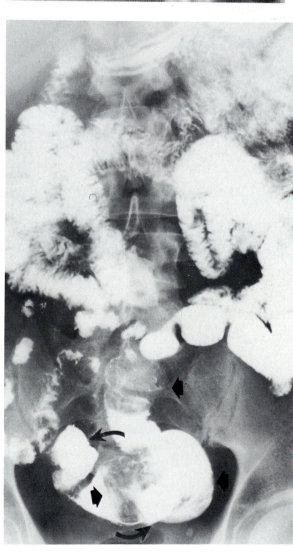

**Fig. 3–119. Metastatic melanoma to small bowel.**
Several bulky polypoid masses involve the mid-small
bowel (black arrows). Some have undergone large ulcerations (curved arrows). (Reproduced from Oddson TA, et al[98])

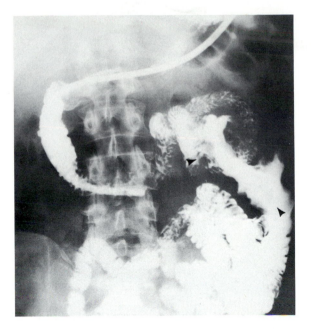

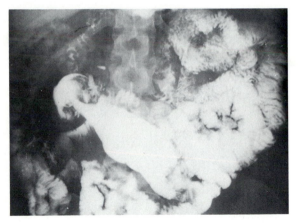

**Fig. 3–121. Metastatic melanoma to small bowel.**
A huge cavitating mass with intussusception is present in the ileum. (Reproduced from Oddson TA, et al[98])

**Fig. 3–120. Metastatic melanoma to small bowel.**
A large cavitating mass is present in the proximal jejunum (arrowheads). (Reproduced from Oddson TA, et al[98])

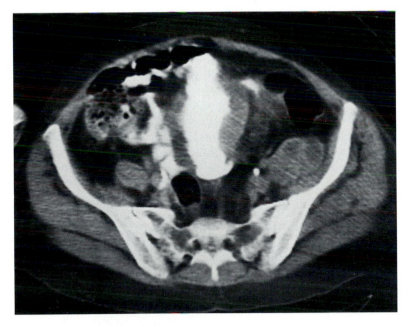

**Fig. 3–122. Metastatic melanoma to small bowel.**
Computed tomography demonstrates aneurysmal dilatation with submucosal masses, a widened lumen, and grossly ulcerated mucosa. Enlarged iliac nodes are also present.

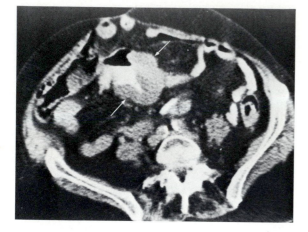

**Fig. 3–123. Metastatic melanoma to small bowel.**
Computed tomography demonstrates an ulcerated
submucosal mass involving an opacified mid-small
bowel loop (arrows).

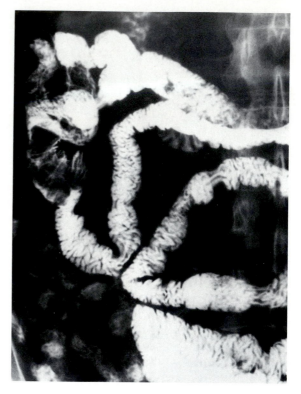

**Fig. 3–125. Metastatic melanoma to small bowel.**
Multiple submucosal masses of approximately equal
size confined to one segment of small bowel indicate
embolic metastases within a discrete arterial distribution.

melanomas may involve any portion of the alimentary tract, they tend to be more numerous
and more frequent in the small bowel. In an
autopsy series of 1000 cases, secondary small
bowel involvement was found in 58%.[101] When
multiple, they may be either widespread (Figs.
3–115 and 3–124) or confined to a segment of
intestine (Fig. 3–125). This reflects their mode
and periodicity of vascular distribution.[1] Diffuse
metastases are infrequently of different sizes
(Figs. 3–124), indicating periodic embolic
showers. At times, the secondary deposits are
present within the field of a specific arterial distribution when, typically, the nodules are of approximately the same size (Figs. 3–125 and 3–
126). A further observation which is useful in

identifying such submucosal masses as embolic
metastases relates to their specific sites on the
bowel wall.[1] When the lesion is localized to one
wall of the bowel, a distinct predilection is
shown for the antimesenteric border. In the

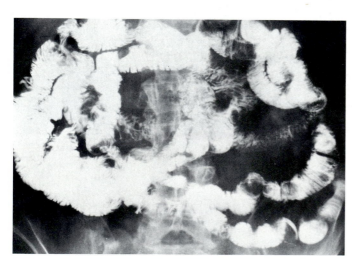

**Fig. 3–124. Metastatic melanoma to small
bowel.**
Numerous submucosal masses are scattered throughout the small intestine. Their
varying sizes indicate probable embolic
metastatic showers at different times.
(From Meyers and McSweeney[1])

**Fig. 3–126. Metastatic melanoma to the ascending colon.**
Its embolic nature is revealed by the two large submucosal masses of approximately equal size on the antimesenteric border in the field of distribution of the right colic artery. (From Meyers and McSweeney[1])

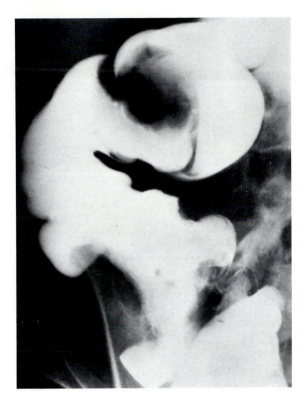

small intestine, this is readily identified as the convex margin of the loop (Fig. 3–127), since the mesentery supports the concave surface. In the ascending and descending colon, the lateral borders constitute the antimesenteric margins (Fig. 3–126). These findings are apparently related to the entrance of the intestinal vessels on the mesenteric border and their intramural ramifications toward the antimesenteric side. They are in agreement with Coman's experimental work, which revealed that strictly mechanical and circulatory factors can account for the distribution of some secondary tumors.[102]

A patient with melanoma with small bowel involvement, a stage III designation, now has available surgical treatment complemented by adjuvant therapy and immunotherapy, with an improved survival rate.[103]

## Breast Metastases

Breast metastases to the gastrointestinal tract result in a different pattern. Autopsy series record an incidence of breast metastases to the gastrointestinal tract as high as 8.2%[104] to 16.4%.[96] The need for surgical intervention for an abdominal complication of the metastasis is not uncommon.[97] Asch and associates[96] collected a group of 18 cases of metastatic breast lesions requiring surgery, often many years after a mastectomy.

The type that gives rise to gastrointestinal metastases and symptoms most often is the poorly differentiated breast cancer that grows in rows of small anaplastic cells.[104] No significant desmoplastic response accompanies the highly cellular secondary deposits. Although all layers of the bowel wall may be diffusely infiltrated, most of the embolic deposits reside in the submucosa,[97] where they are more readily subject to radiologic identification.

While widespread peritoneal metastases may be present, a linitis plastica appearance often dominates the radiologic findings, commonly in the stomach[1,105,106] (Fig. 3–128). Although no desmoplastic response is elicited by breast metastases, the highly cellular submucosal deposits may narrow and deform the lumen, presenting a scirrhous appearance. Rigidity and thickening with markedly diminished or absent peristalsis are associated with spiculation and angulation of the folds. Pseudoulcerations are

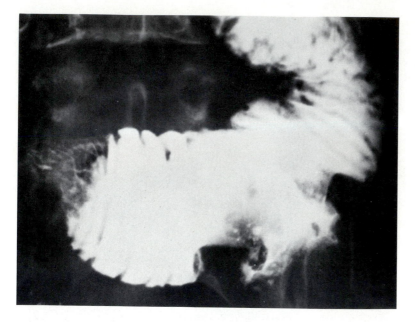

**Fig. 3–127. Metastatic melanoma to small bowel.**
There is a nonobstructing submucosal mass with a large ulcerated excavation in a distal jejunal loop. The hematogenous metastasis is distinctly localized to the antimesenteric border of the loop. (From Meyers and McSweeney[1])

produced by buckling or redundancy of the mucosa. The changes may be diffuse or localized but are more common and prominent in the distal two-thirds of the stomach. Despite the occasional severe circumferential narrowing of the antrum, some degree of luminal patency is maintained so that gastric outlet obstruction is not a characteristic feature. The linitis plastica appearance produced is indistinguishable from that of a primary scirrhous carcinoma or lymphoma. Osteoblastic metastases, however, are frequently present[1,107] (Fig. 3–128a). Secondary ulceration may be encountered as a prominent feature (Fig. 3–129).

Breast metastases to the small bowel may result in alternating areas of narrowing with interval dilatations (Fig. 3–130).

Carcinoma of the breast is the most common source of hematogenous spread to the colon. In a series of 337 autopsies in patients with breast carcinoma, Asch and associates[96] observed metastases to the colon in 4.5%. Of a group of 75 patients with advanced breast carcinoma who had laparotomy or autopsy, Graham[97] noted that 16% demonstrated colonic metastases. These may present clinically many years after a radical mastectomy.[19] The spread to the large intestine may be easily mistaken for primary inflammatory processes, such as granulomatous or ulcerative colitis, both clinically and radiologically.[19] Diarrhea may be a conspicuous clinical presentation, occasionally of several years' dura-

tion, and perhaps associated with some blood and mucus. Characteristic radiologic findings (Figs. 3–131 through 3–136) include mucosal thickening, nodular masses, multiple and eccentric strictures, asymmetric involvement, pseudosacculations, spiculations of contour, and frequent associated terminal ileal involvement.[19] The findings may be limited to the right colon (Figs. 3–131 and 3–132), diffuse (Figs. 3–133 through 3–135), or rarely confined to the rectum (Fig. 3–136). It is apparent that these changes share many common features with inflammatory colitis, particularly Crohn's disease. Deep biopsy and cytologic analysis of any ascitic fluid may be confirmatory.

## Bronchogenic Carcinoma

Metastatic involvement of the large intestine by bronchogenic carcinoma is rare.[108] Luomanen and Watson[109] report that of 676 patients who died of lung cancer, only 2.2% revealed metastases to the colon at autopsy. These were often small, serosal deposits. Metastases may infrequently be seen as mural rigidity or annular narrowing[110] (Figs. 3–137 and 3–138). Occasionally, they result in large mesenteric masses with infiltration of the bowel wall and fixation and angulation of the bowel and its mucosal folds (Figs. 3–139 and 140). In such cases, the findings are indistinguishable from those in widespread intraabdominal metastases from other

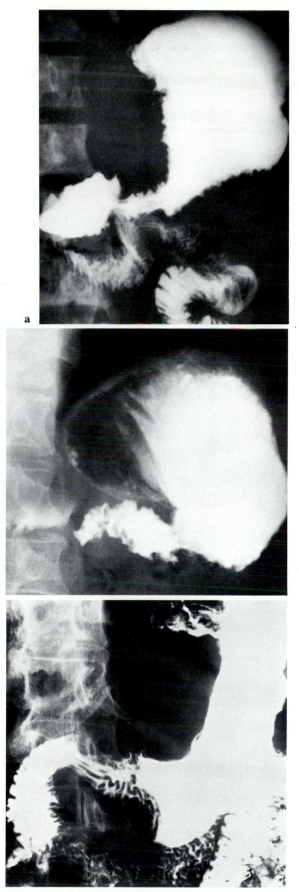

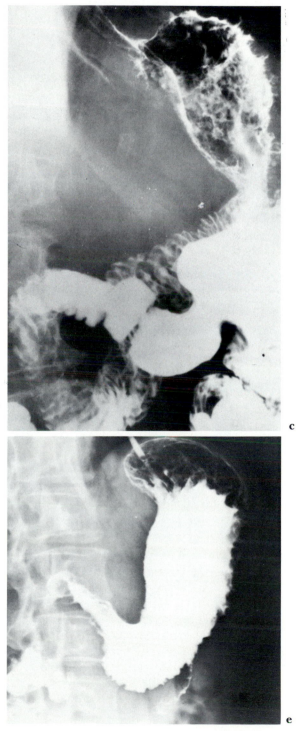

**Fig. 3–128. Different cases of breast metastases to stomach.**
These are characterized by rigidity and narrowing with markedly decreased peristalsis and fixation, spiculation, and angulation of folds. Although any portion of the stomach may be involved, the changes are more common and prominent in the distal two-thirds. The findings are indistinguishable from those of a primary linitis plastica. Note, however, the osteoblastic metastases in (a). (a and b from Meyers and McSweeney[1])

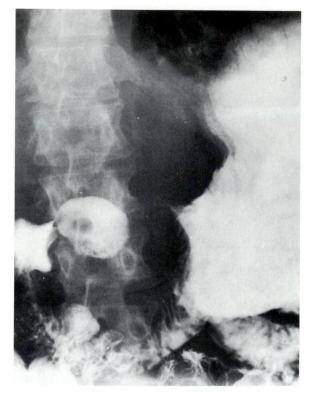

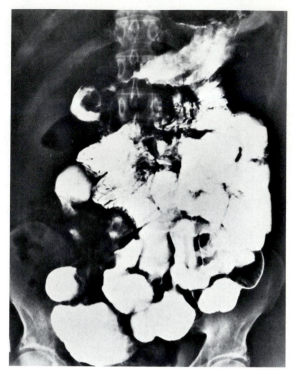

**Fig. 3–130. Metastatic breast carcinoma to small bowel.**
There are multiple skip areas of strictures with intervening dilatation. Diffuse submucosal metastases are also present within the stomach. (From Meyers et al[19])

**Fig. 3–129. Breast metastasis to stomach.**
A large submucosal mass in the distal stomach and antrum has undergone prominent ulceration.

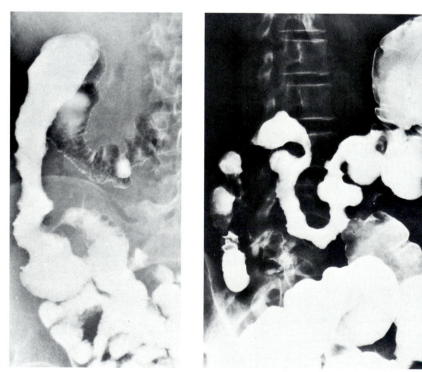

3-131

3-132

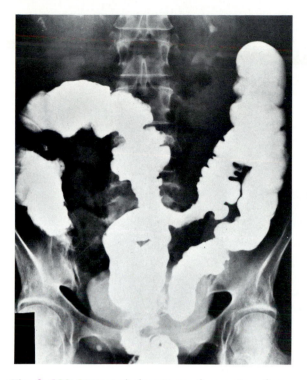

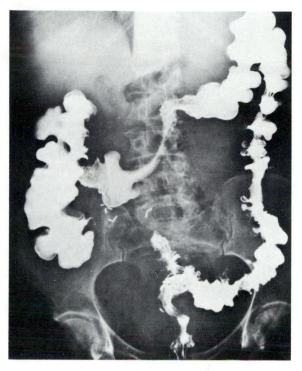

**Fig. 3–133. Metastatic breast carcinoma to colon.**
Skip areas of narrowing with localized loss of haustral and mucosal pattern involving the ascending, transverse, sigmoid, and rectosigmoid colon. Pseudosacculations reflect the asymmetric nature of the process. Deep transverse ulcers appear to project from the narrowed segment in the transverse colon. (From Meyers et al[19])

**Fig. 3–134. Metastatic breast carcinoma to colon.**
The entire large intestine is involved by multiple sites of narrowing and rigidity, with pseudosacculations.

---

**Fig. 3–131. Metastatic breast carcinoma to right colon.**
The entire ascending colon is encased by densely cellular submucosal secondary deposits. It is diffusely and irregularly narrowed, the mucosal and haustral patterns are effaced, and occasional nodular filling defects and serrations resembling minute ulcers are present. The ileocecal valve is widely patulous. The lesion strikingly resembles granulomatous colitis. (From Meyers et al[19])

**Fig. 3–132. Metastatic breast carcinoma to right colon.**
The ascending and proximal transverse colon show asymmetric narrowing, scattered pseudosaccular formation, loss of the normal haustral and mucosal pattern, and the appearance of marginal ulcerations. The terminal ileum is also involved. (From Meyers et al[19])

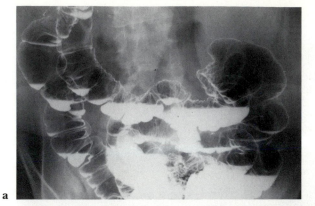

a

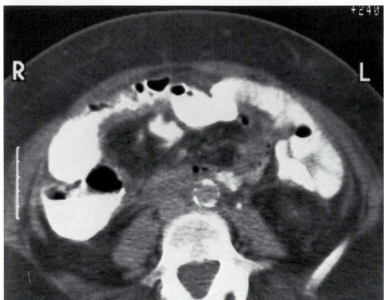

b

**Fig. 3–135. Metastatic breast carcinoma to colon.**
**(a)** Barium enema shows narrowing, angulation, fixation, and buckling of the mucosa in the transverse colon.
**(b)** Computed tomography documents mural thickening with luminal narrowing and mucosal spiculations.
(Courtesy of Michiel Feldberg, MD, University of Utrecht, The Netherlands)

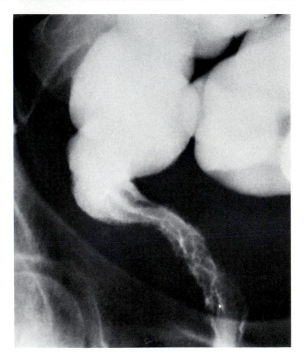

◁

**Fig. 3–136. Metastatic breast carcinoma to rectum.** There is narrowing of the rectum with nodularity and distortion of the mucosal folds and the appearance of multiple cobblestone ulcerations. There is a gradual transition to normal, distended sigmoid segment. (From Meyers et al[19])

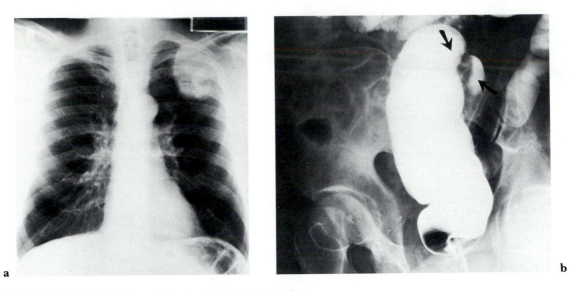

a                                                                                    b

**Fig. 3–137. Metastatic bronchogenic carcinoma to colon.**
**(a)** Chest film shows peripheral left upper lobe squamous cell carcinoma with pleural extension and partial excavation.
**(b)** Barium enema study shows metastatic annular narrowing in the sigmoid colon (arrows).
(Reproduced from Smith HJ, Vlasak, MG[110])

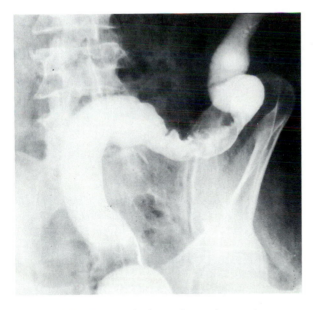

**Fig. 3–138. Metastatic bronchogenic carcinoma to colon.**
Submucosal deposition results in an eccentrically narrowed segment of the sigmoid colon. (From Smith HJ, Vlasak MG[110])

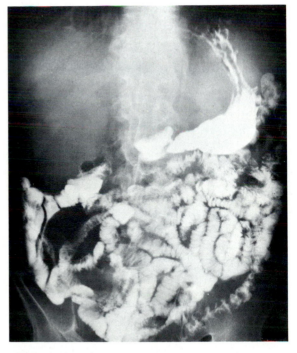

**Fig. 3–139. Metastatic lung carcinoma.**
Large mesenteric and serosal mass displaces distal small bowel and right colon.

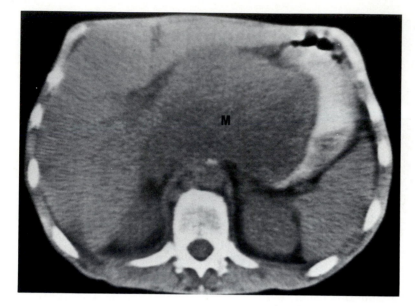

**Fig. 3–140. Metastatic lung carcinoma.**
Computed tomography demonstrates a large mass (M) of metastatic lymph nodes in the gastrohepatic ligament separating and deforming the liver and stomach.

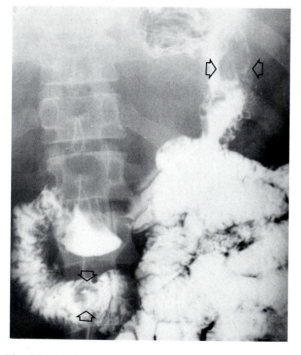

**Fig. 3–141. Hematogenous metastases of carcinoma of lung to stomach and third portion of the duodenum** (arrows).
The duodenal metastasis shows irregular central ulceration. (From Meyers and McSweeney[1])

sources. Rarely, central ulceration may be seen in the submucosal deposits (Fig. 3–141), which may lead to perforation.[108]

## Renal Carcinoma

Hematogenous metastasis to bowel from a renal carcinoma is rare. In some cases, Batson's vertebral venous plexus is a possible route.[111] It typically presents as a solitary bulky intramural lesion.[57]

## References

1. Meyers MA, McSweeney J: Secondary neoplasms of the bowel. Radiology 105: 1–11, 1972
2. Willis RA: The Spread of Tumours in the Human Body. Second edition. Butterworth and Co, London, 1952
3. Meyers MA: Distribution of intra-abdominal malignant seeding: Dependency on dynamics of flow of ascitic fluid. AJR 119: 198–206, 1973
4. Meyers MA: Metastatic seeding along small bowel mesentery: Roentgen features. AJR 123: 67–73, 1975
5. Meyers MA: Intraperitoneal spread of malignancies and its effect on the bowel. Second Annual Leeds Lecture. Clin Radiol 32: 129–146, 1981
6. Meyers MA, Whalen JP: Roentgen significance of the duodenocolic relationships: An anatomic approach. AJR 117: 263–274, 1973
7. De Castro CA, Dockerty MB, Mayo CW: Meta-

static tumors of the small intestines. Int Abstr Surg 105: 159–165, 1957

8. Farmer RG, Hawk WA: Metastatic tumors of the small bowel. Gastroenterology 47: 496–504, 1964

9. Meyers MA, Oliphant M, Berne AS, et al: The peritoneal ligaments and mesenteries: Pathways of intra-abdominal spread of disease. Annual Oration. Radiology. 163: 593–604, 1987

10. Oliphant M, Berne A, Meyers MA: Subperitoneal spread of intraabdominal disease. *In* Computed Tomography of the Gastrointestinal Tract Including the Peritoneal Cavity and Mesentery. Edited by MA Meyers. Springer-Verlag, New York, 1986, pp 95–137

11. Oliphant M, Berne AS: Computed tomography of the subperitoneal space: Demonstration of direct spread of intraabdominal disease. J Comp Assist Tomogr 6(6): 1127–1137, 1982

12. Balfe DM, Mauro MA, Koehler RE, et al: Gastrohepatic ligament: Normal and pathologic CT anatomy. Radiology 150: 485–490, 1984

13. Weinstein JB, Heiken JP, Lee JKT, et al: High resolution CT of the porta hepatis and hepatoduodenal ligament. Radiographics 6(1): 55–73, 1986

14. Dehn CB, Reznek RH, Nockler B, et al: The preoperative assessment of advanced gastric cancer by computed tomography. Br J Surg 71: 413–417, 1984

15. Vaittinen F: Carcinoma of the gallbladder: A study of 390 cases diagnosed in Finland 1953–1967. Ann Chir Gynecol Fenn 29(Suppl 168): 7, 1970

16. Meyers MA, Volberg F, Katzen B, et al: Haustral anatomy and pathology: A new look. I. Roentgen identification of normal pattern and relationships. Radiology 108: 497–504, 1973

17. Meyers MA, Volberg F, Katzen B, et al: Haustral anatomy and pathology: A new look. II. Roentgen interpretation of pathologic alterations. Radiology 108: 505–512, 1973

18. Kajitan T, Kyuno K, Nishi M: Pathology of gastric cancer. Gendaig 35B: 19–81. Nakayamashoten, Tokyo, 1974

19. Meyers MA, Oliphant M, Teixidor H, et al: Metastatic carcinoma simulating inflammatory colitis. AJR 123: 67–83, 1975

20. Rubesin SE, Levine MS: Omental cakes: Colonic involvement by omental metastases. Radiology 154: 593–596, 1985

21. Rubesin SE, Levine MS, Glick SN: Gastric involvement by omental cakes: Radiographic findings. Gastrointest Radiol 11: 223–228, 1986

22. Meyers MA: Roentgen significance of the phrenicocolic ligament. Radiology 95: 539–545, 1970

23. Bachman AL: Roentgen appearance of gastric invasion from carcinoma of the colon. Radiology 63: 814–822, 1954

24. Lee KR, Levine E, Moffat RE, et al: Computed tomographic staging of malignant gastric neoplasms. Radiology 133: 151–155, 1979

25. Moss AA, Schnyder P, Marks W, et al: Gastric adenocarcinoma: A comparison of the accuracy and economics of staging by computed tomography and surgery. Gastroenterology 80: 45–50, 1981

26. Kiyota YK, Mukai H, et al: Endoscopic ultrasonography (EUS) in the diagnosis of upper digestive tract diseases. Determination of the depth of cancer invasion. Gastroenterol Endosc 28: 253–263, 1986

27. Komaki S: Gastric carcinoma. *In* Computed Tomography of the Gastrointestinal Tract: Including the Peritoneal Cavity and Mesentery. Edited by MA Meyers. Springer-Verlag, New York, Tokyo, 1986, pp 23–54

28. Machi J, Takeda J, Sigel B, et al: Normal stomach wall and gastric cancer: Evaluation with high-resolution operative US. Radiology 159: 85–87, 1986

29. Meyers MA, Evans JA: Effects of pancreatitis on the small bowel and colon: Spread along mesenteric planes. AJR 119: 151–165, 1973

30. Treitel H, Meyers MA, Maza V: Changes in the duodenal loop secondary to carcinoma of the hepatic flexure of the colon. Br J Radiol 43: 209–213, 1970

31. Krestin GP, Beyer D, Lorenz R: Secondary involvement of the transverse colon by tumors of the pelvis: Spread of malignancies along the greater omentum. Gastrointest Radiol 10: 283–288, 1985

32. Vieta JO, Blanco R, Valentini GR: Malignant duodenocolic fistula: Report of two cases, each with one or more synchronous gastrointestinal cancers. Dis Colon Rectum 19: 542–552, 1976

33. Diamond RT, Greenberg HM, Boult IF: Direct metastatic spread of right colonic adenocarcinoma to duodenum: Barium and computed tomographic findings. Gastrointest Radiol 6: 339–341, 1981

34. McCort JJ: Roentgenographic appearance of metastases to central lymph nodes of superior mesenteric artery in carcinoma of right colon. Radiology 60: 641–646, 1953

35. Schabel SI, Rogers CI, Rittenberg GM: Duodeno-duodenal fistula—A manifestation of carcinoma of the colon. Gastrointest Radiol 3: 15–17, 1978

36. Jeffrey RB, Federle MP, Goodman PC: Computed tomography of the lesser peritoneal sac. AJR 144: 567–575, 1985

37. Dodds WJ, Foley WD, Lawson TL, et al: Pictorial Essay. Anatomy and Imaging of the Lesser Peritoneal Sac. AJR 144: 567–575, 1985

38. Chun CH, Raff MF, Conteras L, et al: Splenic abscess. Medicine (Baltimore) 59: 50–65, 1980

39. Meyers MA: Peritoneography: Normal and pathologic anatomy. AJR 117: 353–365, 1973

40. Meyers MA: Clinical involvement of mesenteric and anti-mesenteric borders of small bowel. I. Normal pattern and relationships. Gastrointest Radiol 1(1): 41–48, 1976

41. Meyers MA: Clinical involvement of mesenteric and anti-mesenteric borders of small bowel. II. Radiologic interpretation of pathologic alterations. Gastrointest Radiol 1(1): 49–58, 1976

42. Whitley NO, Bohlman ME, Baker LP: CT patterns of mesenteric disease. J Comp Assist Tomogr 6(3): 490–496, 1982

43. Whitley NO: Mesenteric disease. *In* Computed Tomography of the Gastrointestinal Tract Including the Peritoneal Cavity and Mesentery. Edited by MA Meyers. Springer-Verlag, New York, 1986, pp 139–178

44. Mueller PR, Ferrucci JT, Harbin WP, et al: Appearance of lymphomatous involvement of the mesentery by ultrasonography and body computed tomography: The "sandwich sign." Radiology 134: 467–473, 1980

45. Grinnel RS: Lymphatic block with atypical and retrograde lymphatic metastasis and spread in carcinoma of the colon and rectum. Ann Surg 163: 272–280, 1966

46. Moffat RE, Gourley WK: Ileal lymphatic metastases from cecal carcinoma. Radiology 135: 55–58, 1980

47. Perez C, Cacares J, Valls J: Carcinoma of the hepatic flexure with proximal lymphatic invasion mimicking Crohn's disease. Gastrointest Radiol 9: 365–367, 1984

48. Threefoot SA: Gross and microscopic anatomy of the lymphatic vessels and lymphaticovenous communications. Cancer Chemother Rep 52: 1–20, 1968

49. Pressman J, Dunn RF, Burtz M: Lymph node ultrastructure related to direct lymphaticovenous communication. Surg Gynecol Obstet 124: 963–973, 1967

50. Correia JP, Baptista AS, Antonio JF: Slowly evolving widespread diffuse alimentary tract carcinoma (linitis plastica). Gut 9: 485–488, 1968

51. Khilnani MT, Marshak RH, Eliasoph J, et al: Roentgen features of metastases to the colon. AJR 96: 302–310, 1966

52. Wigh R, Tapley Ndu V: Metastatic lesions to the large intestine. Radiology 70: 222–228, 1958

53. Gengler L, Baer J, Finby N: Rectal and sigmoid involvement secondary to carcinoma of the prostate. AJR 125: 910–917, 1975

54. Winter CC: The problem of rectal involvement by prostatic cancer. Surg Gynecol Obstet 105: 136–140, 1957

55. Young HH: The cure of cancer of the prostate by radical perineal prostatectomy (prostato-seminal vesiculectomy). History, literature, and statistics of Young's operation. J Urol 53: 188–252, 1945

56. Kradjian RM, Bennington JL: Renal carcinoma recurrent 31 years after nephrectomy. Arch Surg 90: 192–195, 1965

57. Khilnani MT, Wolf BS: Late involvement of the alimentary tract by carcinoma of the kidney. Am J Dig Dis 5: 529–540, 1960

58. Shoemaker CP, Hoyle CL, Levine SB, et al: Late solitary recurrence of renal carcinoma. Am J Surg 120: 99–100, 1970

59. Meyers MA: The spread and localization of acute intraperitoneal effusions. Radiology 95: 547–554, 1970

60. Sampson JA: Implantation peritoneal carcinomatosis of ovarian origin. Am J Pathol 7: 423–443, 1931

61. Buie LA, Jackman RJ, Vickers PM: Extrarectal masses caused by tumors of the recto-uterine or rectovesical space. JAMA 117: 167–169, 1941

62. Raiford TS: Tumors of small intestine. Arch Surg 25: 321–355, 1932

63. Walther HE: Krebsmetastasen, Benno Schwabe, Basel, 1948

64. Hultborn KA, Morales O, Romanus R: The so-called shelf tumour of the rectum. Acta Radiol Suppl 124: 1955

65. Theander G, Wehlin L, Langeland P: Deformation of the rectosigmoid junction in peritoneal carcinomatosis. Acta Radiol Diagn 1: 1071–1076, 1963

66. Blumer G: Rectal shelf: Neglected rectal sign of value in diagnosis of obscure malignant and inflammatory disease within abdomen. Albany Med Ann 30: 361, 1909

67. Esenstein ML, Shaw SL, Pak HY, et al: CT demonstration of multiple intraperitoneal teratomatous implants. J Comp Assist Tomogr 7: 1117–1118, 1983

68. Feldman GB, Knapp RC: Lymphatic drainage of the peritoneal cavity and its significance in ovarian cancer. Am J Obstet Gynecol 119: 991–994, 1974

69. Simer PH: The drainage of particulate matter from the peritoneal cavity by lymphatics. Anat Rec 88: 175–192, 1944

70. Feldman GB, Knapp RC, Order SE: The role of lymphatic obstruction in the formation of ascites

in a murine ovarian carcinoma. Cancer Res 32: 1663–1666, 1972

71. Higgins GM, Graham AS: Lymphatic drainage from the peritoneal cavity in the dog. Arch Surg 19: 453–465, 1929

72. Bettendorf U: Lymph flow mechanism of the subperitoneal diaphragmatic lymphatics. Lymphology 11: 111–116, 1978

73. French GE, Florey HW, Morris BL: The absorption of particles by the lymphatics of the diaphragm. Q J Exp Biol 45: 88–103, 1960

74. Vock P, Hodler J: Cardiophrenic angle adenopathy: Update of causes and significance. Radiology 159: 395–399, 1986

75. Bergman F: Carcinoma of the ovary: A clinicopathological study of 86 autopsied cases with special reference to mode of spread. Acta Obstet Gynecol Scand 45: 211–231, 1966

76. Rosenoff SH, DeVita VT, Hubbard S, et al: Peritoneoscopy in staging and follow-up of ovarian cancer. Semin Oncol 2(3): 223–228, 1975

77. Dagnini G, Marin G, Caldironi MW, et al: Laparoscopy in staging, follow-up, and restaging of ovarian carcinoma. Gastrointest Endosc 33: 80–83, 1987

78. Ozols RF, Fisher RI, Anderson T, et al: Peritoneoscopy in the management of ovarian cancer. Am J Obstet Gynecol 140: 611–619, 1981

79. Piver MS, Barlow JJ, Lele SB: Incidence of subclinical metastasis in stage I and II ovarian carcinoma. Obstet Gynecol 52: 100–104, 1978

80. Young RC, Decker DG, Wharton JT, et al: Staging laparotomy in early ovarian cancer. JAMA 250(22): 3072–3076, 1983

81. Triller J, Goldnirsch A, Reinhard J-P: Subcapsular liver metastasis in ovarian cancer: Computed tomography and surgical staging. Europ J Radiol 5: 261–266, 1985

82. Jeffrey RB Jr: CT demonstration of peritoneal implants. Am J Roentgenol 135: 323–326, 1980

83. Kalovidouris A, Gouliamos A, Pontifex GR, et al: Computed tomography of ovarian carcinoma. Acta Radiol Diagn 25: 203–208, 1984

84. Seshul MB, Coulam CM: Pseudomyxoma peritonei: Computed tomography and sonography. AJR 136: 803–806, 1981

85. Miller DL, Udelsman R, Sugarbaker PH: Case report: Calcification of pseudomyxoma peritonei following intraperitoneal chemotherapy: CT demonstration. J Comp Assist Tomogr 9: 1123–1124, 1985

86. Mitchell DG, Hill MC, Hill S, et al: Serous carcinoma of the ovary: CT identification of metastatic calcified implants. Radiology 158: 649–652, 1986

87. Pandolfo I, Blandino A, Gaeta M, et al: Calcified peritoneal metastases from papillary cystadeno-

carcinoma of the ovary: CT features. J Comp Assist Tomogr 10(3): 545–546, 1986

88. Solomon A, Rubinstein Z: Importance of the falciform ligament, ligamentum teres, and splenic hilus in the spread of malignancy as demonstrated by computed tomography. Gastrointest Radiol 9: 53–56, 1984

89. Ferenczy A, Talens M, Zoghby M, et al: Ultrastructural studies on the morphogenesis of psammoma bodies in ovarian serous neoplasia. Cancer 39: 2451–2459, 1977

90. Cooper C, Jeffrey RB, Silverman PM, et al: Computed tomography of omental pathology. J Comp Assist Tomogr 10(1): 62–66, 1986

91. Levitt RG, Sagel SS, Stanley RJ: Detection of neoplastic involvement of the mesentery and omentum by computed tomography. AJR 131: 835–838, 1978

92. Meyers MA: Clinical report: A new view of the peritoneal cavity. Mod Med 44(6): 51–56, 1976

93. Dunnick NR, Jones RB, Doppman JL, et al: Intraperitoneal contrast infusion for assessment of intraperitoneal fluid dynamics. AJR 133: 221–223, 1979

94. Meyers MA: Peritoneography: Normal and pathologic anatomy. Chapter 3 in Dynamic Radiology of the Abdomen: Normal and Pathologic Anatomy. Springer-Verlag, New York, 1976.

95. Roub LW, Drayer BP, Orr DP, et al: Computed tomographic positive contrast peritoneography. Radiology 131: 699–704, 1979

96. Asch MJ, Wiedel PD, Habif DV: Gastrointestinal metastases from carcinoma of the breast: Autopsy study and 18 cases requiring operative intervention. Arch Surg 96: 840–843, 1968

97. Graham WP III: Gastrointestinal metastases from carcinoma of the breast. Ann Surg 159: 477–480, 1964

98. Oddson TA, Rice RP, Seiler HF, et al: The spectrum of small bowel melanoma. Gastrointest Radiol 3: 419–423, 1978

99. Goldstein HM, Beydoun MT, Dodd GD: Radiologic spectrum of melanoma metastatic to the gastrointestinal tract. AJR 129: 605–612, 1977

100. Smith SJ, Carlson HC, Gisvold JJ: Secondary neoplasms of the small bowel. Radiology 125: 29–33, 1977

101. Das Gupta T, Brasfield R: Metastatic melanoma: Clinico-pathologic study, Cancer 17: 1323–1339, 1969

102. Coman DR, De Long KP, McCutcheon M: Studies on the mechanism of metastasis: The distribution of tumors in various organs in relation to the distribution of arterial emboli. Cancer Res 11: 648–651, 1951

103. Einhorn LH, Burgess MA, Vallejos C, et al: Prognostic correlations and response to treatment in advanced metastatic malignant melanoma. Cancer Res 34: 1995–2004, 1974

104. Choi SH, Sheehan FR, Pickren JW: Metastatic involvement of the stomach by breast cancer. Cancer 17: 791–797, 1964

105. Eker R, Efskind J: Investigations on the intramural spread of gastric carcinoma. Acta Path Microbiol Scand 30: 371–383, 1952

106. Cormier JC, Gaffey TA, Welch JM, et al: Linitis plastica caused by metastatic lobular carcinoma of the breast. Mayo Clin Proc 55: 747–753, 1980

107. Joffe N: Metastatic involvement of the stomach secondary to breast carcinoma. AJR 123: 512–521, 1975

108. Antler AS, Ough Y, Pitchumoni CS, et al: Gastrointestinal metastases from malignant tumors of the lung. Cancer 49: 170–172, 1982

109. Luomanen RKJ, Watson WL: Autopsy findings. Lung Cancer: A Study of Five Thousand Memorial Hospital Cases, Chapter 20. Edited by WL Watson. CV Mosby, St. Louis, Mo. 1968

110. Smith HJ, Vlasak MG: Metastasis to the colon from bronchogenic carcinoma. Gastrointest Radiol 2: 393–396, 1977

111. Hayes HT, Burr HB: Hypernephroma of the sigmoid colon. Am J Surg 81: 98–100, 1951

# 4 The Extraperitoneal Spaces: Normal and Pathologic Anatomy

## General Introduction

The extraperitoneal portion of the abdomen has always been considered a difficult region in terms of anatomic definitions, clinical evaluation, and radiologic diagnosis. Anatomically, it has been vaguely considered as occupying the posterior half of the abdomen, without well-defined fascial boundaries. Clinically, it is commonly recognized that extraperitoneal effusions are difficult to diagnose. The area is not accessible to the bedside modalities of auscultation, palpation, or percussion. Symptoms and signs may be obscure, delayed, nonspecific, or misleading.

Extraperitoneal tissues do not react as acutely and severely to bacterial contamination as does the peritoneal cavity.[1] Known amounts of bacteria introduced intraperitoneally result in acute peritonitis and dramatic constitutional signs. When introduced into the extraperitoneal tissues, however, they cause a more smoldering infection. This explains the prolonged duration of the symptoms of extraperitoneal abscess before operation or death, often as long as 2 months.[2]

Several reports emphasize the difficulties in clinically recognizing even severe extraperitoneal infection. Indeed, in large series, the diagnosis has been completely overlooked in 25–50% of the patients.[2,3] Unless diagnosed early and treated adequately, extraperitoneal abscess is associated with prolonged morbidity and high mortality.

*Extraperitoneal infection* is usually secondary, a complication of infection, injury, or malignancy in adjacent retroperitoneal or intraperitoneal organs. Only rarely is it a consequence of bacteremia or suppurative lymphadenitis.

The predominant symptoms of an extraperitoneal infection are chills, fever, abdominal or flank pain, nausea, vomiting, night sweats, and weight loss. The clinical course is usually insidious and the initial symptoms are so nonspecific that the correct diagnosis is usually not considered. Constitutional symptoms may be present for weeks to months before localizing signs develop. With pressure on the extraperitoneal nerves, pain may be referred to the groin, hip, thigh, or knee, with little or no complaint of abdominal or back pain. Urologic symptoms are rare, even with perirenal abscess.

A mass or swelling of the flank is palpable about 50% of the time[3] but only if it is large or localizes inferiorly below the costal margin. Almost all patients exhibit tenderness to palpation over the abscess. Scoliosis, psoas spasm, and a sinus tract may be other clinical signs. Although there is invariably leukocytosis, urinalysis may be normal, even in perirenal abscess.

Unusual complications of extraperitoneal abscess include rupture into the free peritoneal cavity and progressive dissection in the soft tissues. Spread may involve the anterior abdominal wall, subcutaneous tissues of the back or flank, subdiaphragmatic spaces, mediastinum, thoracic cavity, psoas muscle, thigh, or hip. A fistula may extend from the kidney into the extraperitoneal portion of the bowel or into a bronchus.

*Extraperitoneal blood* is usually caused by trauma, ruptured aneurysm, malignancy, bleeding diathesis, or overanticoagulation.

Extraperitoneal gas is most often the result of bowel perforation secondary to inflammatory or ulcerative disease, blunt or penetrating trauma, a foreign body, iatrogenic manipulation, or a gas-producing infection originating in extraperitoneal organs. The underlying condition may be chronic, occult, or only suspected clinically. Often it is not until the gas is recognized radiologically that attention is directed to or confirms the presence of an acute process in the abdomen. Extraperitoneal gas is seen as mottled lucencies within the tissues or as linear shadows tracking along fascial planes.

Radiologically, loss of visualization of the lateral margin of the psoas muscle has been considered the hallmark of extraperitoneal effusions. This sign, however, is unreliable since 25–44% of normal individuals show unequal visualization of the psoas borders.[4,5]

An editorial in *Lancet* has woefully highlighted the problem[6]:

> Many a clinical reputation lies buried behind the peritoneum. In this hinterland of straggling mesenchyme with . . . its shadowy fascial boundaries, the clinician is often left with only his flair and his diagnostic first principles to guide him.

It is essential to realize that this is no longer true. Rather, roentgen-anatomic studies by Meyers et al have clarified the fascial relationships that clearly demarcate the region into three distinct compartments.[7–12] Each has specific boundaries and relationships that can be recognized. Radiologic identification by retroperitoneal pneumography of the renal fascia enclosing the contents of the perirenal space was described by Meyers,[13] and the structure was subsequently noted on urography and nephrotomography[11,12,14–16] and then definitively on computed tomography.[7,17–19] The pathways of flow, preferential routes of spread from various sites, and margination of infection or other effusions within a particular extraperitoneal compartment are guided primarily by the fixed fascial planes and paths of least resistance. This information permits the recognition of the presence, extent, and localization of fluid and gas collections in the extraperitoneal tissues and often pinpoints the precise site of origin and nature of the fluid.

# Anatomic Considerations

Basic to an understanding of the clinical and radiologic criteria is precise knowledge of the anatomy of the extraperitoneal fascial planes, compartments, and relationships. Figure 4–1 shows that the retroperitoneal space is bounded anteriorly by the posterior parietal peritoneum and posteriorly by the transversalis fascia. It extends from the pelvic brim inferiorly to the diaphragm superiorly. The major organs and structures within it include (a) the adrenal glands, kidneys, and ureters; (b) the descending, transverse, and ascending portions of the duodenum, and the pancreas; (c) the great vessels and branches; and (d) the ascending and descending colon.

The anatomic sections further illustrate that the intraperitoneal structures do not simply occupy the anterior half of the abdomen and the extraperitoneal structures the posterior half. Rather, the extraperitoneal space is mildly C-shaped, with its convexity projecting anteriorly in the midline. This is a function of both the particular relationships of the abdominal organs and their accommodation to the lordotic curvature of the lumbar spine. In this way, segments of the extraperitoneal region (e.g., the body of the pancreas and the duodenal loop) lie considerably anterior to portions of intraperitoneal viscera (e.g., the spleen and posterior aspects of the liver).

## The Three Extraperitoneal Compartments and Perirenal Fasciae

More detailed evaluation shows that the extraperitoneal region, rather than being composed of amorphous "straggling mesenchyme," is distinctly demarcated by well-defined fascial planes. Figure 4–2a is an enlarged horizontal cross-section through the flank at the lower pole of the kidney. Central to the division of the extraperitoneal region are the conspicuous anterior and posterior layers of renal fascia. (The posterior renal fascia was first described by Zuckerkandl[20] and the anterior renal fascia subsequently by Gerota,[21] but the two layers have since been known collectively as Gerota's fascia.)

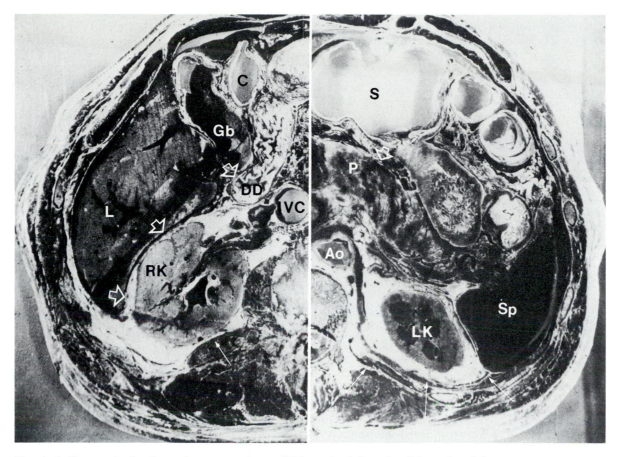

**Fig. 4–1. Composite horizontal cross-section at T11 on the left and at L2 on the right.**
The extraperitoneal region extends from the posterior parietal peritoneum in front (open arrows) to the transversalis fascia behind (long arrows). Within it are the right and left kidneys (RK and LK), descending duodenum (DD), pancreas (P), aorta (Ao), and inferior vena cava (IVC). SP = spleen, S = stomach, C = colon, Gb = gallbladder, L = liver. (From Meyers et al[12])

The renal fascia is a dense, collagenous, elastic connective tissue sheath that envelops the kidney and perirenal fat. Its two layers fuse behind the ascending or descending colon to form the single lateroconal fascia, which then continues around the flank to blend with the peritoneal reflection forming the paracolic gutter. Figure 4–2b illustrates these important fascial relationships by computed tomography. In this way, I have defined precisely three individual extraperitoneal compartments. Their major fascial marginations are illustrated in Figure 4–2c.

1. The *anterior pararenal space* extends from the posterior parietal peritoneum to the anterior renal fascia. Significantly, it is confined laterally by the lateroconal fascia.

2. The *perirenal space* encompasses the kidney and its investing fat. A conspicuous anatomic feature is the perirenal fat, which is most abundant behind and somewhat lateral to the lower pole of the kidney. This becomes of practical importance in the diagnosis of coalescent perirenal abscesses and hematomas.

3. The *posterior pararenal space* extends from the posterior renal fascia to the transversalis fascia. It consists of a thin layer of fat and its most notable feature is that it continues uninterruptedly external to the lateroconal fascia as the properitoneal fat of the abdominal wall (Fig. 4–3). It is important to recognize that it is the posterior pararenal fat, as it courses laterally external to the lateroconal fascia and deep to the transversalis fascia, that is radiologically visualized as the "flank stripe" (Figs. 4–4 and 4–5).

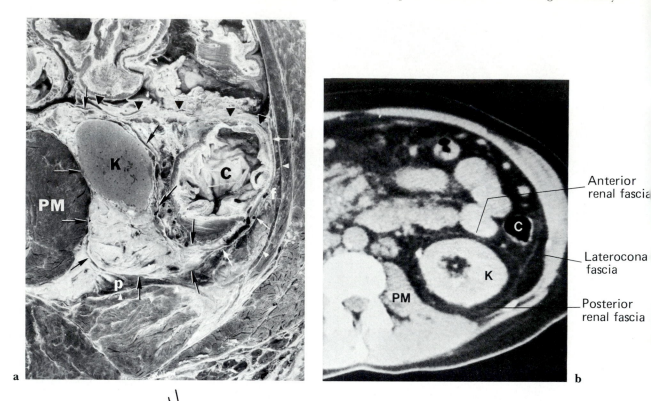

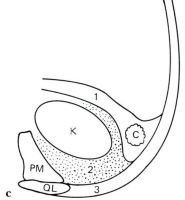

**Fig. 4–2. Extraperitoneal anatomy of the flank.**
**(a) Transverse cross-section.** The anterior and posterior renal fasciae (black arrows) envelop the kidney (K) and perirenal fat. From their line of fusion, the lateroconal fascia (white arrows) continues behind the descending colon (C) to the parietal peritoneum (black arrowheads). The posterior pararenal fat (p) is continuous with the flank fat (f) deep to the transversalis fascia (white arrowheads). PM = psoas muscle.
**(b) Computed tomography** demonstrates the anterior and posterior renal fasciae and the lateroconal fascia, which demarcate the extraperitoneal fat. Note their relationships to the kidney (K) and descending colon (C).
**(c) The three extraperitoneal spaces:** 1 = the anterior pararenal space, 2 = the perirenal space, 3 = the posterior pararenal space. QL = quadratus lumborum muscle.
(Modified from Meyers[9])

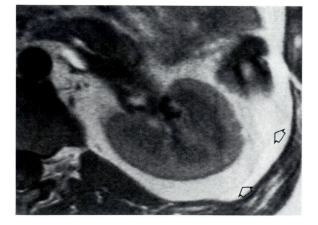

**Fig. 4–3. Posterior renal fascia seen by magnetic resonance imaging** (arrows) on transverse plane. Note that the perirenal and posterior pararenal fat have different signal intensities.

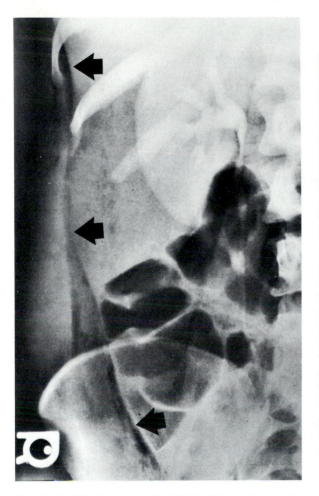

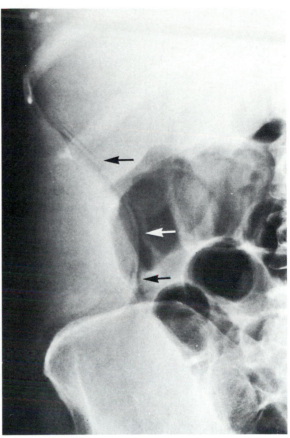

**Fig. 4–4. Flank stripe highlighted by air post-laparoscopy.**
Following laparoscopy, air inadvertently entering the anterior abdominal wall is seen as it courses around the flank extraperitoneally (arrows). Here, it lies deep to the transversalis fascia, within the flank extension of the posterior pararenal fat.

**Fig. 4–5. Flank hematoma.**
The blood is seen as a prominent soft-tissue mass displacing the intact flank stripe medially (arrows). These features localize the hematoma to be superficial to the transversalis fascia and therefore subcutaneous in position.

Figure 4–6a is a horizontal diagram illustrating the major relationships and components of the three extraperitoneal compartments.

The *anterior pararenal space* includes the ascending and descending colon, the duodenal loop, and the pancreas. In other words, the extraperitoneal portions of the alimentary tract reside within this compartment. While the space is potentially continuous across the midline, I have observed that collections of fluid or gas are generally confined to their side of origin. A notable exception includes pancreatic extravasations, probably for two reasons: (a) the pancreas itself straddles the midline and (b) liberated pancre-

atic enzymes, particularly trypsin, dissect the fascial planes and permit freer dissemination. Ventrally, the anterior pararenal space is anatomically continuous wth the roots of the small bowel mesentery and transverse mesocolon.[22]

The *perirenal spaces* generally have no continuity across the midline. Medially, the posterior fascial layer fuses with the psoas or quadratus lumborum fascia,[23] and the anterior renal fascia blends into the dense mass of connective tissue surrounding the great vessels in the root of the mesentery and behind the pancreas and duodenum[24] (Fig. 4–7). Originally, Gerota[21] claimed bilateral continuity of the perirenal compart-

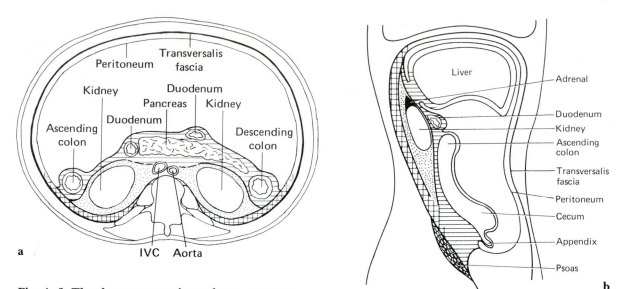

**Fig. 4–6. The three extraperitoneal compartments.**
Striped areas = anterior pararenal space, stippled areas = perirenal space, cross-hatched areas = posterior pararenal space. (From Meyers[8])

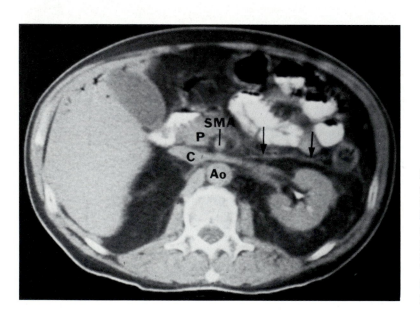

**Fig. 4–7. Midline termination of the anterior renal fascia.**
CT shows thickened anterior renal fascia (arrows) blending into tissues near the midline around the renal pedicle in relationship to the superior mesenteric artery (SMA). There is no evidence of continuity across the midline. Ao = aorta, P = pancreas, C = inferior vena cava.

ments deep to the anterior renal fasciae. A thin connecting pathway at the lower lumbar level has been thought to be observed by CT in one report.[24a] However, most precise dissections and injection experiments and meticulous CT observations have shown that the two perirenal spaces have no actual or potential direct communications.[8,9,12,17] At the level of the renal hilum, CT seems to confirm the work of Martin,[25] namely

that the anterior and posterior ipsilateral fasciae occasionally fuse and blend with the hilar vessels, preventing communications between both perirenal spaces across the midline[17] (Fig. 4–8).

The *posterior pararenal space* is demarcated on each side of the body by the fusion of the transversalis fascia medially with the muscle fascia. It is therefore limited by and parallels the margin of the psoas muscle. The space is open laterally

**Fig. 4–8. Medial fascial closure of the perirenal space.**
CT demonstrates accentuated renal fascial planes fusing medially around the renal pedicle (arrows). (Courtesy of Michiel Feldberg, MD, University of Utrecht, The Netherlands)

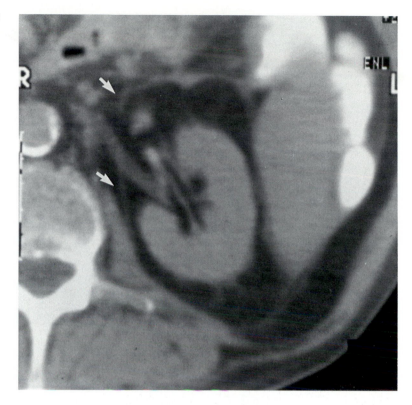

toward the flank and inferiorly toward the pelvis. Bilaterally they are potentially in communication only via the properitoneal fat of the anterior abdominal wall deep to the transversalis fascia. As opposed to the other two extraperitoneal spaces, the posterior pararenal spaces contain no organs.

Figure 4–6b is a sagittal view of a few more anatomic features that have particular diagnostic significance:

(a) the lines of fusion of the anterior and posterior renal fascial layers are unique and contribute distinctly to the spread and confinement of extraperitoneal effusions. The perirenal space on each side narrows as it extends inferiorly, resembling an inverted cone. (For this reason, the single layer of fascia extending laterally from the cone of renal fascia has been designated as the lateroconal fascia.) Inferiorly, the layers fuse weakly or blend with the iliac fascia; as they narrow medially, they also blend loosely with the periureteric connective tissue. Although the apex of the cone is open anatomically toward the iliac fossa, most infections are confined to the perirenal space by early inflam-

matory sealing of this potential outlet. Superiorly, the two layers are firmly fixed to each other above the adrenal glands to the diaphragmatic fascia.

(b) At the level of the iliac crest, below the cone of renal fascia, the anterior and posterior pararenal spaces are in potential communication.

(c) At this same level, the lateroconal fascia disappears as a distinct boundary so that the anterior pararenal space communicates laterally with the properitoneal fat of the flank stripe.

(d) Superiorly, posterior pararenal fat continues as a thin subdiaphragmatic layer of extraperitoneal fat.

At the level of the renal hilum, the posterior renal fascia terminates at the midportion of the psoas muscle. Further down it withdraws toward the quadratus lumborum muscle (Fig. 4–9), only to fuse again with the posterolateral margin of the psoas muscle at the level of the inferior apex of the cone.[17,23,25,26]

The normal thickness of the fascial planes is 1–2 mm. On computed tomography the posterior renal fascia is normally seen far more often

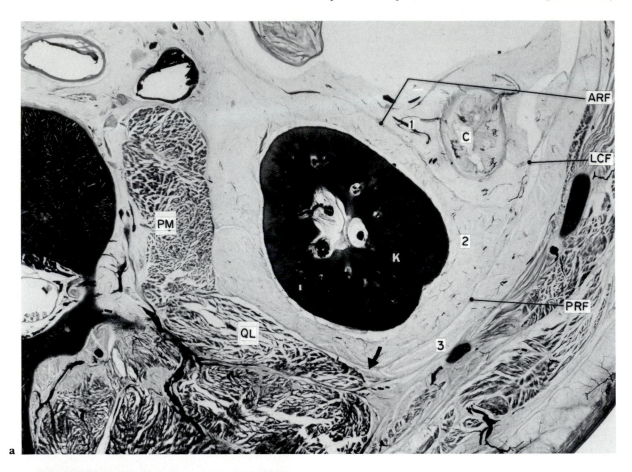

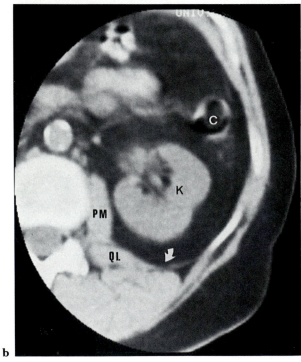

Fig. 4–9. **Medial insertion of posterior renal fascia.** Anatomic cross-section (a) and CT (b) below mid-level of left kidney (K) show termination of the posterior renal fascia in relationship to the quadratus lumborum muscle (arrow). The quadratus lumborum has variable width and thus the medial extent of the posterior pararenal space varies from patient to patient.[34] PM = psoas muscle, C = descending colon, ARF = anterior renal fascia, LCF = lateroconal fascia, PRF = posterior renal fascia, 1 = anterior pararenal space, 2 = perirenal space, 3 = posterior pararenal space.

**Fig. 4–10. Localized thickening of the renal fascia** (arrow) at the site of a pyelonephritic cortical scar. (Courtesy of Roger Parienty, MD, Neuilly, France)

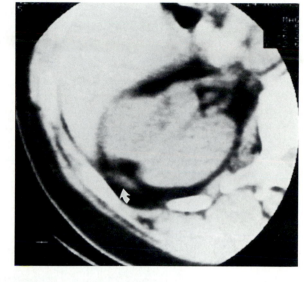

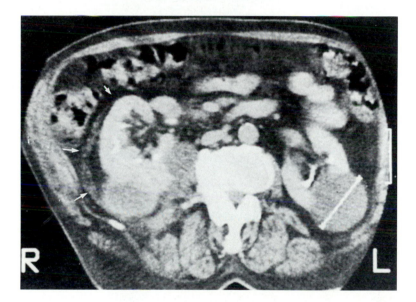

**Fig. 4–11. Thickening of the renal fascia** (arrows) in conjunction with an infected right renal cyst. An uninvolved simple renal cyst is present on the left. (Courtesy of Roger Parienty, MD, Neuilly, France)

than the anterior. A fascia that is focally thickened or greater than 2–3 mm in width is usually abnormal[19,27] (Figs. 4–10 and 4–11). Renal fascial thickening may be caused by edema, hyperemia fibrosis, or lipolysis.[28] It has been reported in a large variety of pathologic conditions[27,29,30] including inflammatory, malignant, and traumatic processes, and is further nonspecific in not allowing diagnostic localization to a primary extraperitoneal site since it may be related to disease in the kidney, perirenal space, or pararenal compartments.[7,8,11,19]

Rarely, the appearance of thickened fascia may be simulated on CT supine scans by intraperitoneal fluid within posterior peritoneal recesses, particularly on the left.[17,31,32] Fluid layering in a deep left paracolic gutter may mimic thickening of the lateroconal fascia and a portion of the posterior renal fascia. As the fluid continues superiorly into the inferior extension of the splenorenal recess, and perhaps to some degree medially within the unusual variant of a retropancreatic recess, the appearance of a thickened anterior renal fascia may result (Fig.

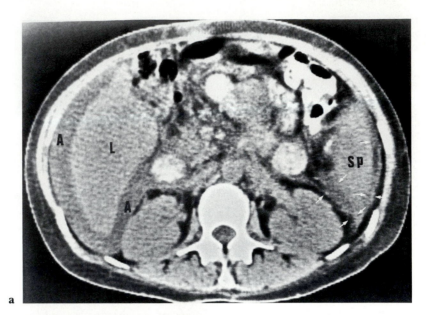

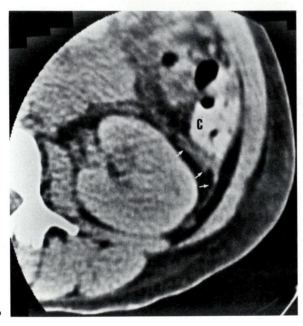

**Fig. 4–12. Thickened fascia simulated by intraperitoneal fluid.**
CT scan **(a)** and magnified view **(b)** at lower level. Ascitic fluid (A) surrounds the liver (L). A small amount of ascites around the spleen (Sp) in the splenorenal recess (arrows) results in the appearance of a thickened left anterior renal fascia. C = descending colon.

4–12). In those cases where distinction from intrinsic involvement of the anterior pararenal space may be difficult,[32] two further findings may be of value: (1) intraperitoneal fluid would be expected to shift position on decubitus or prone CT scans; and (2) although there is some variability in the peritoneal fixation of the descending colon[33] (Fig. 4–13), evidence of involvement of the extraperitoneal attachment of the descending colon indicates fluid in the anterior pararenal space (Fig. 4–14).

The posterior renal fascia has been shown by dissection studies to be divided into two laminae at a variable point from the kidney.[34] The thinner anterior leaf extends anteriorly to be continuous with the anterior renal fascia. The thicker posterior lamina becomes the lateroconal fascia. Figures 4–15 and 4–16 clearly display these laminae in two different patients. A potential space between the two laminae is thus anatomically continuous with the anterior pararenal space.[34]

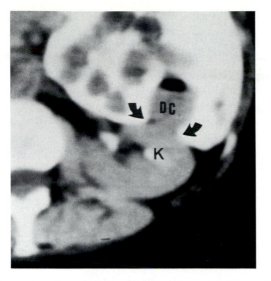

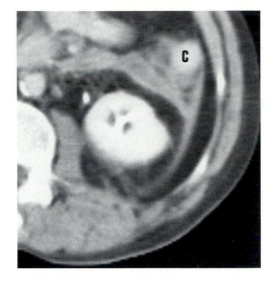

**Fig. 4–13. The peritoneal reflection over the descending colon** (arrows) is shown on this CT study by intraperitoneal contrast medium. The bare area of the descending colon (DC) is contiguous with the adipose tissue of the anterior pararenal space ventral to the left kidney (K).

**Fig. 4–14. Involvement of descending colon's extraperitoneal bare area.**
In a case of thickened renal fascia secondary to acute pancreatitis, CT demonstrates inflammatory involvement of the extraperitoneal fat related to the bare area of the descending colon (C). This localizes the process to the anterior pararenal space and distinguishes the changes from intraperitoneal fluid.

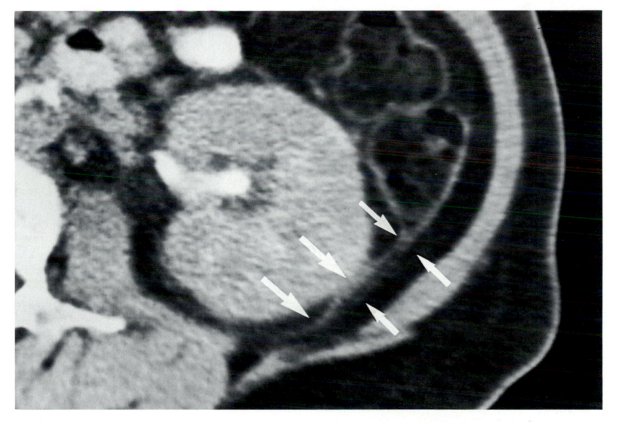

**Fig. 4–15. In vivo identification of the two layers of the posterior renal fascia.**
CT demonstrates an enlarged left kidney, secondary to acute pyelonephritis, abutting the posterior renal fascia and the presence of a double line of the posterior renal fascia (arrows). The inner line adjacent to the kidney is thickened, and the potential space between the two leaves of the posterior renal fascia is now seen. (Courtesy of Michael Oliphant, M.D., Syracuse, N.Y.)

189

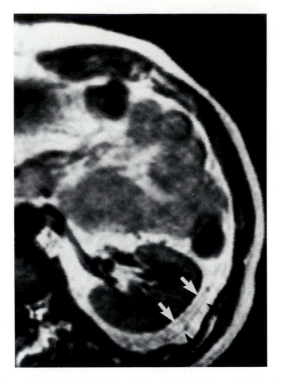

**Fig. 4–16. Two layers of the posterior renal fascia** (arrows) shown discretely by magnetic resonance imaging.

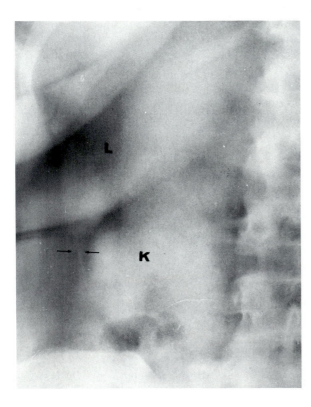

On plain films of the abdomen, the lateroconal fascia sometimes appears as a thin line lateral to the kidney (Fig. 4–17). It is more commonly seen on the right, where it projects inferior to the hepatic angle. Characteristically, it is slightly angled medially as it extends inferiorly. The lateral fusion of the renal fascial layers at the level of the lateroconal fascia demarcates the perirenal fat medially from the posterior pararenal fat laterally as it extends into the flank stripe. These fascial layers are more frequently visualized in nephrotomography. In the past, this fascial line has been mistaken for the peritoneal reflection itself, leading to considerable confusion in the radiologic localization of disease processes. Its significance lies in the fact that it is truly an extraperitoneal structure that provides a boundary.

Variations in the origin of the lateroconal fascia may explain the uncommon occurrence of retrorenal colon or extension of ascitic fluid.[35–37]

Kunin has called attention to three groups of bridging connective tissue septa which may divide the perirenal space into relatively discrete compartments. These include fibrous lamellae that connect the renal capsule to the perirenal fascia and some that connect the anterior and posterior renal fasciae, but the most commonly visible in well-fatted patients is the posterior renorenal bridging septum.[38] This is attached only to the renal capsule and runs parallel to the surface of the kidney. It is variable in extent somewhere between the posteromedial and posterolateral margins. The septa may course over a considerable distance (Fig. 4–18) and may thicken in response to the same stimuli that cause thickening and increased visibility of the anterior and posterior renal fasciae[39,40] (Figs. 4–19 through 4–21). Venous collaterals in the perirenal fat secondary to renal vein occlusion[27,41] or simply the hypervascularity associated with a neoplasm[27] should be distinguished from thickened bridging renal septa (Fig. 4–22).

◁————————————————————

**Fig. 4–17. Plain film demonstration of the edge of the lateroconal fascia** (arrows).
This projects as a thin density inferior to the angle of the liver (L) and lateral to the kidney (K). This demarcates the extraperitoneal adipose tissue into the perirenal fat medially and posterior pararenal fat laterally, extending into the flank fat. (From Meyers et al[12])

**Fig. 4–18. Perirenal bridging septa.**
**(a–c)** CT shows the posterior lamella (arrows) over a vertical extent of 4.5 cm.

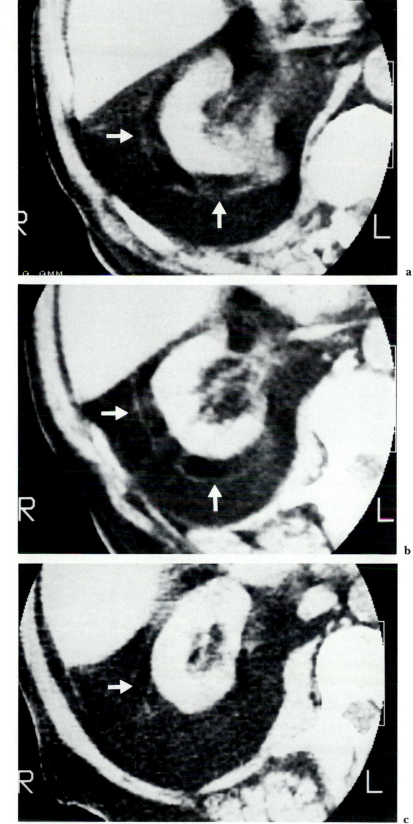

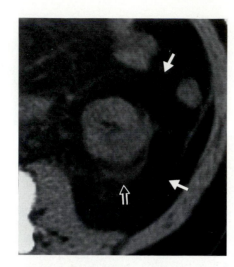

**Fig. 4–19. Bridging renal septa.**
The most conspicuous one is a thickened posterior renorenal septum (open arrow). Gerota's fascia is evident (closed arrows).

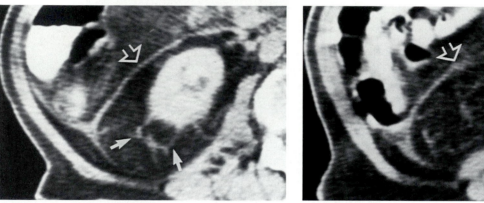

a                                                                                                        b

**Fig. 4–20. Bridging renal septa.**
(a) Among multiple bridging septa, the most conspicuous is a dorsal renorenal septum (arrows). These are associated with a thickened anterior renal fascia (open arrow).
(b) At a level below the lower renal pole, the septa continue within the fat in the cone of fascia.

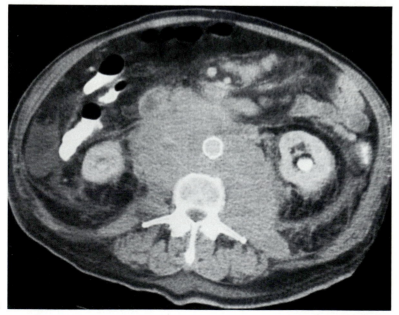

**Fig. 4–21. Lymphatic stranding through the extraperitoneal spaces.**
(a) In a patient with non-Hodgkin's lymphoma with gross paraaortic/paracaval adenopathy, CT demonstrates extraperitoneal lymphedema with thickening of fasciae and septa.
(b) Within the perirenal space the process extends below the level of the kidneys.

a

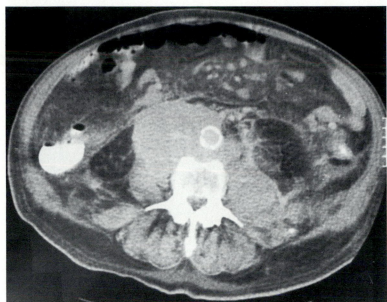

4–21                                                                                                                                                  b

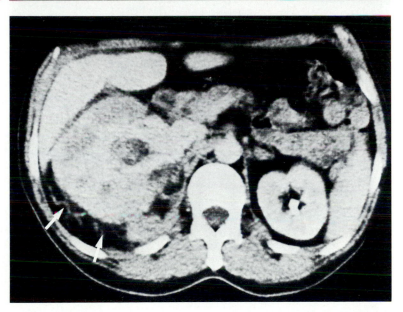

**Fig. 4–22. Collateral perirenal venous drainage.**
CT demonstrates a right renal carcinoma with tumor thrombus of the main renal vein extending into an enlarged inferior vena cava. Drainage through enlarged capsular veins in the perirenal fat (arrows) should not be mistaken for bridging septa on a single transaxial section. (Courtesy of Roger Parienty, MD, Neuilly, France)

## The Psoas Muscle

I have clarified the radiographic anatomy of the psoas muscle by anatomic sections through the extraperitoneal tissues at different levels.[8] The upper and lower segments of the psoas muscle are visualized by virtue of the contrast provided by different aspects of the extraperitoneal fat.

At the level of the kidney, it is the perirenal fat that predominantly marginates the lateral border of the psoas muscle. However, below the kidney, secondary to the lines of fusion of the cone of renal fascia, posterior pararenal fat provides the contrast margination of the muscle.

Loss of visualization of the complete muscle border is often misleading and must be carefully evaluated. It is often not seen unilaterally in normal individuals.[4,5] Furthermore, the psoas outline may disappear with only very minimal rotation or scoliosis of the lumbar spine,[42] and extraperitoneal fat may be scanty in emaciated patients or in those who have lost weight.

A reliable sign, however, is *segmental* loss of visualization of the psoas border. Such asymmetry in properly centered films immediately localizes a fluid collection to a specific extraperitoneal compartment. Thus, localized perirenal processes tend to obliterate only the upper mar-

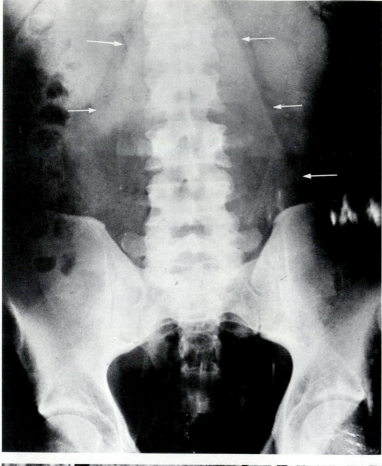

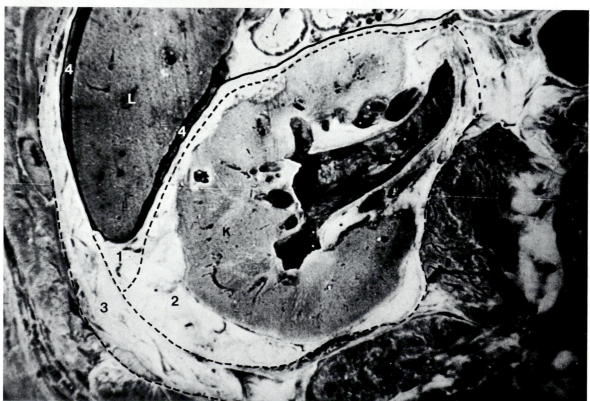

4–24

gin, whereas fluid collection in the posterior pararenal spaces obliterates the psoas muscle in its lower segment (Fig. 4–23) or throughout, depending on its extent. Two qualifications must be appreciated: (a) on frontal films, a large collection within the anterior pararenal space may, by superimposition of the density, obscure the psoas border, but well-penetrated oblique projections will nevertheless demonstrate its intact margin; (b) extraperitoneal gas localized within the posterior pararenal compartment will sharply outline the lateral border of the psoas muscle at all levels.

## The Hepatic and Splenic Angles

The hepatic and splenic angles, the posterior and inferior contours of these intraperitoneal organs, are outlined normally by the contrast provided by the subjacent extraperitoneal fat.[43] Figure 4–24 shows that the lateral aspects of the angles are adjacent to the lateral extension of the posterior pararenal fat, while the medial aspects are related to the anterior pararenal and perirenal fat. Loss of their visualization, however, is a nonlocalizing abnormality. Either intraperitoneal (subhepatic) fluid collections or infiltration within any of the three extraperitoneal compartments may act as a mass to displace the angle out of the bed of fat.

# Anterior Pararenal Space

## Roentgen Anatomy of Distribution and Localization of Collections

Selective opacification of the anterior pararenal space in the cadaver permits identification of the preferential pathway of spread and the characteristic localizing features as shown in Figure 4–25. Preferential flow is downward to the iliac fossa, and the collection demonstrates several diagnostic features:

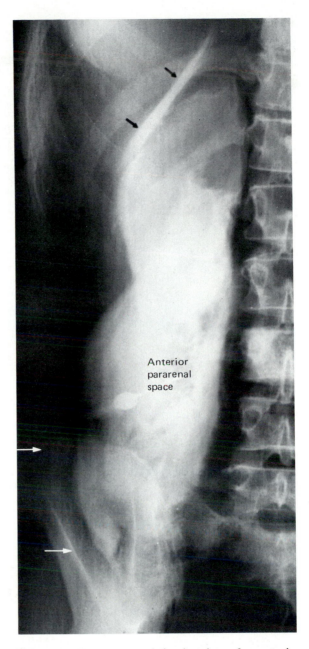

Anterior pararenal space

**Fig. 4–25. Postmortem injection into the anterior pararenal space.**
The collection has a generally vertical axis. Laterally, the lucent flank stripe is intact (white arrows). Medially, spread approaches the spine over the psoas muscle. Superiorly, it follows the obliquity of the kidney and there is extension to the bare area of the liver at the site of reflection of the coronary ligament (black arrows). (From Meyers et al[12])

◁ ——————————————————————————————————
**Fig. 4–24. Transverse anatomic section shows the hepatic angle embedded in extraperitoneal fat.**
Infiltration of any of the three compartments as well as of the intraperitoneal space may result in loss of radiographic visualization of the hepatic angle. 1 = anterior pararenal fat, 2 = perirenal fat, 3 = posterior pararenal fat, 4 = intraperitoneal space, K = kidney, L = liver.

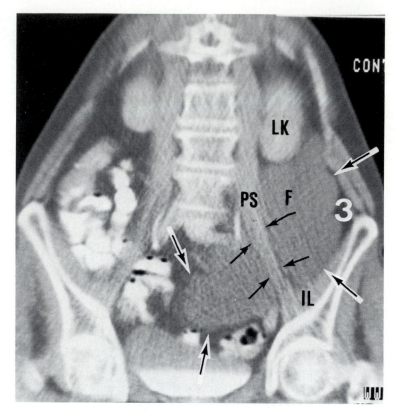

**Fig. 4–26. Fluid in the anterior pararenal space.**
Direct coronal CT section reveals a fluid collection (F) in the left anterior pararenal space (arrows) with a vertical axis and medial extension inferiorly. The outlines of the kidney and of the psoas muscle (PS) are preserved (black arrows) and the flank fat (3) of the posterior pararenal space is not infiltrated. The descending colon is not visible since it has been displaced ventrally. LK = left kidney, IL = iliacus muscle. (Reproduced from Feldberg[17])

1. The general axis is vertical.
2. Medially, the collection overlaps the lateral border of the psoas muscle and approaches the spine.
3. Laterally, the lucent flank stripe is preserved, since flow is restricted by the lateroconal fascia.
4. Superiorly, the renal outline remains demarcated where the space lies anterior to the kidney. The hepatic or splenic outline, displaced from its bed of contrasting extraperitoneal fat, is lost. On the right, communication may be established across the reflections of the coronary ligament to the bare area of the liver. (The occasional development of abscess in the bare area of the liver secondary to extraperitoneal infection, most commonly from appendicitis, is explained by this anatomic continuity with the anterior pararenal space.)

Figure 4–26 exquisitely confirms these findings in vivo. Figure 4–27 clarifies these relationships in the horizontal plane.

The significant criteria for the radiologic localization and distinction of collections within the anterior pararenal space are outlined in Table 4–1.

## Sources of Effusions

The anterior pararenal compartment is the most common site of extraperitoneal infection. Of 160 patients with extraperitoneal abscess reviewed by Altemeier and Alexander,[3] the process was confined to the anterior pararenal

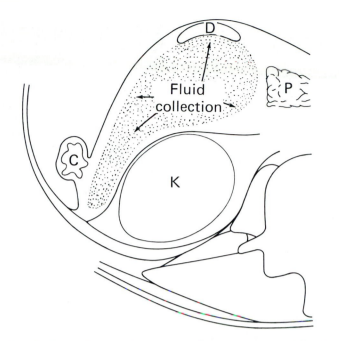

**Fig. 4–27. Fluid collection in the right anterior pararenal compartment with viscus displacement.**
K = kidney, P = pancreas, D = duodenum, C = colon. (From Meyers et al[12])

**Table 4–1.** Radiologic criteria for localizing extraperitoneal effusions

| Radiologic features | Anterior pararenal space | Perirenal space | Posterior pararenal space |
|---|---|---|---|
| Perirenal fat and renal outline | Preserved | Obliterated | Preserved |
| Axis of density | Vertical | Vertical (acute) Inferomedial (chronic) | Inferolateral (parallel to psoas margin) |
| Kidney displacement | Lateral and superior | Anterior, medial, and superior | Anterior, lateral, and superior |
| Psoas muscle outline | Preserved | Upper half obliterated | Obliterated in lower half or throughout |
| Flank stripe | Preserved | Preserved | Obliterated |
| Hepatic and splenic angles | Obliterated | Obliterated | Preserved or obliterated |
| Displacement of ascending or descending colon | Anterior and lateral | Lateral | Anterior and medial |
| Displacement of descending duodenum or duodenojejunal junction | Anterior | Anterior | Anterior |

space in 84 (52.5%). Most arise from primary lesions of the alimentary tract, especially the colon, extraperitoneal appendix, pancreas, and duodenum. The exudates originate from perforating malignancies, inflammatory conditions, penetrating peptic ulcers, and accidental or iatrogenic trauma.[3,44] I have also recognized localization to this compartment in hemorrhage from hepatic and splenic arteries and in some cases of spontaneous extraperitoneal bleeding.

## Extraperitoneal Perforations of the Colon and Appendix

Figure 4–28 illustrates that extraperitoneal perforations of the colon can be identified as clearly localized to the anterior pararenal space, even on plain films. The extraperitoneal collection of mottled gaseous lucencies is oriented with a general vertical axis, medially overlaps the psoas muscle and approaches the spine, and does not

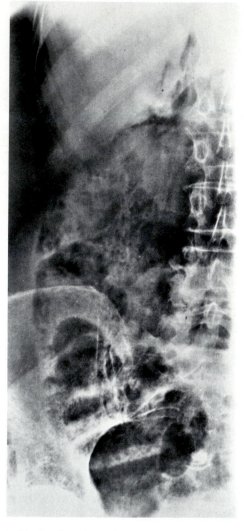

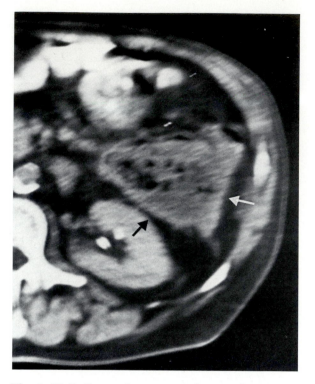

**Fig. 4–29. Left anterior pararenal space abscess** secondary to a perforated diverticulum of the mid-descending colon. The gas-producing infection has coalesced deep to the peritoneum between the anterior renal fascia and the lateroconal fascia (arrows).

**Fig. 4–28. Perforation of the hepatic flexure.**
Mottled lucent areas on the right represent collections of gas extending medially over the psoas muscle and approaching the spine. The flank stripe is intact. These changes localize the extraperitoneal gas to the anterior pararenal space.

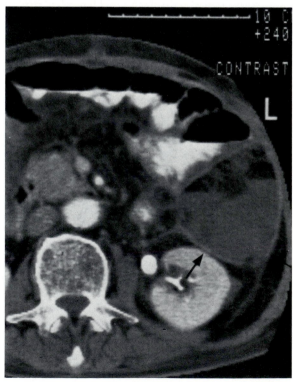

▷

**Fig. 4–30. Left anterior pararenal abscess** following left hemicolectomy. The gas-producing infection is bounded by thickened anterior renal and lateroconal fasciae (arrows).

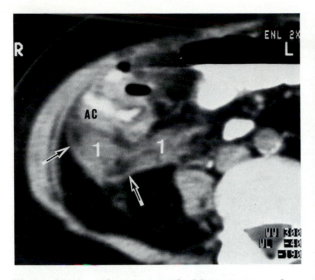

**Fig. 4–31. Anterior pararenal phlegmon secondary to extraperitoneal appendicitis.**
CT shows infiltrate in right anterior pararenal space (1) in an ascending retrocecal position. There is thickening of the lateroconal and anterior renal fasciae (arrows). The ascending colon (AC) shows bowel wall thickening. (Reproduced from Feldberg[17])

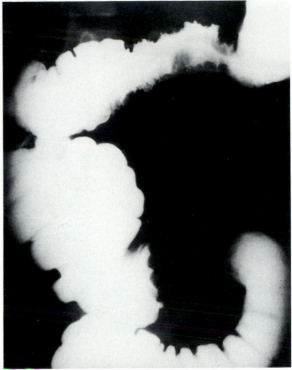

**Fig. 4–32. Large anterior pararenal space abscess originating from extraperitoneal appendicitis.**
Note deformity of the medial contour of the cecum and the abscess extending to the transverse colon. (From Meyers[8])

obscure the flank stripe laterally. In this patient, who developed fever after numerous scattered polyps were removed by colonoscopic cautery, the characteristic findings localize the site of perforation to the ascending colon.

Abscesses secondary to perforated lesions of the ascending or descending colon are localized by the characteristic fascial boundaries[45] (Figs. 4–29 and 4–30).

The appendix in an ascending retrocecal position is frequently an extraperitoneal structure.[46] Perforation then leads to an abscess localized within the right anterior pararenal space[18,47] (Fig. 4–31).

Because the structures and connective tissue behind the anterior pararenal space are relatively unyielding, massive accumulations within it tend to distend the space anteriorly, bulging forward into the peritoneal cavity and displacing small intestinal loops. Figure 4–32 illustrates a huge abscess originating from a perforated extraperitoneal appendicitis. Its dimensions in an anterior–posterior plane approach its vertical extent from the cecal area to the transverse colon.

In children, extraperitoneal appendicitis and its associated abscess within the anterior para-

renal space commonly produce pressure on the right ureter after it has emerged from the cone of the renal fascia. This typically occurs at the L5 or lumbosacral level, producing localized obstruction and hydronephrosis (Fig. 4–33). In adults, similar changes may be due to perforated carcinoma or diverticulitis of the colon but more frequently are secondary to granulomatous ileocolitis[48] with extension of the infection into the anterior pararenal space (Fig. 4–34). Indeed, this localization explains the ureteral complications of Crohn's disease.

I have confirmed by postmortem injections the anatomic continuity of the right anterior pararenal space with the nonperitonealized bare area of the right lobe of the liver (Fig. 4–25) at the site of reflection of the right coronary ligament.[12] This pathway permits the spread of disease from extraperitoneal perforations of the bowel precisely to the bare area of the liver[22] (Fig. 4–35).

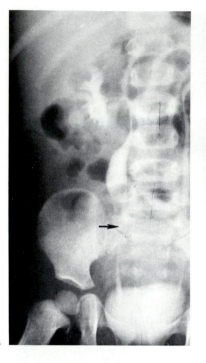

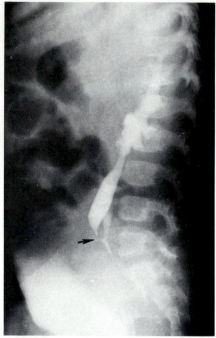

a

b

**Fig. 4–33. Extraperitoneal appendicitis.**
The associated abscess within the anterior pararenal space partially obstructs the right ureter (arrow).

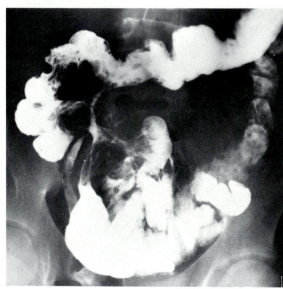

a

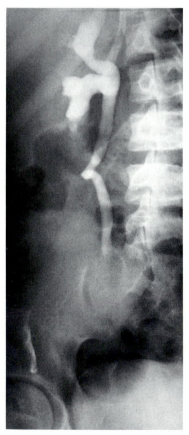

b

**Fig. 4–34. Anterior pararenal space abscess from granulomatous ileocolitis.**
(a) Barium enema reveals severe ileoileal, ileocolic, and colocolic fistulas secondary to Crohn's disease.
(b) The associated abscess within the anterior pararenal space obstructs the right ureter after it has exited from the cone of renal fascia at the level of L5–S1.
(From Meyers[8])

## Perforation of the Duodenum

Perforation of the duodenum is usually caused by blunt trauma to the abdomen and is now being encountered as an automobile lap-belt deceleration injury. The duodenum bears the brunt of the injury because of its firm attachment, acutely angled flexures, and compression against the vertebral column. Comparatively few patients are greatly inconvenienced by the original trauma. Only when the effects of the extravasation become evident, do the symptoms become marked. Rupture usually occurs at the junction of the second and third portions; multiple perforations are possible and there may be accompanying traumatic pancreatitis. Early recognition is important because unrecognized duodenal perforation has a 65% mortality rate as opposed to a 5% mortality rate in those patients operated upon within the first 24 hours after injury.[49]

The extraperitoneal gas with the extravasated bile and pancreatic juices is limited to the right anterior pararenal space and takes a characteristic distribution (Figs. 4–36 and 4–37). CT is considerably more sensitive than plain films in detecting the extraluminal gas.[50]

Figure 4–38 illustrates another striking finding. Only when the infection progresses inferiorly, below the apex of the cone of renal fascia and the limitation of the lateroconal fascia, can the gas proceed directly to the properitoneal fat. Gaseous lucencies can then be identified in the extraperitoneal tissues, with local extension into the flank, specifically at the level of the iliac crest and progressing cephalad. The finding is typical of gaseous spread down the right anterior pararenal compartment and is seen most commonly in perforation of the extraperitoneal duodenum.

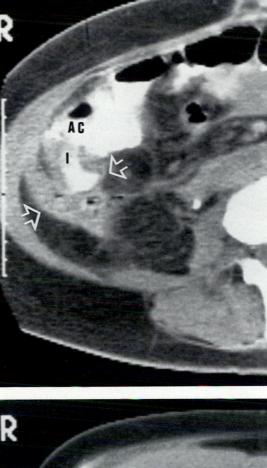

a

b

**Fig. 4–35. Extension of anterior pararenal inflammation to bare area of liver.**
**(a)** After an ileocecal resection for Crohn's disease, inflammatory changes (arrows) within the anterior pararenal space surround the anastomotic site between the ileum (I) and the ascending colon (AC).
**(b)** The inflammatory changes have extended cephalad within the anterior pararenal extraperitoneal space to the bare area of the liver (arrows).
(Reproduced from Meyers et al[22])

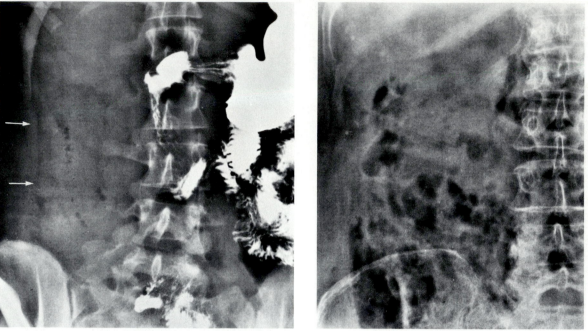

4-36                                                                                                                   4-37

**Fig. 4–36. Extraperitoneal perforation of the duodenum after blunt trauma.**
Several gas bubbles associated with a fluid soft-tissue density are present in the right anterior pararenal space.
These cause loss of the hepatic angle, but the flank stripe (arrows) is intact. The upper GI series shows medial
displacement of the descending duodenum but does not demonstrate the site of extravasation.

**Fig. 4–37. Extraperitoneal perforation of the descending duodenum following blunt trauma, with spread
through the right anterior pararenal space.**
The mottled gas shadows continue over the psoas muscle medially but do not extend into the flank fat
laterally. (From Meyers[9])

An upper gastrointestinal series may demonstrate the perforation site (Fig. 4–38a), but not
always (Fig. 4–36).

Violation of the fascial boundaries in cases of
blunt retroperitoneal duodenal rupture may
result in the appearance of gas surrounding the
right kidney[51,52] and is associated with other
findings that indicate extensive retroperitoneal
cellulitis. However, CT has shown that the exudate may not truly enter the perirenal space but
extend from the anterior to the posterior
pararenal space around the renal fascial
cone[18,50] (Fig. 4–39).

### Retroduodenal Hematoma

Blunt trauma or acute deceleration may also
cause rupture of the small blood vessels behind
the fixed second portion of the duodenum. The
hematoma resides within the right anterior
pararenal space. It results in a characteristic
spiculation of the mucosal folds of the posterior

margin of the descending duodenum and may
displace that structure anteriorly (Fig. 4–40).

Confirmation of its presence, precise localization, and extent is readily shown by computed
tomography which is also useful in follow-up to
document the usual course of spontaneous resolution of the hematoma (Figs. 4–41 and 4–42).

### Pancreatitis

The fascial reactions in acute pancreatitis have
been meticulously studied by computed tomography.[17] Thickening of the anterior renal fascia
is commonly seen (Fig. 4–43) and the inflammatory process often extends to involve
typically the anterior pararenal space[7,8,12,54–59]
(Figs. 4–44 through 4–46). This usually spreads
to the left from the tail of the pancreas. Reactive
thickening of Gerota's fascia and perhaps the
lateroconal fascia may remain after resolution
of the pancreatitis (Fig. 4–47).

On plain films, in the presence of an exudate

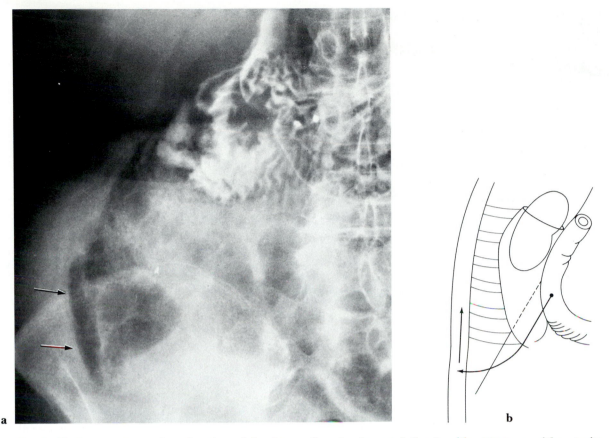

a                                                                                          b

**Fig. 4–38. Extraperitoneal perforation of the descending duodenum following blunt trauma with anterior pararenal space infection.**
(a) Gastrografin gastrointestinal series shows extravasation from the duodenum. Mottled gaseous lucencies extend inferiorly and laterally. Below the level of the cone of the renal fascia and the lateroconal fascia, the infection reaches and then ascends the flank fat (arrows).
(b) Pathway of spread inferior to the lateroconal fascia to communicate with the flank fat.
(From Meyers[8])

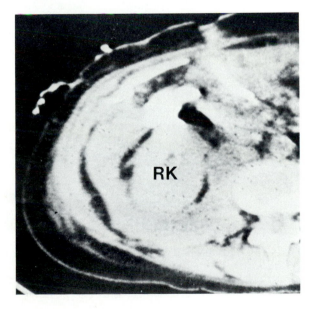

**Fig. 4–39. Extraperitoneal perforation of the duodenum and traumatic pancreatitis.**
CT scan shows the collection digesting across fascial boundaries from the anterior to the posterior pararenal space on the right. The perirenal fat around the right kidney (RK) is maintained.

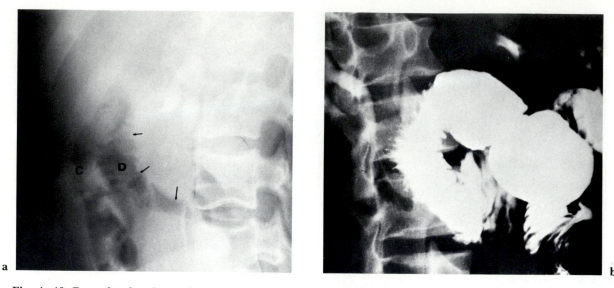

**Fig. 4–40. Retroduodenal anterior pararenal hemorrhage.**
**(a)** Lateral excretory urogram shows a mass separating the right kidney from the anteriorly displaced descending duodenum (D). C = colon.
**(b)** Upper gastrointestinal series shows spiculation of mucosal folds along the posterior aspect of the descending duodenum.
(From Meyers et al[12])

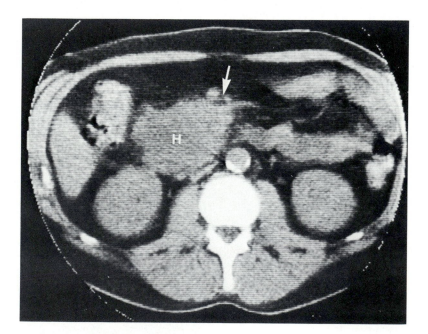

**Fig. 4–41. Paraduodenal hematoma in anterior pararenal space.**
CT scan demonstrates a 6-cm hematoma (H) in the right anterior pararenal compartment posterior to the mesenteric vessels (arrow). Pancreas appeared normal on higher level scans. A follow-up scan 4 weeks later showed spontaneous reduction in the size of the hematoma. (Reproduced from Sagel SS et al[53])

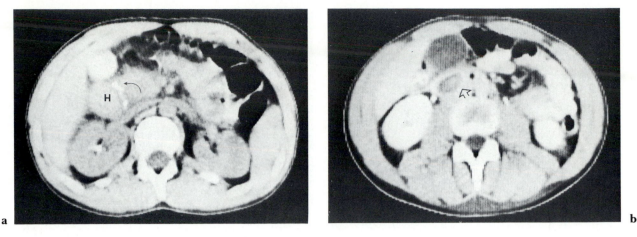

**Fig. 4–42. Intramural hematoma of duodenum and anterior pararenal hemorrhage.**
**(a)** CT scan following blunt trauma to the abdomen demonstrates a prominent anterior pararenal space hematoma (H), compressing the lateral aspect of the contrast-filled duodenum (curved arrow).
**(b)** Contrast-enhanced scan 3 weeks later shows partial liquefaction of the resolving hematoma (arrow). Note that the perirenal fat is maintained.
(Reproduced from Love et al[7])

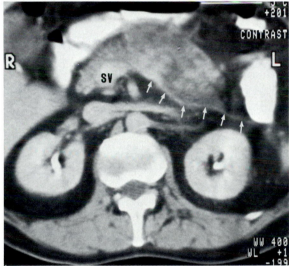

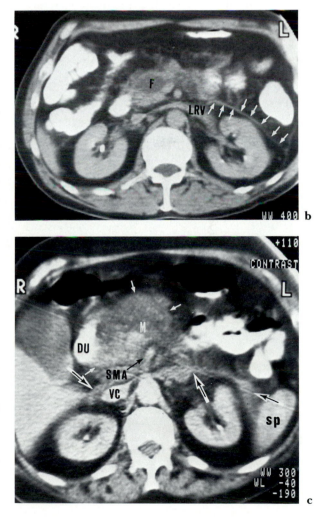

**Fig. 4–43. Anterior renal fascial reactions in pancreatitis in three different patients.**
**(a)** A thickened left anterior renal fascia converges behind the pancreas (arrows) which is swollen with intrapancreatic fluid. SV = splenic vein.
**(b)** Intrapancreatic fluid collection (F) with thickened left anterior renal fascia blending into posterior pancreatic tissue (arrows). LRV = left renal vein.
**(c)** Inflammatory pancreatic mass (M) with very thickened anterior renal fascial planes bilaterally (black-white arrows). DU = duodenum, SMA = superior mesenteric artery, SP = spleen, VC = vena cava.
(Reproduced from Feldberg[17])

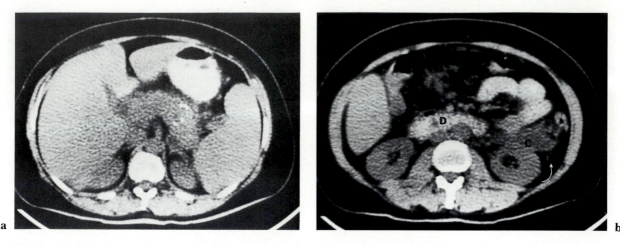

a                                                                                                b

**Fig. 4–44. Acute recurrent pancreatitis localized to anterior pararenal space.**
**(a)** CT scan in patient with persistent pain and increased serum amylase demonstrates evidence of chronic calcific pancreatitis.
**(b)** Scan at a lower level shows fluid collection (C) in the anterior pararenal space on the left. There is mild thickening of Gerota's fascia (curved arrow), but the perirenal space and flank fat are intact. These changes represent acute recurrent pancreatitis. A follow-up scan 2 months later after conservative management demonstrated resolution. D = opacified third duodenum.

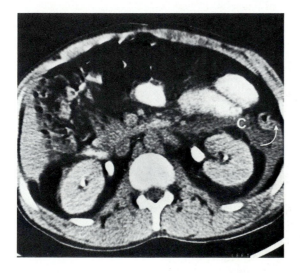

**Fig. 4–45. Pancreatitis extending through anterior pararenal space.**
CT scan shows fluid collection (C) extending from tail of pancreas through the anterior pararenal space on the left. Note its continuation to the bare area posteriorly of the descending colon (curved arrow), where it is bounded laterally by the lateroconal fascia. There is fluid interposition within the posterior renal fascia, but the perirenal space and flank fat remain uninvolved.

in the left anterior pararenal space, a radiolucent halo about the left kidney may rarely be evident, secondary to enhanced visualization of the peripheral margin of the uninvolved perirenal fat.[59,60]

Extraperitoneal spread of a pancreatic abscess may be extensive but usually follows recognizable planes.[56] Drainage from the head of the pancreas tends to be downward and to the right. Figure 4–48 illustrates the typical localization found at surgery in cases of extensive pancreatic infections within the anterior pararenal compartment. The large abscess pictured has come into contact with the ascending colon and has not crossed the midline. Figure 4–49 demonstrates identical characteristic features in vivo. Figure 4–50 shows the operative findings when the process has continued inferiorly to the level of the iliac crest. The drainage here has led to a discrete collection external to the peritoneum. Although this pathway has not been previously explained in the surgical literature, it is clearly the result of the process extending below the level of the lateroconal fascia and then gaining immediate access to the properitoneal flank fat. This is basically the same pathway as outlined in Figure 4–38.

Emphysematous or fulminating pancreatitis is a principal exception to unilateral confine-

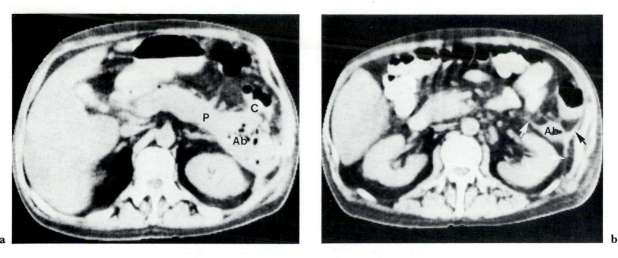

**Fig. 4–46. Abscess of the tail of the pancreas with extension within the anterior pararenal space.**
**(a)** CT scan in an alcoholic male who developed high fever demonstrates a gas-containing pancreatic abscess (Ab) extending from the tail of the pancreas (P) within the anterior pararenal space. It displaces the descending colon (C) anteriorly. Gerota's fascia is segmentally obliterated and thickened, but the perirenal and posterior pararenal spaces are intact.
**(b)** At a lower level, the abscess is smaller and the thickened Gerota's fascia (white arrows) and lateroconal fascia (black arrow) are more clearly identified.
(Reproduced from Love et al[7])

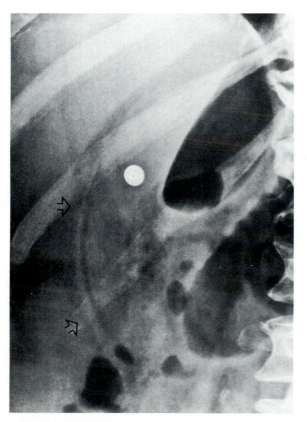

**Fig. 4–47. Thickened renal fascia** (arrows).
This is identified on plain film as a curvilinear soft-tissue band separated by lucent perirenal fat from the lateral contour of the kidney. This finding persisted after resolution of acute pancreatitis.

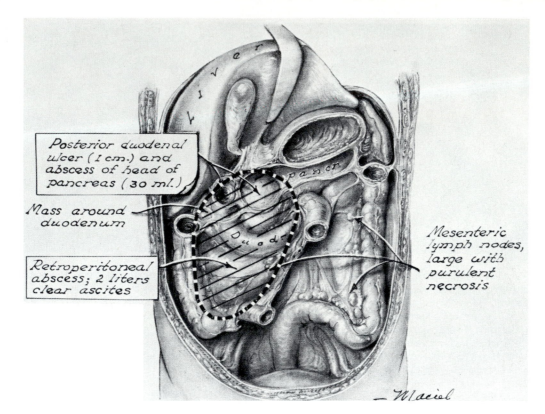

**Fig. 4–48. Inferior drainage of infection from pancreatic abscess within anterior pararenal space** secondary to penetration of a posterior duodenal ulcer. (Reproduced from Wulsin[63])

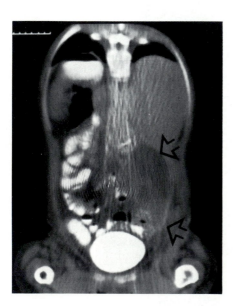

**Fig. 4–49. Inferior extension of abscess from head of pancreas within right anterior pararenal space** (arrows) shown in a coronal CT section. (Courtesy of Michiel Feldberg, MD, University of Utrecht, The Netherlands)

**Fig. 4–51. Gas-producing infection of the pancreas.** Mottled lucencies are present diffusely throughout the pancreas and progress down both sides within the anterior pararenal spaces (arrows), overlying the psoas muscle. The flank stripes are maintained. (From Meyers[9])

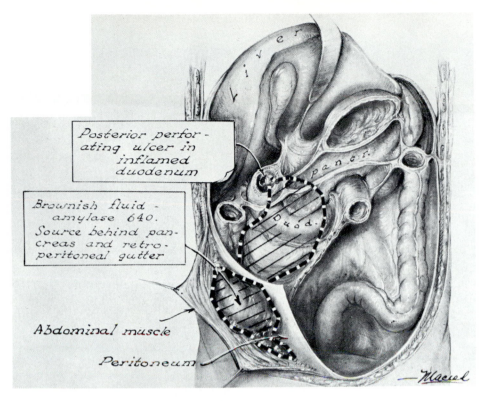

**Fig. 4–50. Pancreatitis secondary to duodenal ulcer.**
The anterior pararenal extension reaches the flank fat external to the peritoneum below the level of the cone of renal fascia. (Reproduced from Wulsin[63])

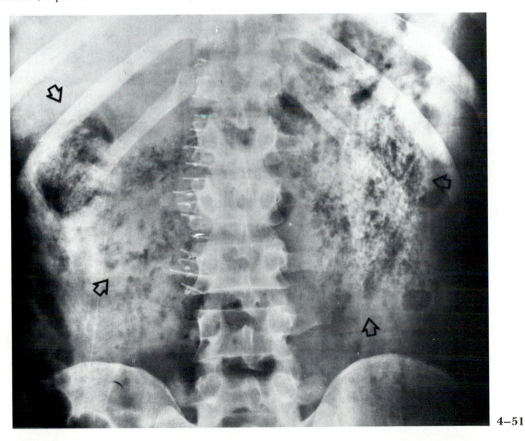

4–51

209

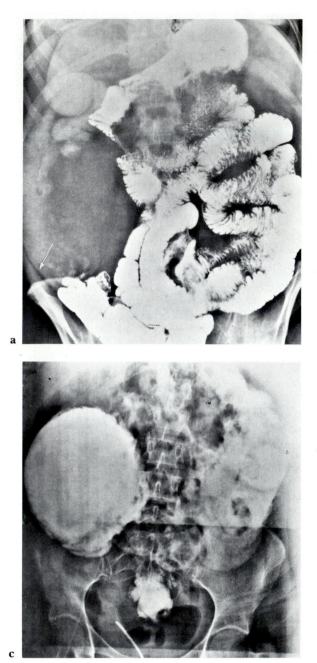

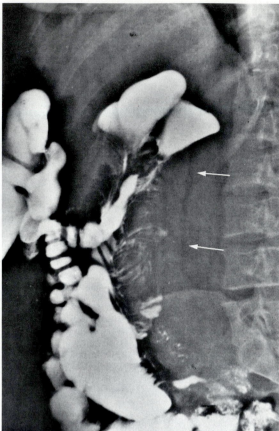

Fig. 4–52. **Bilateral infected pancreatic pseudocysts within the anterior pararenal compartments.**
**(a)** On the right a large mass with a vertical axis displaces bowel toward the midline. The flank stripe is intact (arrow). Another extraperitoneal abscess is present on the left, draping small bowel loops.
**(b)** Steep oblique projection shows bowel displaced anteriorly and intact perirenal fat on right (arrows).
**(c)** Contrast injections of the huge pseudocysts verify their bilateral anterior pararenal compartmentalization.

ment within the anterior pararenal space from a process arising in the upper abdomen. Figure 4–51 illustrates a gas-producing infection of the pancreas with spread downward within both sides of the compartment. The gaseous lucencies overlie the psoas muscles, but there is no evidence of direct continuity across the midline. This indicates that the infection has dissected separately down both sides from the pancreas. Figure 4–52 shows similar bilateral changes of large infected pseudocysts of the pancreas in an alcoholic male. Yet, the anatomic planes of the anterior pararenal space may allow direct extension across the midline (Fig. 4–53), particularly in cases of liberated pancreatic enzymes (Fig. 4–54).

A potential space into which fluid collections from the anterior pararenal space can extend is created by the division of the posterior renal fascia into two laminae. In moderate to severe cases of pancreatitis, retrorenal extension of pancreatic effusion or phlegmon into this potential space is common.[34] Raptopoulos and colleagues have emphasized the typical appearance of this posterior extension of pancreatitis as a widening of the posterior renal fascia that tapers posteriorly[34] (Fig. 4–45). However, I have observed that variability in the origin of the division into two leaves in the horizontal plane as well as apparently in the vertical dimensions of the cleavage account for the varied appearances of fluid accumulation in this plane (Figs. 4–55 and 4–56).

Posteriorly these collections at some axial level generally become contiguous with the lateral edge of the quadratus lumborum muscle. In the flank, communication may be established to the posterior pararenal space and to the structures of the abdominal wall (Figs. 4–56 through 4–58). I have shown[12] that these pathways provide an anatomic–radiologic explanation for the classic clinical sign of subcutaneous discoloration in the costovertebral angle (Grey-Turner's sign) which may be associated with acute pancreatitis.[61,62]

The liberated digestive enzymes of severe pancreatitis may dissect within fascial planes to result in an interesting extension to the posterior pararenal space from the anterior pararenal space without the contamination of the intervening perirenal compartment. This may be a consequence either of violation of the latero-

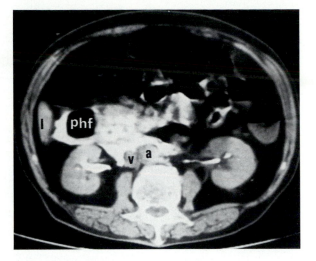

**Fig. 4–53. In vivo opacification of right anterior pararenal space.**
This occurred from extravasation of contrast medium from a ruptured pseudocyst in the head of the pancreas during ERCP. Note that there is extension in this plane across the midline. Laterally, the extravasate is in relationship to the posterior hepatic flexure (phf) and angle of the liver (l). a = aorta, v = inferior vena cava.

conal fascia[7,18] or the process spreading from the pancreas down the anterior pararenal space and then rising posterior to the cone of renal fascia within the posterior pararenal space[8,12] (Fig. 4–59). The kidney and colon are pushed forward and the psoas muscle and flank stripe obliterated.

Despite the digestive effects of pancreatic fluid, the renal fascia almost invariably is not transgressed so that the perirenal fat and kidney retain their integrity. Indeed, in acute pancreatitis, CT documentation of extrapancreatic fluid collections with perirenal spread and without renal involvement is rare.[31,63a,63b]

## Bleeding from Hepatic or Splenic Artery

The hepatic and splenic arteries are located anatomically within the anterior pararenal compartments. When these vessels rupture from trauma or aneurysm, the bleeding may be discretely localized to the extraperitoneal space on the side of origin (Fig. 4–60).

Bleeding from the hepatic artery is clearly shown in the following case history: A 70-year-old man was examined because of a 1-month history of colicky right upper quadrant pain.

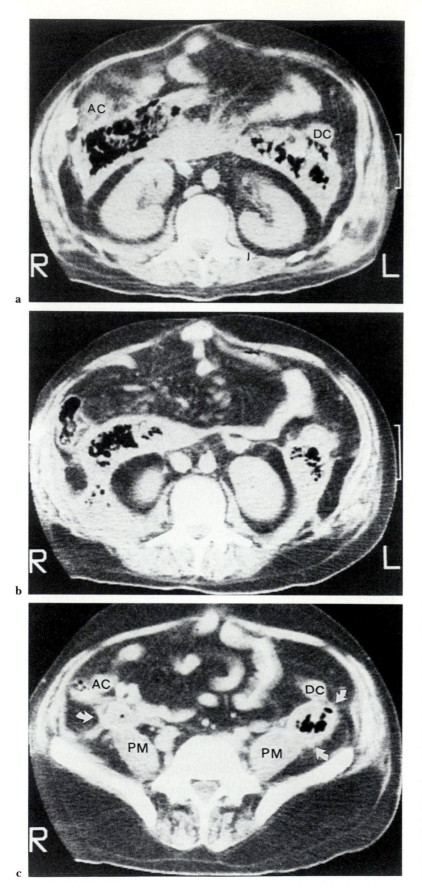

**Fig. 4–54. Bilateral spread of emphysematous pancreatitis within anterior pararenal spaces.**
(a) CT displays a gas-producing pancreatic phlegmon extending across the midline throughout both anterior pararenal spaces. AC = ascending colon, DC = descending colon.
(b) More inferiorly, the collection has fused into the anterior and posterior pararenal spaces.
(c) At the level of the iliac crests, CT shows the apex of the renal fascial cones (arrows), where anterior and posterior pararenal spaces communicate, just in front of and slightly lateral to the psoas muscles (PM) and immediately behind the ascending (AC) and descending colon (DC).
(Courtesy of Roger Parienty, MD, Neuilly, France)

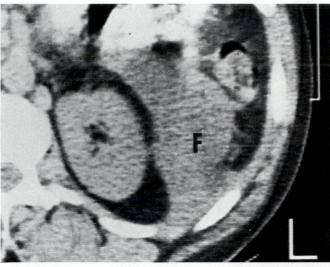

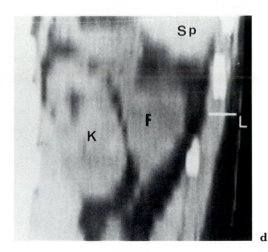

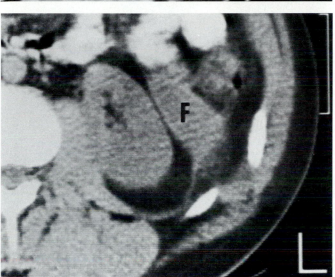

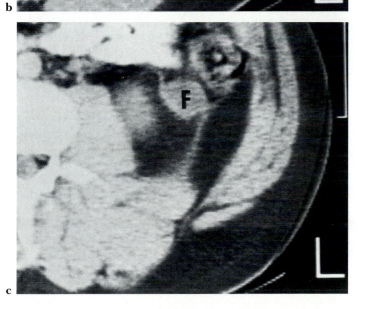

**Fig. 4–55. Pancreatitis extending from anterior pararenal space to within the leaves of the posterior renal fascia.**

(a–c) Three axial CT levels demonstrate pancreatic fluid collection (F) spreading from the left anterior pararenal space to the potential space between the bilaminated posterior renal fascia. Inferiorly the collection tapers to remain as a small loculated intrafascial collection. Dissection through the posterior renal fascia thus appears most prominent in the portion related to the upper renal pole.

(d) Reconstructed CT image demonstrates in the coronal plane the size, position, and relationships of the fluid collection within the posterior renal fascia. K = left kidney, Sp = spleen.

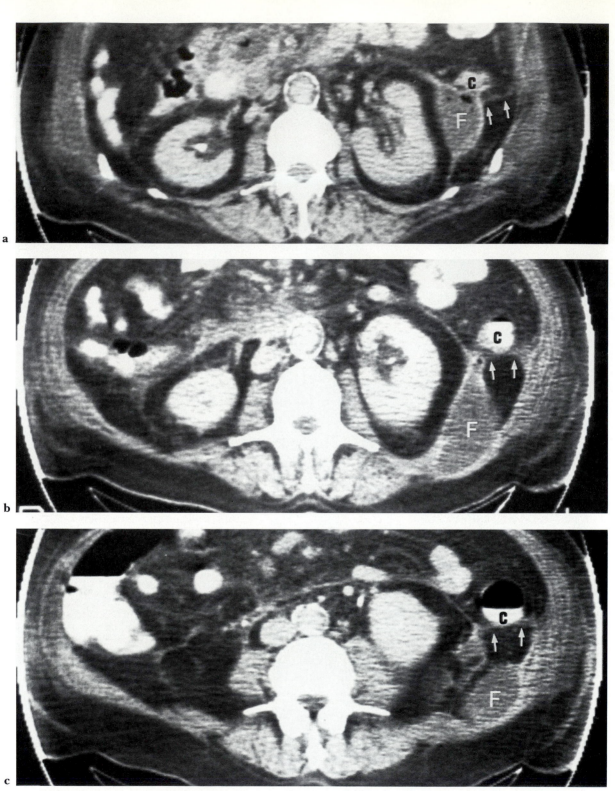

**Fig. 4–56. Extension of pancreatitis to posterior abdominal wall.**
**(a)** Accompanying thickening of the renal fasciae and of the lateroconal fascia (arrows), there is a loculation of fluid (F) between the leaves of the posterior renal fascia immediately behind the descending colon (C).
**(b)** At a lower level, the fluid collection has dissected more posteriorly and comes into relationship with the posterior abdominal wall, presumably effacing the intervening segment of the posterior pararenal space.
**(c)** More inferiorly, while some fluid distention of the posterior renal fascia remains evident, a loculated fluid collection intrudes upon the flank lateral to the quadratus lumborum muscle.

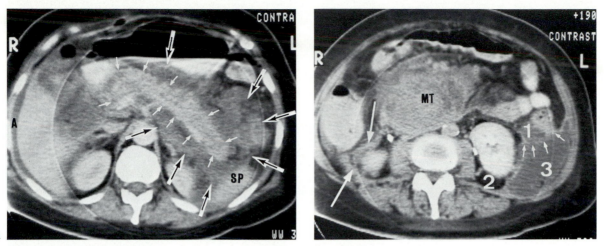

**Fig. 4–57. Extension of pancreatitis to posterior pararenal space.**
**(a)** Extensive phlegmonous infiltrate in anterior pararenal space (black-white arrows) surrounds pancreas whose preserved contours are identifiable after bolus contrast injection (white arrows). A = ascitic fluid, Sp = spleen.
**(b)** The extrapancreatic inflammatory process with fluid has extended from the anterior pararenal space (1) to the posterior pararenal space (3). At this particular level, the lateroconal fascia remains visible (small arrows). The perirenal space (2) is preserved. On the right renal fasciae are also thickened (large arrows). Pancreatic abscess extends into small bowel mesentery (MT).
(Reproduced from Feldberg[17])

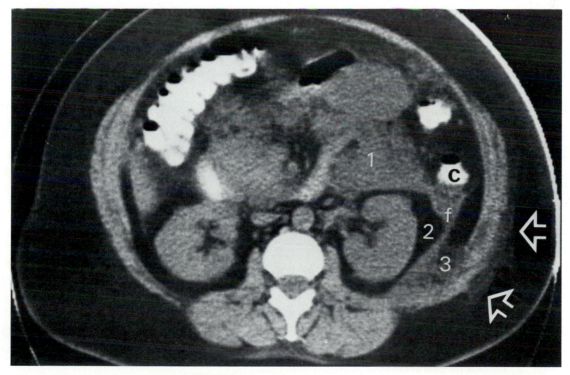

**Fig. 4–58. The Grey-Turner sign secondary to pancreatitis.**
Extravasated pancreatic fluid in the left anterior pararenal space (1) dissects between the leaves of the posterior renal fascia with a loculated fluid collection (f) near the descending colon (c). The perirenal space (2) is maintained.

Inflammatory changes have reached an adjacent portion of the posterior pararenal space (3) and the subcutaneous tissues in the left flank (arrows) at the clinical site of discoloration.

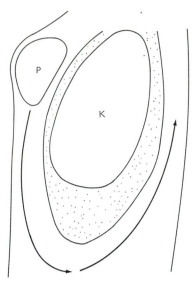

**Fig. 4–59. Pancreatic extravasation with extension down the anterior pararenal space and then upward into the posterior pararenal compartment.**
Diagram illustrates fluid collection in the left anterior pararenal space from the pancreas (P), and continuity under and around the cone of renal fascia into the posterior pararenal compartment. (From Meyers[8])

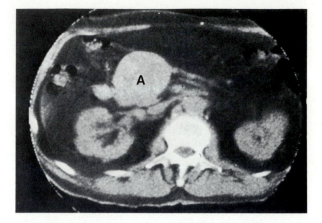

**Fig. 4–60. Hepatic artery aneurysm.**
Unenhanced CT scan shows the relationships and size of an aneurysm (A) of the proximal hepatic artery, subsequently confirmed by arteriography. Bleeding from such an aneurysm characteristically extends through the right anterior pararenal space. (Courtesy of David H Stephens, MD, Mayo Clinic, Rochester, Minn.)

His past medical history included acute rheumatic fever at the age of 5 and an episode of acute staphylococcal endocarditis at the age of 56. Oral cholecystography revealed moderate opacification of the gallbladder and the hepatic angle, flank fat, and psoas muscle were clearly visualized (Fig. 4–61a) at this time. However, 24 hours later, the patient's colicky right upper quadrant pain increased suddenly, with abdominal distention. Initial diagnostic considerations included acute cholecystitis, acute pancreatitis, and penetrating peptic ulcer. An abdominal radiograph now showed a density throughout the right abdomen, with loss of the hepatic angle, although the flank fat was clearly maintained (Fig. 4–61b). These changes indicated an acute fluid collection extraperitoneally, specifically within the anterior pararenal compartment. On

the basis of these plain-film abnormalities, a ruptured hepatic artery aneurysm was diagnosed radiologically. The patient's condition deteriorated rapidly, however, and he died on the second hospital day. Postmortem examination revealed a 10-cm aneurysm involving the proximal hepatic artery and celiac axis (Fig. 4–61c), containing a laminated bland thrombus. Rupture had occurred with massive hemorrhage extraperitoneally on the right.

Bleeding from the splenic artery assumes a similar distribution, but a frequent associated finding is a localized change in the region of the splenic flexure of the colon, especially along its lateral margin (Fig. 4–62a). This is secondary to extension of the hemorrhage into the phrenicocolic ligament[64] at this level (Fig. 4–62b).

A specific structural lesion can be identified ultimately in most instances of bleeding into the anterior pararenal space. I have only rarely encountered a case of spontaneous, nontraumatic

**Fig. 4–61. Acute bleeding in right anterior pararenal space.**
**(a)** At the time of initial oral cholecystogram, extraperitoneal fat is intact, allowing visualization of the hepatic angle and flank stripe (arrows) and psoas muscle.
**(b)** Film obtained the next day during abdominal catastrophe documents acute loss of the hepatic angle associated with a diffuse density throughout the right abdomen. Significantly, the flank stripe (arrows) is preserved.
**(c)** Gross specimen. Ruptured hepatic artery aneurysm, thrombus removed.

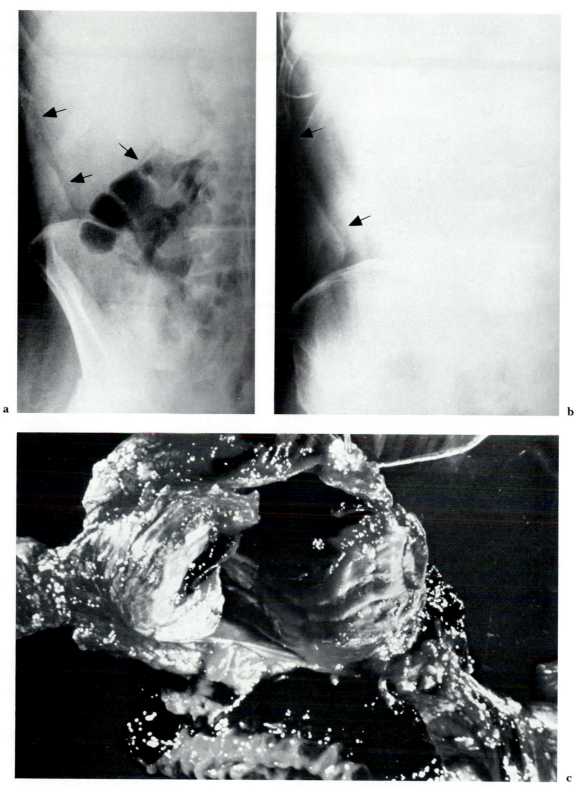

4–61

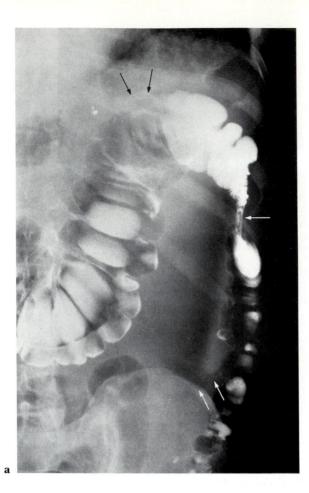

a

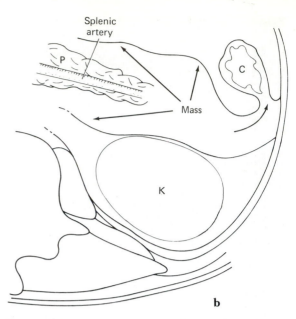

b

Fig. 4–62. Anterior pararenal hemorrhage from a ruptured calcified splenic artery aneurysm (black arrows).

(a) The fluid mass displaces the descending colon laterally as it extends downward within the anterior compartment (white arrows). The prominent localized changes of hematoma in the phrenicocolic ligament on the anatomic splenic flexure of the colon (single white arrow) further localize the effusion to the anterior pararenal space.

(b) Extension from ruptured splenic artery into the anterior pararenal space and into the phrenicocolic ligament. C = colon, P = pancreas, K = kidney. (From Meyers[64])

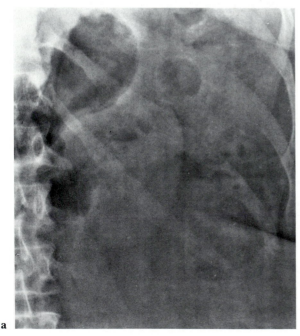

a

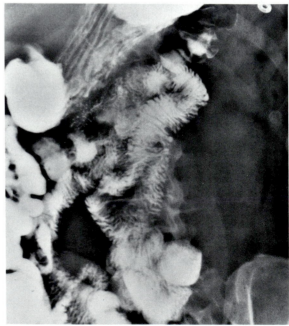

b

4–63

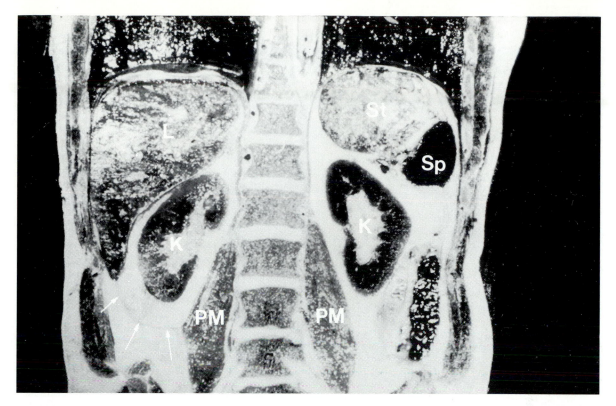

**Fig. 4–64. Coronal anatomic section.**
The cone of renal fascia (arrows) envelops the adrenal gland, kidney (K), and perirenal fat. Medially it blends with the fascia of the psoas muscle (PM). The perirenal fat is particularly abundant in relationship to the lower pole of the kidney. The hepatic angle abuts on pararenal and perirenal fat. L = liver, St = stomach, Sp = spleen. (Courtesy of Manuel Viamonte, Jr. MD, Mt. Sinai Hospital, Miami Beach, Fla.)

hemorrhage in which neither a vascular source nor a bleeding dyscrasia could be diagnosed (Fig. 4–63).

# Perirenal Space

## Roentgen Anatomy of Distribution and Localization of Collections

The perirenal space on each side is distinctly defined by the cone of renal fascia (Figs. 4–64 through 4–66).

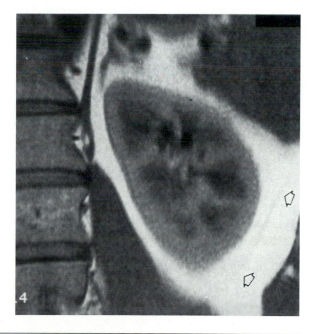

**Fig. 4–65. The edge of the cone and lateroconal fascia (arrows) seen by magnetic resonance imaging on coronal plane.**

**Fig. 4–63. Spontaneous left anterior pararenal hemorrhage** in a middle-aged female with a fall in hematocrit from 34 to 20% within 10 days. No specific etiology could be identified.
**(a)** A left-sided mass is evident but the contours of the kidney and psoas muscle are clearly maintained.
**(b)** Small bowel series. Oblique view demonstrates that the intestine is displaced anteriorly.

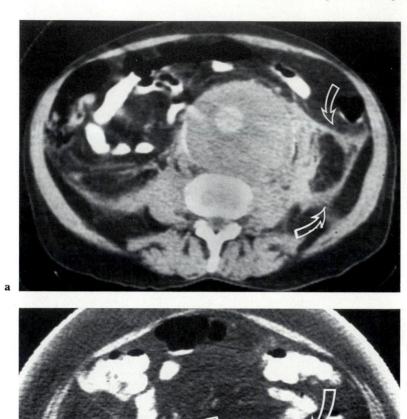

**Fig. 4–66. The lower cone of renal fascia.**
CT shows the narrowed cone of renal fascia on the left near its inferior apex just above the level of the iliac crests (arrows) in two different patients.

Thickening and adjacent changes render it visible secondary to (**a**) a leaking abdominal aortic aneurysm and (**b**) pancreatitis.

Selective opacification of this compartment in the cadaver permits identification of the preferential pathway of spread and the characteristic localizing features. This is shown in Figure 4–67. The space is surprisingly capacious and distention yields a typical outline. The injection study demonstrates that the lower border of the distended cone of renal fascia presents a diagnostic silhouette, inferiorly convex, overlying the region of the iliac crest. Some acute traumatic episodes provide an *in vivo* model and confirm these investigational observations (Figs. 4–68 and 4–69). This outline is the hallmark of perirenal collections and its identification,

therefore, on plain films as well as on other studies (Fig. 4–70) serves reliably to localize a disease process immediately.

The significant criteria for the localization and distinction of collections within the perirenal space are outlined in Table 4–1.

## Sources of Effusions

The overwhelming majority of perirenal *abscesses* are secondary to a renal infection. The underlying condition is most often pyelonephritis, tuberculosis, or carbuncle. Perforation

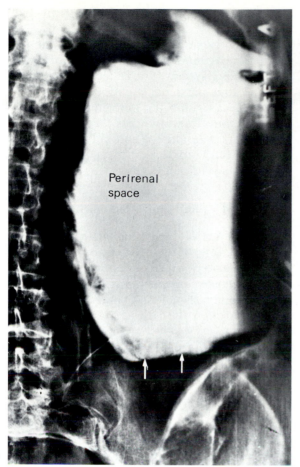

Perirenal
space

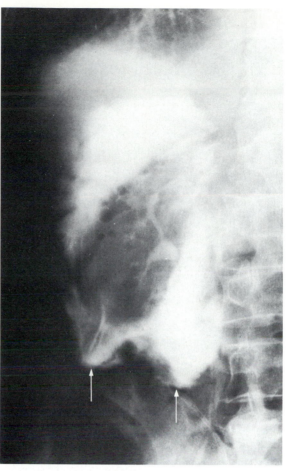

4-67

4-68

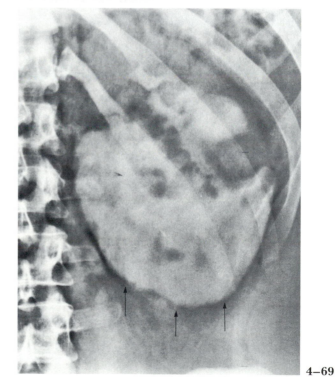

4-69

**Fig. 4-67. Postmortem injection into the perirenal space.**

After the introduction of 450 ml of contrast medium, the distended cone of renal fascia is vertical and presents an inferiorly convex border overlying the iliac crest (arrows).

This contour is highly characteristic of acute fluid distention of the perirenal space. (From Meyers et al[12])

**Fig. 4-68. Opacification of the perirenal space, occurring as a complication of attempted selective renal venography.**

The distended cone extends to the level of the iliac crest. At this level, pressure from the overlying hepatic flexure disrupts the typical inferiorly convex border (arrows).

**Fig. 4-69. Opacification of the perirenal space.**

Gross extravasation during high-dose urography in a case of traumatic fracture of the kidney opacifies the distended perirenal space, demonstrating its convex lower contour (arrows).

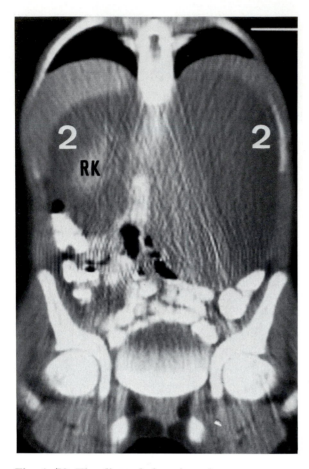

**Fig. 4–70. The distended perirenal space.**
Direct coronal CT section reveals fluid collections in
both perirenal spaces (2). The distended cone of renal fascia on the left extends more inferiorly to the
level of the iliac crest. RK = right kidney. (Reproduced from Feldberg[17])

of the renal capsule then leads to contamination
of the perirenal space.

Two predominant forms are encountered.
An acute gas-producing infection can diffusely
involve the perirenal compartment. It is secondary to *Escherichia coli, Aerobacter aerogenes,* or
rarely, *Clostridium,* and develops especially in di-
abetics. Or, the infection may localize within the
perirenal fat as a coalescent abscess. The offending organism is usually *E. coli, B. proteus,* or
a streptococcus. Bilateral involvement is rare
and is secondary to bilateral renal infections. In
children, hematogenous spread occasionally occurs to the perirenal fat from remote sites of
infection, such as furunculosis, wound infection, or upper respiratory disease.[68a]

Chronic extravasation of *urine* into the perirenal compartment is a result of perforation of
the collecting system. The collection develops as
a uriniferous perirenal pseudocyst (urinoma).

*Hematomas* within the perirenal space as well
as within the subcapsular zone, are secondary to
trauma or to lesions of the kidneys and their
blood vessels, ranging from neoplasms to periarteritis nodosa.

## Perirenal Gas-Producing Infection

The radiologic features of a perirenal space gas-
producing infection are distinctive. Their recognition is related directly to an understanding of
the characteristic appearance of the acutely distended cone of renal fascia and the preferential
spread through the rich perirenal fat dorsal to
the kidney.

The gas may encircle the kidney or present as
a mottled collection of radiolucencies within the
shadows of the perirenal fat. Figure 4–71 illustrates the typical distribution in a diabetic female. Three characteristic features localize the
infection to the perirenal space:

(a) associated exudate distends the cone of
renal fascia so that its lower border can be identified as an inferiorly convex shadow overlying
the iliac crest;

(b) the gas is most prominent within the rich
fat posterior to the kidney; and

(c) inflammatory thickening of the renal fascia itself may be seen.

The inferiorly convex border of the distended perirenal space is a highly reliable localizing sign (Fig. 4–72). Figure 4–73a demonstrates this finding at an early stage in a diabetic
patient with pyelonephritis and fever. Twenty-
four hours later (Fig. 4–73b), a diffuse gas-producing infection of the perirenal space becomes
apparent. When localization occurs, it preferentially develops posterior to the kidney (Fig.
4–74).

Fulminating infection may disrupt the perirenal fascial boundaries, allowing the gas to
escape to other compartments. Figure 4–75
demonstrates acute fascial violation with direct
extension into the flank fat. The resulting decompression of the perirenal space may not distend it to the level of the iliac crest, but it tends
to maintain a diagnostic silhouette with an inferiorly convex lower border.

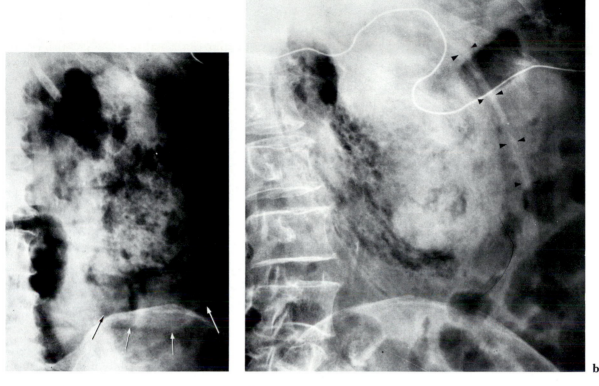

a                                                                                                                             b

**Fig. 4–71. Acute gas-producing left perirenal abscess.**
(a) In addition to the mottled gaseous radiolucencies, fluid distention of the renal fascial cone overlies the iliac crest, presenting a typical convex inferior border (arrows).
(b) Oblique view demonstrates the preponderance of gas and fluid in the perirenal fat dorsal to the kidney. Inflammatory thickening of the anterior renal fascia is shown as a striplike density (arrowheads). (From Meyers[8])

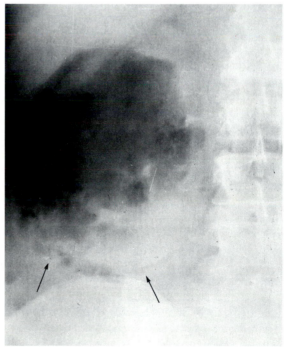

**Fig. 4–72. Right perirenal gas-producing infection in a diabetic.**
A convex lower border (arrows) at the level of the iliac crest characterizes the distended cone of renal fascia.

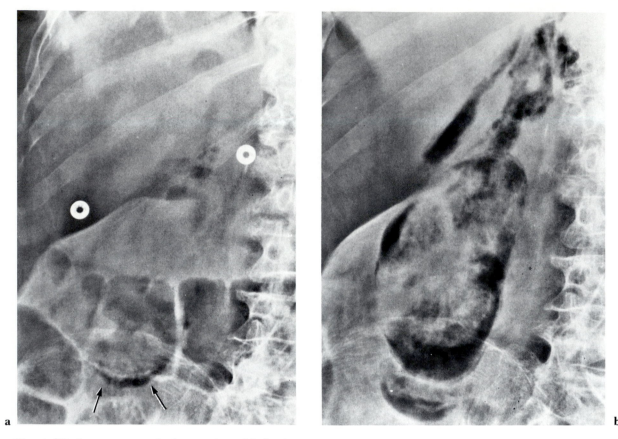

**Fig. 4–73. Acute gas-producing perirenal infection.**
**(a)** In addition to a few ill-defined mottled lucencies in the right flank, a crescentic gas collection (arrows) overlies the iliac crest.
**(b)** The next day, extensive infection has developed throughout the perirenal space.

Bilateral perirenal gas-producing infections are unusual but their contours are again distinctive (Fig. 4–76). In such instances septic emboli or retrograde pyelonephritis from the bladder should be particularly considered.

## Perirenal Abscess

Initially, fluid introduced into the perirenal space is evenly dispersed throughout the perirenal fat. Preferential flow then seeks the abundant fat dorsolateral to the lower pole of the kidney[8,12] (Figs. 4–77 and 4–78). The exudate is guided by gravity along the path of least resistance. This natural drainage is also illustrated in Figure 4–79, in which a portion of a large staghorn calculus has eroded through the kidney to ultimately seek out the area of rich fat behind and lateral to the lower pole. It is important to understand that the coalescence at this

particular site forms the basis for the radiologic identification of most perirenal abscesses.[8,12]

As a rule, a single finding is nonspecific because it may be due to some other disease. But in combination, radiologic signs usually permit the correct diagnosis.[66]

For practical application, roentgen signs may be divided into primary and secondary groups. *Primary roentgen signs* include the following (see Figs. 4–80 through 4–85):

1. *Loss of definition of the lower renal outline* with increased density or an identifiable discrete mass in the region of the kidney.

2. *Displacement and, perhaps, axial rotation of the kidney.* The lower pole is displaced medially, upward and anteriorly, and the kidney may be rotated about its vertical axis.

On frontal supine films, the affected kidney

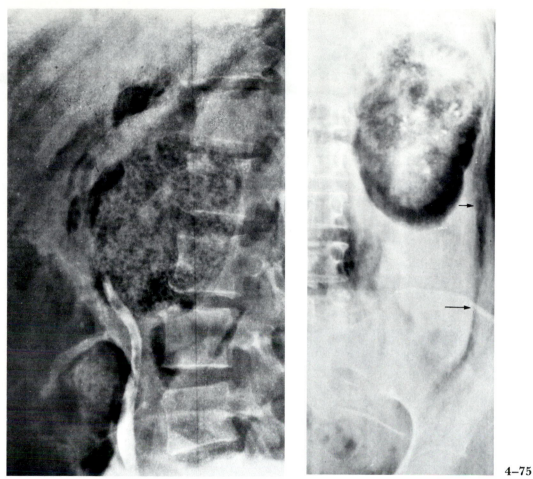

4–74                                                                              4–75

**Fig. 4–74. Localized gas-producing perirenal infection.**
The process has localized behind the kidney, displacing it anteriorly (lateral view, retrograde study).

**Fig. 4–75. Perirenal gas-producing infection.**
The process has broken into and extends down the flank fat (arrows). Lateral view, retrograde study.

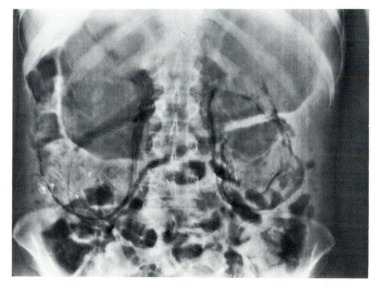

Fig. 4–76. Bilateral perirenal gas-producing infections.

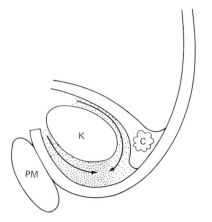

**Fig. 4–77. Coalescence of perirenal effusions.**
This typically develops behind and somewhat lateral to the lower pole of the kidney. K = kidney, C = colon, PM = psoas muscle.

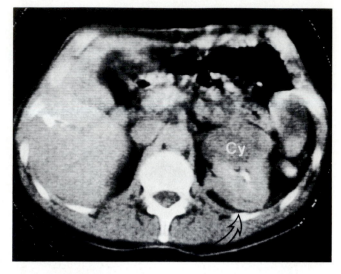

△

**Fig. 4–78. Perirenal hematoma.**
Following percutaneous puncture of a left renal cyst (Cy), CT scan shows a collection of blood (arrow) localized to the perirenal fat behind the kidney.

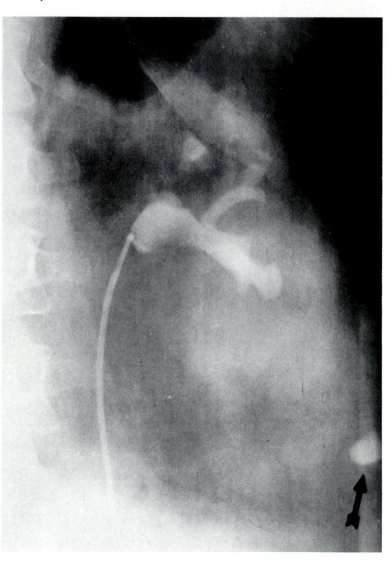

**Fig. 4–79. Chipped piece of staghorn calculus** (arrow).
This has gravitated to the rich perirenal fat behind and lateral to the lower pole of the kidney. Plain film with opaque ureteral catheter.

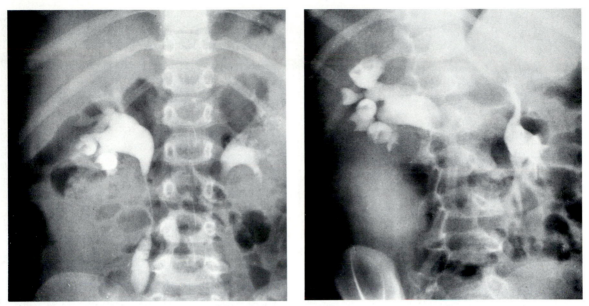

**Fig. 4–80. Right perirenal abscess.**
The infection is localized behind the lower pole, resulting in anterior, medial, and superior displacement of the kidney.
**(a)** The affected kidney appears larger because of the magnification resulting from its anterior displacement. There is loss of the renal outline and the hepatic angle. Extension of the infection along the ureter has caused mild ureteropelvic obstruction.
**(b)** On oblique projection, the abscess itself is visualized as a mass density.
(From Meyers[8])

**Fig. 4–81. Right perirenal abscess.**
The collection in the dorsolateral fat near the lower pole displaces the kidney upward and medially, deflects the upper ureter medially, and obscures the proximal psoas margin. Note the loss of contrast of the perirenal fat and renal outline.
(From Evans et al[66])

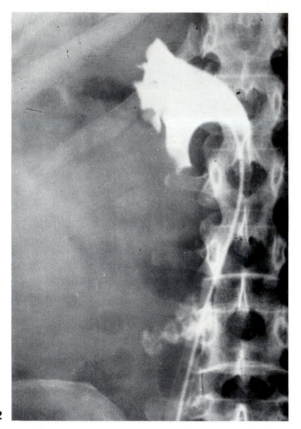

4–82

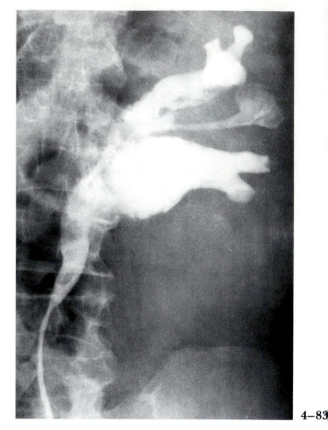

4–83

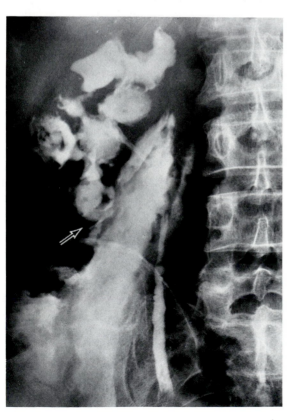

4–84

**Fig. 4–82. Perirenal abscess.**
Retrograde pyelogram shows characteristic upward
and medial displacement of the kidney and proximal
ureter with axial rotation of the kidney by a large
mass. There is loss of visualization of the renal outline and psoas margin. (From Evans et al[66])

**Fig. 4–83. Large left perirenal abscess.**
This displaces the lower pole anteromedially and
results in renal magnification. Gross inflammatory
disease involves the collecting system. (From Meyers[8])

**Fig. 4–84. Extensive perirenal abscess draining into
the iliac fossa beyond the confines of the renal fascia.**
The abscess originated from a lower calyx (arrow) in
a kidney involved by severe pyonephrosis.

may appear larger because of magnification; a lateral film will then document its anterior displacement. The suspected side should be dependent for the lateral view since in this position a kidney in its normal location does not project anterior to the lumbar spine.

3. *Loss of the upper segment of the psoas muscle margin.*

4. *Extrinsic compression of the renal pelvis and proximal ureter.* The mass tends to press from the lateral aspect so that the proximal ureter may also be displaced anteriorly over the psoas muscle as well as medially. Compression may be severe enough to cause dilatation of the upper collecting system.

5. *Fixation of the kidney.* Normal renal mobility of 2–6 cm can be shown on erect views or with respiratory excursions.[67] A perirenal process tends to fix the kidney in most patients.

6. *Extravasation into the perirenal space.* Communication of the collecting system with the perirenal compartment is presumptive evidence of a perirenal abscess in all but the most acute circumstances. The extravasation may be demonstrated by retrograde pyelography or fistulography.

7. *Displacement of contiguous bowel.* A collection of pus in the perirenal compartment may produce a mass effect on adjacent intestine. On the right, the descending duodenum may be displaced medially and anteriorly and the hepatic flexure of the colon downward. On the left, the distal transverse colon may be displaced superiorly or inferiorly and the duodenojejunal junction medially.

8. *Arteriographic findings.* Arteriography may be of particular value in cases where the conventional radiographic findings are uncertain or where primary renal infection is suspected to extend through the capsule. The angiogram may define the size and location of the abscess. Characteristically, the findings include an increased number and size of perforating arteries extending from the kidney, stretching of tortuous and prominent capsular and, perhaps, pelvic arteries around the margin of the abscess, and a contrast blush.

9. *Infiltration of flank stripe.* This indicates fulminating and widespread extension into the adjacent tissues.

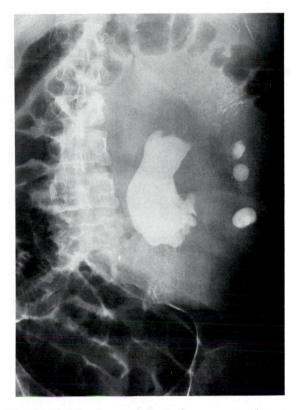

**Fig. 4–85. Massive perirenal abscess secondary to calculous pyonephrosis.**
Plain film shows increased density, loss of kidney outline, and numerous renal calculi. The abscess has displaced the transverse and descending colon.

*Secondary roentgen signs* include the following:

1. *Scoliosis.* This occurs in less than half the patients with perirenal abscess.

2. *Restriction of diaphragmatic motility and pulmonary basilar changes.* Nesbit and Dick[68] showed that of 85 patients with perirenal abscess, 14 (16.5%) had pulmonary complications. These may vary from a minimal pleuritis to effusion, pneumonia, and nephrobronchial fistula. Excursion of the ipsilateral hemidiaphragm, especially its posterior segment, may be restricted or absent.

Treatment of perirenal abscesses is included in the discussion on page 249.

## Uriniferous Perirenal Pseudocyst (Urinoma)

A unique type of perirenal collection is acutely extravasated urine secondary to ureteral ob-

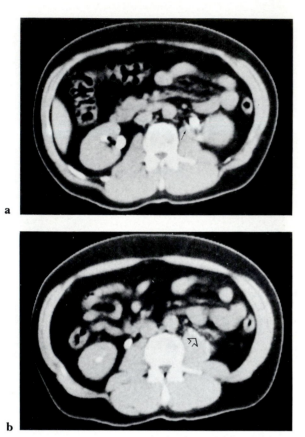

**Fig. 4–86. Periureteral urine extravasation, secondary to an obstructing calculus.**
(**a** and **b**) Enhanced CT scan shows opacified urine extravasating around the proximal ureter (arrow) within the cone of renal fascia. Its inclination along the lateral border of the psoas muscle (open arrow) explains the latter's radiographic loss of visualization which ordinarily occurs in such situations. (From Love et al[7])

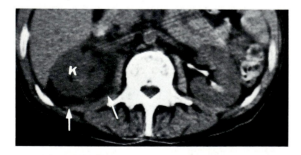

**Fig. 4–87. Early development of uriniferous perirenal pseudocyst.**
CT scan at level of both kidneys shows right kidney (K) with mild hydronephrosis displaced anteriorly by perirenal urine collection (arrows). This occurred as a consequence of pyelosinus backflow secondary to partial distal ureteral obstruction from a retroperitoneal mass.

struction (Figs. 4–86 and 4–87). It has been long established that chronic partial obstruction with repeated pyelosinus backflow may lead to uriniferous pseudocyst formation.[69]

The chronic extravasation of urine into the extraperitoneal tissues around the kidney and upper part of the ureter, leading to an encapsulated collection, is a distinct clinical and radiologic entity. The condition has been given a variety of confusing names, including pseudohydronephrosis, hydrocele renalis, perirenal cyst, perinephric cyst, pararenal pseudocyst, and urinoma. Unfortunately, each of these terms is misleading, nonspecific, or inaccurate. The most accurate designation for this condition should be uriniferous perirenal pseudocyst.[10]

Since the chronic urine extravasation occurs into the perirenal space, with aseptic inflammation and dissolution of its fat, the contents of the pseudocyst are confined by the cone of renal fascia which comes to constitute its walls.[10]

*Etiology and Pathogenesis.* Most cases of chronic urinary extravasation are secondary to accidental or iatrogenic trauma. Early reports stress renal and ureteral trauma from automobile accidents, football injuries, blows, falls, etc. At the time of clinical presentation, the nature of the original injury may not be recognized or may be remote in nature. More recently, instances are being encountered after surgical operations on the kidney or ureter, diagnostic cystoscopic procedures with perforation of the ureter or renal pelvis, or inadvertent trauma to the lower ureter during pelvic operations. In infants and children, a congenital obstruction in the urinary tract may be an underlying factor.[70]

Three factors are necessary to produce the lesion[71]:

1. A transcapsular tear of the renal parenchyma must extend into the calyx or pelvis. Perforations of the pelvis or ureter alone are often sufficient.
2. The injury must fail to heal or fail to be sealed off with a blood clot before leakage of urine in any quantity can take place. Urinary extravasation into the perirenal fat results in rapid lipolysis and a definite fibrous sac (false capsule or pseudocyst) is formed within 12 days.[72] Pseudocysts of up to 2500 ml of urine have been reported. There may also be fatty, fibrous, or oily

debris, altered blood clot, or deposits of urinary salts.

3. Ureteral obstruction must be present. It may be caused by a previous pathologic condition, by a transient blood clot within the ureter or a periureteral hematoma, or from fibrosis secondary to the injury. Indeed, the tissue reaction itself results in a continuing element of obstruction establishing a vicious cycle. The ureter may be bound down by scar tissue as it lies embedded in the newly formed sac wall. The necessarily slow development of scar tissue readily explains the typically delayed formation of the mass. The hydrokinetic system then reaches stability only when autonephrectomy occurs.

*Clinical Signs and Symptoms.* The usual clinical presentation of a uriniferous perirenal pseudocyst is a palpable flank mass associated with some degree of abdominal distress, often mild in nature. The mass is generally only slightly tender to palpation and there is little, if any, increase in temperature. Urinalysis is often completely negative. A typical sequence is general improvement after the original abdominal trauma, followed by the delayed appearance of a flank mass. The latent period between the traumatic episode and the appearance of symptoms and a mass is often 1 to 4 months.[73] The mass has occasionally been noted to increase rapidly in size.[71,74] Sauls and Nesbit[75] observed a latent period of 2 years, and Johnson and Smith reported an unusual case of a calcified pseudocyst diagnosed 37 years after the presumed trauma.[76]

*Radiologic Findings.* Since perirenal effusions localize according to the effect of gravity and planes of least resistance, extravasated urine seeks out the portion of the cone of renal fascia caudad to the kidney. Basic to an appreciation of the characteristic complex of radiographic abnormalities is the fact that the pseudocyst typically conforms to the axis and dimensions of the cone of renal fascia (Fig. 4–88), as encountered at surgery (Fig. 4–89). Slow, persistent effusion within the cone of renal fascia distends

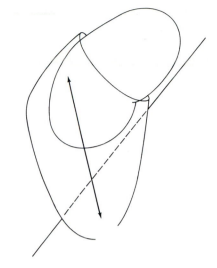

**Fig. 4–88. Cone of renal fascia.**
The two layers of renal fascia completely envelop the kidney and perirenal fat. They fuse in such a manner that the perirenal space bears an axis inferiorly (to the level of the iliac crest) and medially (overlying the lower segment of the psoas muscle). (From Meyers[8])

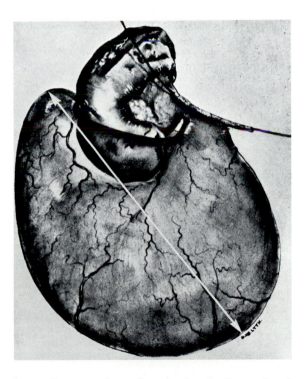

**Fig. 4–89. Surgical specimen of uriniferous perirenal pseudocyst and nonfunctioning hydronephrotic kidney.**
Operation was performed 3 months after a traumatic pelvilithotomy. Note that the findings show massive urine distention of the thickened cone of renal fascia, which nevertheless maintains its characteristic axis downward and medially. (Reproduced from Pyrah and Smiddy[77])

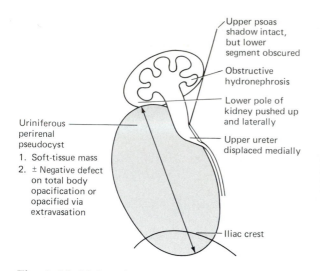

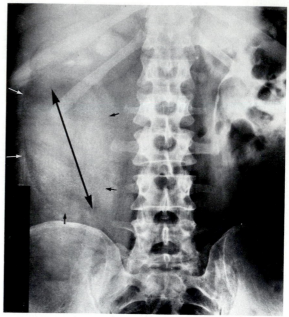

**Fig. 4–90. Major characteristic radiologic changes secondary to uriniferous perirenal pseudocyst.**
Basic are the axis and relationships of the chronically distended cone of renal fascia. (From Meyers[10])

**Fig. 4–91. Uriniferous perirenal pseudocyst post-pelvilithotomy.**
Intravenous urogram shows the lower pole of the partially obstructed right kidney displaced upward and laterally by a large elliptical soft-tissue mass (small arrows). The axis of the mass is characteristically oriented inferomedially. Its contours are further highlighted by the contrast provided by posterior pararenal fat into which it bulges posteriorly. The proximal ureter is displaced medially and is dilated, associated with caliectasis and a mild obstructive nephrogram.

Incision and drainage of 1500 ml of urine, nephrostomy, and a splinted ureterostomy were followed by marked improvement. (From Meyers[10])

the perirenal space but allows it to retain its characteristic axis. This phenomenon accounts for the diagnostic changes[10] (Fig. 4–90).

The characteristic complex of radiographic abnormalities involves features of the soft tissue mass of the pseudocyst and its effects on the kidney and ureter (Figs. 4–91 through 4–95). In addition, extravasation into the pseudocyst may confirm the actual point of leakage or indicate gross communication with the collecting system.

The most typical and consistent feature of the pseudocyst is that its axis conforms to the distended cone of renal fascia. Thus, it is elliptical in outline and obliquely oriented inferomedially. Its upper border is lateral in the flank as it comes into relationship to the lower pole of the kidney and its lower border is more medial as it overlaps the psoas muscle near the level of the iliac crest. Its contours may be further outlined on plain films by the contrast of other extraperitoneal fat (specifically within the posterior pararenal compartment) into which the pressure of the pseudocyst bulges. With huge collections, the cone of renal fascia may become so distended that its axis appears more vertical.

The pseudocyst can be identified as a soft-tissue density or as a lucent defect during the phase of total body opacification. Needle opacification of the pseudocyst may outline precisely its contour, size, and characteristic axis.

The kidney is usually displaced upward and its lower pole characteristically deviated laterally. The fat immediately around the kidney and upper third of the psoas muscle can be visualized intact, but the lower margin of the psoas muscle is obscured by the pseudocyst. The involved kidney shows poor and delayed function or absent excretion on intravenous urography. Hydronephrosis is apparent on delayed films or on retrograde pyelography. The upper ureter is usually deviated medially, occasionally across the midline, but this may require retrograde studies for demonstration. The catheter is often arrested in the upper third of the ureter.

Extravasation into the area of the pseudocyst may be seen on excretory urography or on retrograde pyelography. Opacification of the mass may be noted at the same time as the nephrogram during intravenous urography or as the

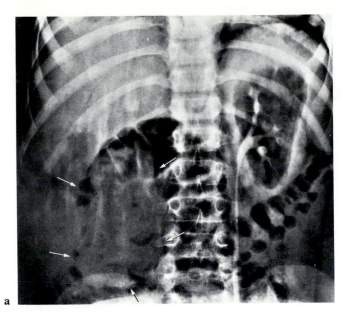

a

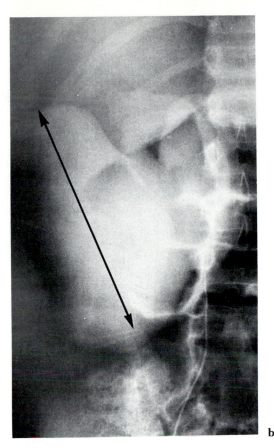

b

**Fig. 4–92. Uriniferous perirenal pseudocyst postpelvilithotomy.**

**(a)** Total body opacification during intravenous urography outlines a lucent mass (arrows). The right kidney is partially obstructed and is displaced upward and laterally.

**(b)** Contrast opacification of pseudocyst through drainage needle confirms its inferomedial axis. Residual contrast from retrograde pyelography shows obstructive uropathy proximal to the strictured and displaced ureter. (From Meyers[10])

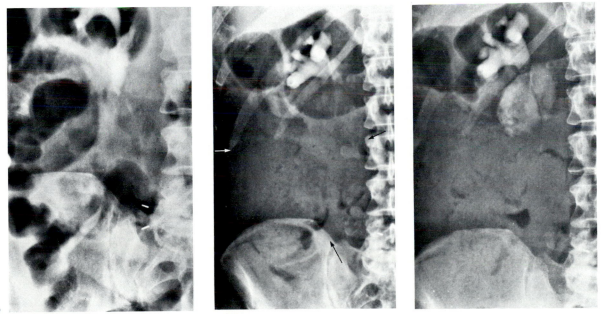

a,b

c

**Fig. 4–93. Uriniferous perirenal pseudocyst.**

**(a)** Following accidental partial interruption of the right ureter at the time of retroperitoneal lymph node dissection, intravenous urography demonstrates extravasation of urine.

**(b)** Three weeks later, there is evidence of a large encapsulated mass (arrows) extending to the level of the iliac crest, with obstruction of the proximal right ureter and hydronephrosis. The lower pole of the kidney is displaced superiorly and laterally.

**(c)** Later radiograph shows localized extravasation into the pseudocyst. (From Meyers[10])

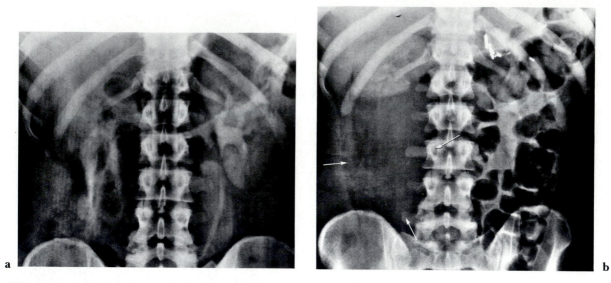

**Fig. 4–94. Uriniferous perirenal pseudocyst.**
**(a)** Following abdominal trauma from an automobile accident, intravenous urography demonstrates extravasation from a poorly functioning right kidney.
**(b)** Ten days later, after emergency gastrectomy and splenectomy, there is evidence of a large soft-tissue mass (arrows) displacing the obstructed kidney upward and laterally and the colon medially. The mass is oriented somewhat inferomedially, extends to the level of the iliac crest, and is outlined as relatively lucent by the effect of total-body opacification.
(From Meyers[10])

patient's position is changed from supine to prone.

Arteriography demonstrates no inflammatory or neoplastic hypervascularity associated with the mass and may be helpful in further evaluating the position and state of function of the kidney.

Ultrasonography may demonstrate the cystic nature of the mass, its size and position, as well as the presence of hydronephrosis and the level of obstruction.[78,79] Isotopic studies may also reveal the characteristic findings[79,80] (Fig. 4–96).

Computed tomography clearly demonstrates the size, position, and relationships of the pseudocyst and may document continuing extravasation by virtue of its opacification[81] (Figs. 4–97 through 4–101).

Unusual sites of development of uriniferous pseudocyst may be a consequence of surgery, instrumentation, or penetrating injury with interruption of anatomic planes.[81]

*Treatment.* It is important to diagnose the condition early so that it can be corrected surgically before inoperable damage to the kidney occurs. The best results have been obtained when surgi-

cal intervention occurred within 2 to 3 weeks after injury. Later, marked fibrosis of the tissues and cicatrization of the ureter make it difficult or impossible to repair or bridge the defect. Nephrostomy drainage with intubation of the repaired ureter is the procedure of choice.[82] If renal function has been lost and the contralateral kidney is normal, nephrectomy is advisable.

## Distinction Between Perirenal and Subcapsular Collections

Abscesses or hematomas in the perirenal space and in the subcapsular region of the kidney can simulate each other and a host of other conditions closely. Identification of their specific localization may be very important in the clinical diagnosis and in determining the most appropriate therapy. Advances in establishing the characteristic features of abscesses or hematomas are based on the anatomic structures that define their collection.[11]

*Anatomic Considerations.* The renal capsule (Fig. 4–102) is a thin tunic that forms an intimate, firm, smooth investment for the kidney. It is composed predominantly of fibrous tissue, but

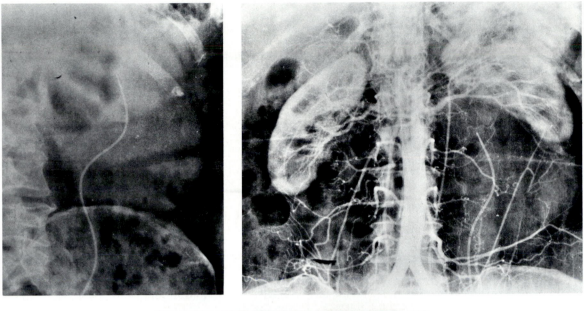

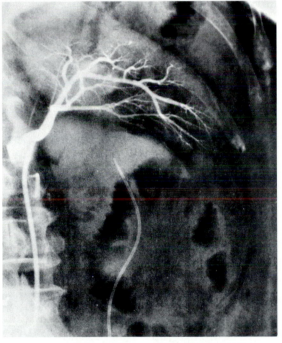

**Fig. 4–95. Uriniferous perirenal pseudocyst 5 weeks after a hysterectomy.**
(a) Plain film. Large soft-tissue mass extends to the level of the iliac crest. Ureteral displacement is shown by the opaque catheter, which could not be passed beyond the UP junction.
(b) Abdominal aortogram. The mass shows no hypervascularity and displaces the lower pole of the left kidney upward and laterally.
(c) By the time the left renal artery is selectively catheterized, extravasation into the pseudocyst becomes evident.
(From Meyers[10])

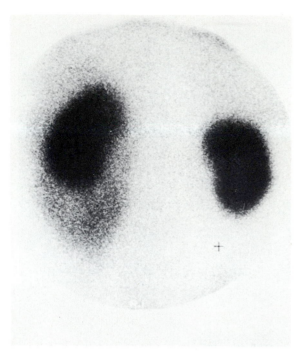

**Fig. 4–96. Uriniferous perirenal pseudocyst,** secondary to obstruction from recurrent invasive carcinoma of the rectum. Posterior radionuclide image demonstrates the left kidney elevated and its lower pole deviated laterally by an elliptical extrarenal urine collection of lesser activity. The axis of this is obliquely oriented inferomedially. (Reproduced from Suzuki et al[80])

◁

**Fig. 4–97. Uriniferous perirenal pseudocyst.**
**(a)** CT scan after intravenous injection of contrast medium shows encapsulated pseudocystic collection of extravasated urine (Ps) displacing the left kidney (LK) laterally.
**(b)** At a lower level, it distends the cone of renal fascia medial to the descending colon (DC). The anterior and posterior pararenal fat and the lateroconal fascia (arrow) remain intact. At this stage in the study, there is no opacification of the extravasated urine.
**(c)** Delayed radiograph demonstrates opacification of the pseudocyst which bears a typical axis and renal displacement.

▽

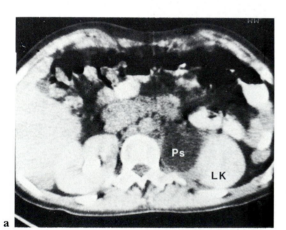

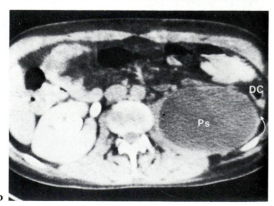

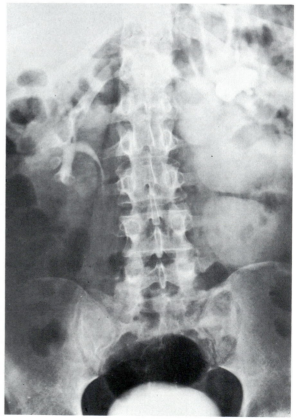

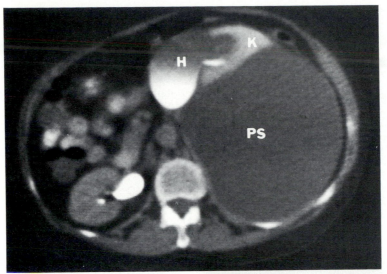

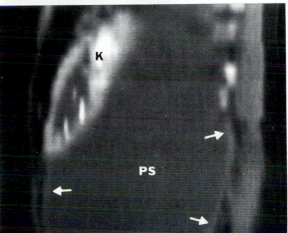

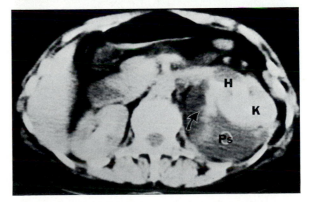

**Fig. 4–98. Uriniferous perirenal pseudocyst** presenting two months after a fall.
**(a)** CT shows large uriniferous pseudocyst within the left perirenal space (Ps), anterior displacement of the kidney (K), and a severely hydronephrotic renal pelvis (H).
**(b)** Sagittal reconstruction demonstrates anterior and superior displacement of the kidney (K) by the large uriniferous pseudocyst (Ps) confined within the cone of thickened renal fascia (arrows).
(Reproduced from Healey et al[81])

there is some smooth muscle within its inner layer. No adipose tissue is found between the renal parenchyma and the capsule. The capsule can be stripped off easily; when this is done, numerous fine processes of connective tissue and small blood vessels are torn through.

The capsular arteries course through and supply primarily the perirenal fat, which is located between the renal capsule and the renal fascia. The somewhat confusing designation of these vessels as "capsular" is apparently derived from the old nomenclature of the perirenal fat as the "adipose capsule of the kidney." They are composed of three basic pathways: superior, middle (recurrent and perforating), and inferior capsular arteries. A prominent arterial arcade is formed within the perirenal fat lateral to the kidney that communicates with renal branches perforating through the capsule.

**Fig. 4–99. Uriniferous perirenal pseudocyst.**
CT in a patient with recurrent carcinoma of the cervix and paraaortic adenopathy demonstrates the left kidney (K) with hydronephrosis (H) displaced anteriorly and laterally by a uriniferous perirenal pseudocyst (Ps). There is extravasation of contrast medium (arrow) into the encapsulated urine collection, decompressing the hydronephrosis.

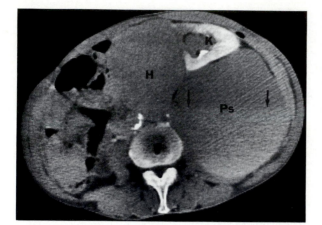

**Fig. 4–100. Uriniferous perirenal pseudocyst.**
CT in a 60-year-old woman 10 weeks after a "fall"
demonstrates a large uriniferous pseudocyst within
the perirenal space (Ps), with contrast medium in its
dependent portion (arrows). Anterior displacement
of the left kidney (K) and a severely hydronephrotic
renal pelvis (H) are also present. (Reproduced from
Healey[81])

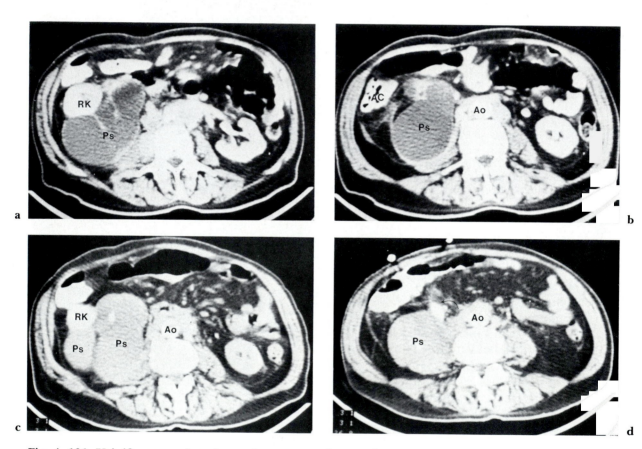

**Fig. 4–101. Uriniferous perirenal pseudocyst,** secondary to obstruction from metastatic carcinoma of the
urinary bladder.
**(a** and **b)** CT scans after intravenous injection of contrast medium show large pseudocystic collection of
extravasated urine (Ps) extending from the right kidney (RK) which it displaced laterally and anteriorly from
the medial border of the psoas muscle. As it extends inferiorly, it remains confined within the cone of renal
fascia medial to the ascending colon (AC). Adhesions or bridging renal septa within the pseudocyst contribute
to mild septation. Metastatic tumor in lymph nodes around the calcified abdominal aorta (Ao) and inferior
vena cava is seen as soft-tissue masses.
**(c** and **d)** Six-hour delayed scans demonstrate a significantly higher CT number within the pseudocyst reflecting active extravasation. It is because of this decompression that although the right ureter is dilated (curved
arrow), the collecting system does not appear obstructed.

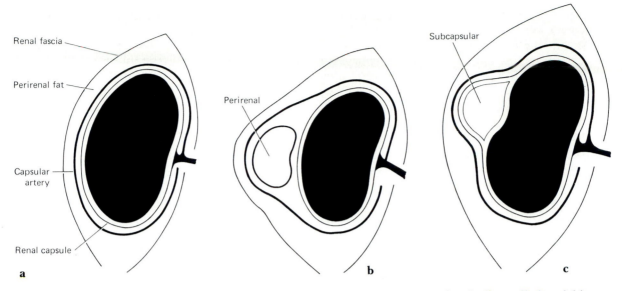

**Fig. 4–102. Normal relationships of investing structures of kidney and major findings distinguishing a perirenal from a subcapsular collection.**
Note particularly the relationships of the displaced renal capsule, perirenal fascia, and capsular arteries at the borders of the mass. Flattening of the underlying renal parenchyma is more commonly found in subcapsular collections. (From Meyers et al[11])

*Etiology and Pathogenesis.* Perirenal *abscesses,* as we have seen, are almost invariably secondary to a site of renal infection that perforates through the capsule to contaminate the perirenal fatty compartment.

Extrarenal *hematomas,* whether subcapsular or perirenal in location, are generally considered either traumatic or spontaneous (nontraumatic). Polkey and Vynalek[65] reported a comprehensive study of the causes of spontaneous hematomas. Of 178 cases reviewed, the location was subcapsular in 18.5% and extracapsular (perirenal or pararenal or a combination of the two) in 81.5%. Lesions of the kidneys and its blood vessels accounted for 92% of the cases. The underlying etiologies, in the order of their relative frequencies, included nephritis, neoplasms, aneurysms of the renal artery, arteriosclerosis, hydronephrosis, periarteritis nodosa, tuberculosis, renal cysts, and blood dyscrasias. Percutaneous renal biopsy results in significant perirenal hematomas in only approximately 0.6%[83] (Fig. 4–103).

In recent years, an increasing number of cases of extrarenal hemorrhage due to periarteritis nodosa and occult, often surprisingly small renal tumors have been reported.[84–87] Many of the earlier cases diagnosed as nephritis

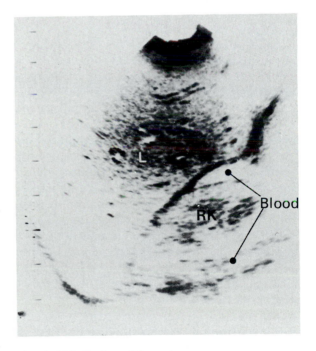

**Fig. 4–103. Perirenal hematoma.**
Parasagittal ultrasonogram after a renal biopsy demonstrates blood within the perirenal space surrounding the right kidney (RK). L = liver.

may have actually been periarteritis nodosa or lupus erythematosus.

Rarely, metastatic disease to the kidneys, especially from vascular tumors such as choriocarcinoma, can cause perirenal hemorrhage.[88] Melanoma and lung cancer tend to involve the kidney and perirenal space contiguously,[89,90] but these do not tend to hemorrhage.

One mechanism of hematoma formation begins with cortical infarcts.[86] The hemorrhage may be confined by the relatively rigid capsule; at other times the blood breaks through the capsule immediately but is confined within the dimensions of the renal fascia. A hematoma within the distensible perirenal compartment can develop to an enormous size before pressure becomes sufficient to cause tamponade of the bleeding site.

The spread of hemorrhage from ruptured abdominal aortic aneurysms depends upon the anatomic level and site of leaking and the amount of extravasated blood. At the level of the kidneys, the aorta lies behind the anterior renal fascia. Thus aortic bleeding may occur directly into the perirenal space.[91,92]

*Clinical Signs and Symptoms.* The clinical diagnosis of subcapsular or perirenal abscess or bleeding is rarely made. Signs and symptoms are often subtle, delayed, nonspecific, or misleading.

With acute bleeding, the clinical picture may consist of pain, tenderness, and rigidity, which may be associated with nausea, vomiting, and abdominal distention. Concomitant signs of internal bleeding may be present, but this may be manifested only by a drop in hemoglobin or hematocrit. A mass may not be palpable, especially if the hematoma lies posteriorly to the kidney. If the hematoma is subcapsular, it may not become particularly large because of the confining effect of the renal capsule, but occasionally the collection may approximate the size of the kidney itself. With sudden and profuse hemorrhages, many types of retroperitoneal and intraperitoneal catastrophes may be mimicked. If the hematoma extends downward in the retrocecal region, the patient may be explored for an acute appendicitis.[93] Rarely, perforation into the peritoneal cavity may occur, causing a generalized peritonitis or a massive intraperitoneal hemorrhage.

With subacute or chronic bleeding, pain may not be a conspicuous feature and the principal findings may be only anemia and, perhaps, a palpable mass.

Hypertension may result from the constrictive renal effects of a large subcapsular[11,94–96] or less commonly a perirenal hematoma, producing the *Page kidney*.[97] If the condition is not particularly chronic, the hypertension may be easily corrected by decompression or nephrectomy.

*Radiologic Findings.* Supcapsular or perirenal hemorrhage or abscess can be indicated on plain films or intravenous urography, and can be clearly documented by nephrotomography or angiography. I have shown that localization of the process to a specific extrarenal compartment is based on recognizing characteristic changes involving the renal capsule, renal fascia, kidney margin, and capsular arteries[11] (Fig. 4–102):

1. *Visualization of the displaced renal capsule or fascia.* Either of these structures, displaced outward from the renal margin, can be seen as a striplike density 1–4 mm thick. The renal fascia can be visualized by plain film roentgenography and urography in cases of perirenal abscess or hematoma (Figs. 4–104 through 4–106). In diffuse processes of the perirenal space, it can be recognized over a considerable length. At times a displaced renal capsule may be demonstrated by urography (Fig. 4–107).

Opacification of the displaced renal capsule (Fig. 4–108) and fascia is achieved in nephrotomography and arteriography,[11,85,98,99] presumably because of their vascularity. Contrast is further afforded by the nonopaque abscess or hematoma on one side and radiolucent fat on the other.

I have noted a type of displacement, which, when present, distinguishes subcapsular from perirenal collections. The renal capsule is sharply deflected over the margin of a subcapsular mass. Even with huge collections, its point of displacement intimately conforms to the border of the hematoma (Fig. 4–108). It appears that this is a consequence of the relatively rigid inelastic nature of the renal capsule. In contrast, renal fascia is often displaced laterally from the margin of the kidney at some distance from a coalescent perirenal collection. Its maximum deflection is at the site of the perirenal hematoma or abscess but it can be seen to depart from close to the renal border both above and below

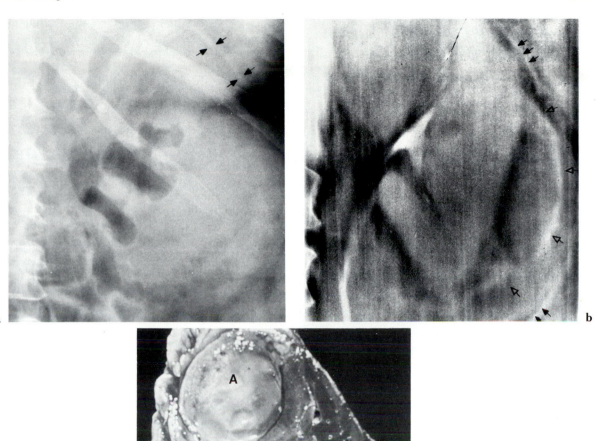

**Fig. 4–104. Multiple perirenal abscesses.**
**(a)** Plain film shows a large mass in relationship to the lower pole of the left kidney. Displaced renal fascia is seen as a striplike density (arrows) lateral to the upper pole.
**(b)** Nephrotomogram demonstrates perirenal mass displacing the renal fascia (solid arrows) and flattening the renal margin. In its upper portion, the displaced renal fascia approaches the renal contour (upper arrows). The thickened lateral wall of the perirenal mass itself is seen (open arrows). Another nonopaque mass compresses the upper pole medially.
**(c)** Gross specimen. Three large perirenal abscesses (A) compress the kidney (K) and displace the thickened renal fascia (arrowheads). Displacement is maximal over the largest abscess but the fascia can be seen to be deflected laterally at some distance from this. This feature is clearly demonstrated radiologically.
(From Meyers et al[11])

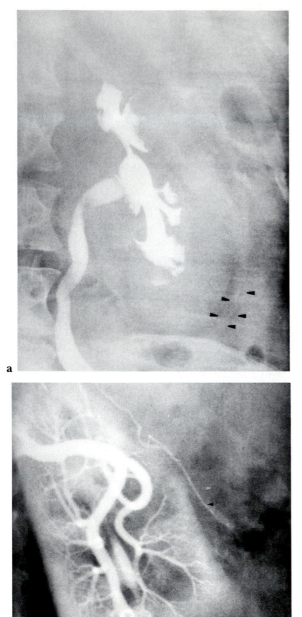

a

**Fig. 4–105. Perirenal abscess communicating with infected renal cysts.**

(a) Intravenous urogram. Mass impressions on lateral minor calyces of the upper pole are secondary to renal cysts. In addition, the renal fascia is seen as a striplike density (arrowheads) lateral to the lower pole.

(b and c) Renal arteriogram. Arterial and nephrogram phases reveal multiple cysts within the left kidney. They appear most confluent within the lower pole where the margin is disrupted. Here the thickened fascia (arrowheads) is displaced laterally. While the superior capsular artery is in close apposition to the upper margin of the kidney, it is displaced outward as it approaches the midportion (upper arrowheads). Some flattening and compression of the renal parenchyma is present at this site.

At surgery, pus was immediately apparent when the renal fascia was opened. There was considerable adherence of the renal fascia and perirenal fat to the kidney. Multiple loculations of pus were found in the perirenal fat. These originated from at least three infected renal cysts. These cysts measured 2–3 cm in diameter, were on the surface of the kidney, and contained thick pus. The perirenal abscesses were drained.

(From Meyers et al[11])

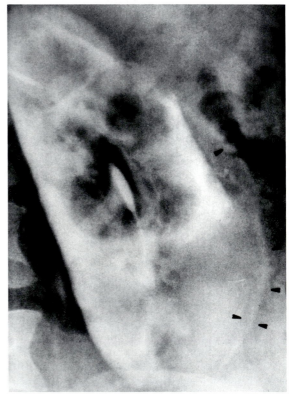

b                                                                                                    c

---

**Fig. 4–106. Perirenal hemorrhage secondary to occult renal tumor.**

(a) Intravenous urogram. Renal fascia is seen as a striplike density (arrows) displaced laterally by a large mass. This also results in loss of definition of the lateral and inferior borders of the kidney.

(b) Renal arteriogram. Perforating capsular arteries extend through the mass to its lateral limit by the dis-

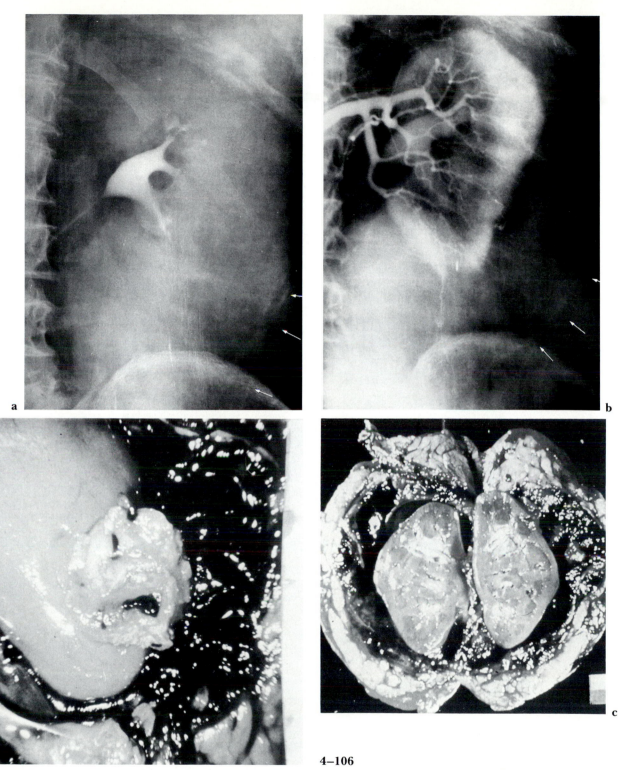

**4–106**

placed renal fascia (arrows). No definite abnormal intrarenal vasculature is identified.

(c) At surgery, a large collection of blood distended the perirenal space, contained within the cone of renal fascia.

Nephrectomy was performed and the pathologic examination disclosed a 3 × 5 × 4 cm infiltrating papillary adenocarcinoma of the lower renal pole.

(d) Bivalved specimen. Extension through the renal capsule had resulted in gross perirenal hemorrhage within the thickened cone of renal fascia.

(From Meyers et al[11])

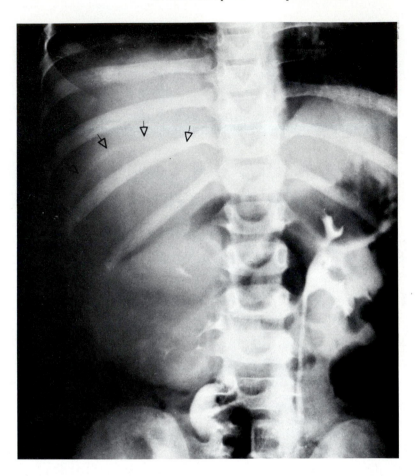

**Fig. 4–107. Subcapsular abscess.**
On the right, the calyces are displaced by a large, relatively lucent mass in the lower half of the kidney. The renal capsule (arrows) is displaced superiorly by a prominent collection that also results in mild compression of the underlying renal margin. The apparent enlargement of the right kidney is secondary to magnification since the kidney is also pushed forward. Decreased function is evident.

At surgery, a large subcapsular abscess containing creamy white pus and some old blood clot was found. The abscess had clearly dissected the capsule off the kidney. It communicated with a large infected thick-walled intrarenal cyst through a small tract along the lateral border of the kidney. It was evident that the cyst accounted for the calyceal deformity and the subcapsular collection also posterior to the kidney accounted for the renal magnification. Drainage and excision of both were accomplished. (From Meyers et al[11])

**Fig. 4–108. Subcapsular hematoma resulting in hypertension ("Page kidney").**
(a) Intravenous urogram. The right kidney is displaced medially. Dilatation of the collecting system and ureter is present.
(b) Nephrotomogram demonstrates the displaced and thickened renal capsule (arrowheads) confining a nonopaque mass that is compressing the lateral contour of the kidney.
(c) Renal arteriogram, arterial phase. The avascular mass compresses the renal parenchyma and vessels, producing a pronounced concave lateral border to the kidney, and displaces the superior capsular artery.

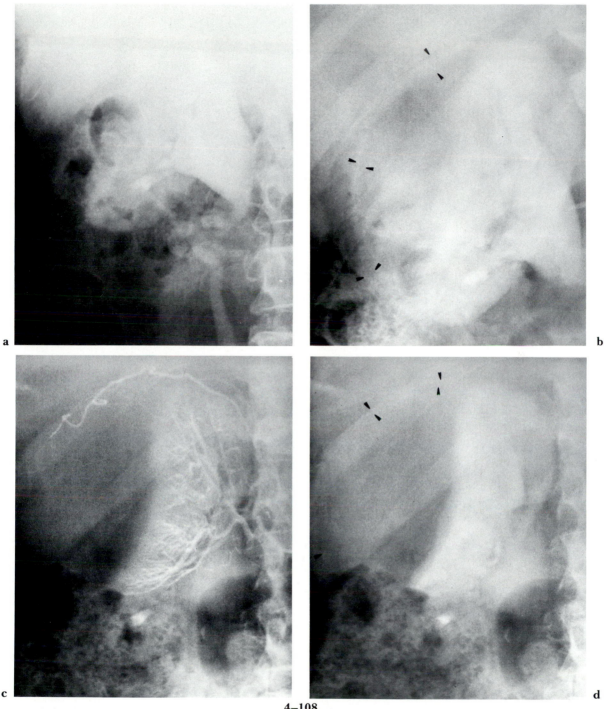

**4–108**

(d) Renal arteriogram, nephrogram phase. The renal capsule (arrowheads) is displaced to the same extent as the capsular artery. The renal parenchyma, while markedly compressed, appears intrinsically intact.

At surgery, a large subcapsular hematoma was confirmed and deep pyelonephritic scars were evident on the surface of the kidney. A right nephrectomy was performed. Pathologic examination confirmed a large, partially organized subcapsular hematoma. A thickened capsule measuring up to 8 mm was present. A 1.2-cm resolving abscess in the midportion of the kidney communicated with the hematoma. Hydronephrosis and generalized pyelonephritis were present. Blood pressure returned to normal after operation. (From Meyers et al[11])

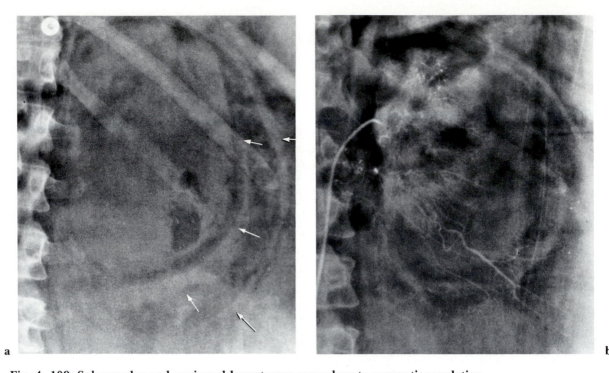

**Fig. 4–109. Subcapsular and perirenal hematomas secondary to overanticoagulation.**
**(a)** Plain film. Two discrete curvilinear densities are seen external to an apparently enlarged renal silhouette. These represent displaced renal capsule (inner arrows) and renal fascia (outer arrows).
**(b)** Renal arteriogram. The kidney itself is not enlarged but rather is compressed by a prominent subcapsular hematoma. Blood in the perirenal space also displaces the renal fascia.

(Fig. 4–104). It is a reflection of the yielding perirenal fat and renal fascia.

At times, simultaneous displacement of both the renal capsule and fascia can be identified (Fig. 4–109).

2. *Visualization of the hematoma or abscess.* The subcapsular or perirenal collection is easily seen as a nonopaque mass between the opacified renal parenchyma on one side and the elevated renal capsule or fascia on the other. This is most often seen in relationship to the lower pole posterolaterally.

3. *Flattening and compression of the kidney.* While this may occur with tense perirenal collections, it is more typical of subcapsular hematoma. The pressure exerted by a confined subcapsular hematoma typically causes flattening of the subjacent renal parenchyma.

4. *Displacement of capsular arteries.* The capsular arteries may be displaced externally in either condition. Examples of conspicuous arcuate displacements and stretching of the capsular artery system in cases of both subcapsular and perirenal hematomas and abscesses have been amply documented in the literature. Rather, I have noted that the level of displacement of the capsular arterial arcade is the angiographic key to the differential diagnosis. If the vessel conforms closely to the border of the mass, a subcapsular collection is indicated (Fig. 4–108c). If deviation of the capsular artery begins at some distance from the extrarenal mass, a perirenal collection is indicated (Fig. 4–105b).

As a differential point, it must be recognized that the capsular arteries will be separated from the cortical margin in cases of renal atrophy[100] (Fig. 4–110). Perirenal adipose replacement in instances of acquired shrinkage of the kidney tends to increase the distance between the capsular artery and the atrophied kidney. This separation can be distinguished easily from a subcapsular or perirenal mass displacing the capsular artery.

The marked increase in intrarenal vascular resistance produced particularly by a large subcapsular hematoma may result in striking slow-

**Fig. 4–110. Chronic atrophic pyelonephritis.**
The nephrographic phase of a selective renal arteriogram shows the capsular arcade (arrows) widely separated from the shrunken renal parenchyma. (From Meyers et al[11])

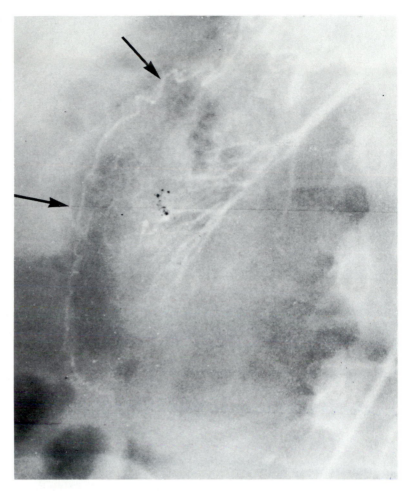

**Fig. 4–111. Right perirenal hematoma and left psoas hematoma.**
CT scan during bolus injection in a patient on anticoagulant therapy shows retroperitoneal hemorrhage (H) of the left psoas muscle which deviates the kidney laterally. The perirenal and posterior pararenal spaces are intact.

On the right side, the hemorrhage (H) is perirenal in location and displaces the kidney ventrally and medially. The posterior pararenal space is intact. (Reproduced from Love et al[7])

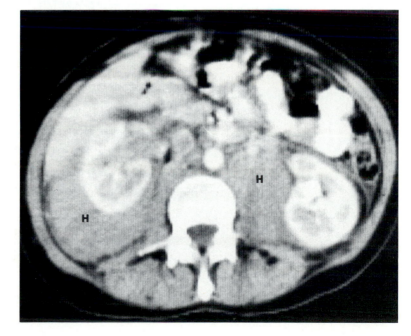

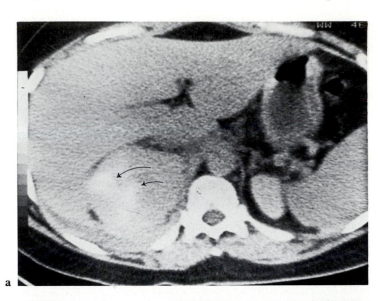

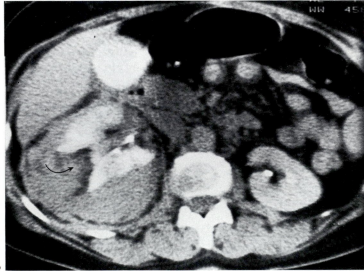

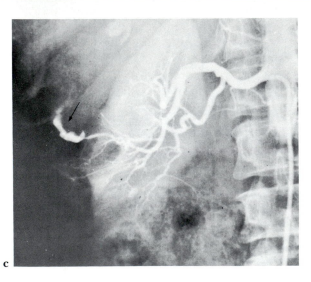

**Fig. 4–112. Perirenal hemorrhage secondary to renal angiomyolipoma.**

(a) CT scan after intravenous contrast medium demonstrates active bleeding (arrows) into hemorrhagic collection within right perirenal space.

(b) At a lower level, blood distends the perirenal space. A structure of low attenuation density (arrow) corresponds to a defect in the nephrogram. This represents the fatty nature of the parenchymal tumor from which bleeding has occurred.

(c) Selective right renal arteriogram demonstrates active bleeding (arrow) into the perirenal space from vessels associated with the tumor mass.

(Courtesy of Daniel Wise, MD, Toronto Western Hospital, Toronto, Canada)

**Fig. 4–113. Intrarenal rupture of abdominal aortic aneurysm.**
Enhanced CT scan shows a low-density tubular mass extending from the aorta directly into the left renal hilus. This originated from a localized aortic aneurysm which ruptured along the renal vascular pedicle. The posterior peri- and pararenal spaces are intact. This case indicates that the renal vascular pedicle may provide an avenue for dissection of blood into the perirenal space. (Reproduced from Gavant[129])

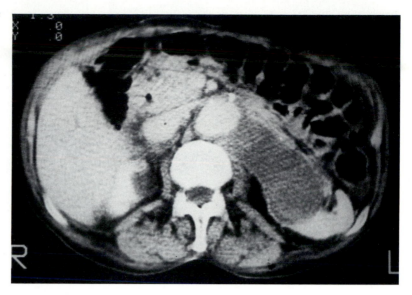

ing of arterial flow with failure of opacification of the small intrarenal and capsular vessels.[86]

5. *Structure and function of the renal collecting system.* Distortion of the calyces and renal pelvis may accompany any gross displacement of the kidney itself. Since perirenal abscesses result from a site of renal infection that has perforated through the capsule, chronic inflammatory changes involving the calyces may be evident. An intrarenal abscess or hematoma may produce mass displacement upon the collecting system.

Failure of excretion of contrast medium on the involved side ("unilateral anuria") can result from the compression of either a perirenal or subcapsular hematoma.[101]

Computed tomography provides a rapid, noninvasive, and highly accurate method to evaluate and distinguish the presence of subcapsular and perirenal bleeding.[7,102–104] By virtue of its ability to discriminate very small differences in tissue density, CT confirms and readily makes apparent the characteristic anatomic features permitting localization of the collections (Figs. 4–111 through 4–116).

*Bridging Renal Septa.* The distribution of perirenal fluid may be limited by the bridging renal septa. Compartmentalization of a fluid collection by this internal architecture of the perirenal fat, particularly the posterior renorenal bridging septum, may mimic a subcapsular collection[38] (Figs. 4–117 and 4–118). At times, on CT,

a black line separating the renal parenchyma from the hematoma may be seen, perhaps representing the swollen renal capsule.[38] I have observed two further differential features in that fluid may further extend within continuous branching septa and the collection may taper to a beak-shape along one contour at the site of traction by an attached septum (Fig. 4–118).

*Treatment.* These observations on the localization of subcapsular and perirenal collections are of considerable help in planning the most appropriate therapy. Whether the underlying cause is predominantly unilateral kidney disease or a systemic condition involving both kidneys must be considered.[105] With the recognition that most extrarenal abscesses are secondary to an infection of the kidney, conservative treatment perhaps with surgical drainage or nephrectomy is determined by the extent of involvement. In subcapsular or perirenal hematoma in the presence of a renal tumor, hydronephrosis, renal artery aneurysm, lithiasis, or unilateral renal tuberculosis, nephrectomy does not present any significant long-term problem. On the other hand, if the etiology is nephritis, arteriosclerosis, periarteritis nodosa, or a blood dyscrasia and nephrectomy must be performed as a life-saving procedure, careful follow-up observation of the remaining kidney must be maintained. If the hematoma is not large and adequate visualization of the bleeding site can be obtained, so that it can be controlled with sutures, a biopsy of the

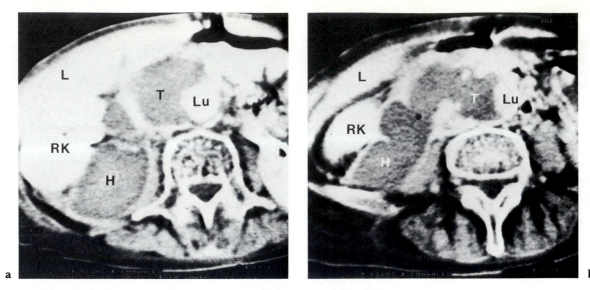

**Fig. 4–114. Perirenal hemorrhage from ruptured aneurysm of the abdominal aorta.**
**(a** and **b)** Enhanced CT demonstrates chronic hemorrhage (H) localizing in the posteromedial portion of the perirenal space displacing the right kidney (RK). There is thickening of Gerota's fascia. An inflammatory pseudomembrane has developed between the hematoma and the kidney. There is no involvement of the posterior pararenal fat in continuity with the flank fat.

The blood originates from a rupture of a large calcified aneurysm of the abdominal aorta. It contains a large thrombus (T) and only the residual lumen (Lu) is opacified. At the lower level, the precise site of leakage (*) from the aneurysm is shown. L = liver.

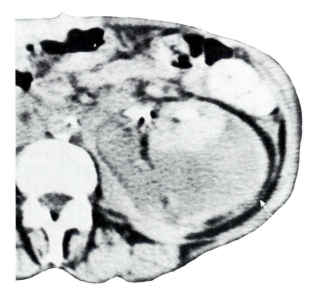

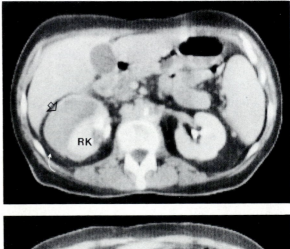

**Fig. 4–115. Subcapsular hematoma.**
CT scan demonstrates that a tense collection of blood has stripped the renal capsule on the left and displaces the kidney anteriorly. The perirenal fat, including the portion outlining the lateral border of the psoas muscle, and Gerota's fascia (curved arrow) are clearly maintained.

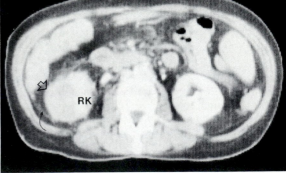

**Fig. 4–116. Subcapsular hematoma.**
**(a** and **b)** Enhanced CT scans shows a large collection of blood which strips the thickened capsule (open arrows) and compresses the lateral aspect of the right kidney (RK). Gerota's fascia is maintained (curved arrow). (From Love et al[7])

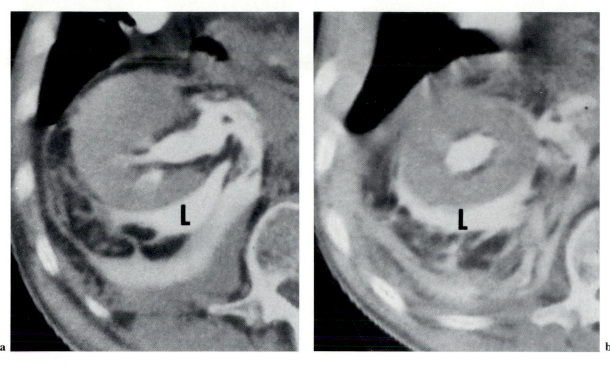

**Fig. 4–117. Contrast extravasation during percutaneous nephrostomy outlines bridging perirenal septa.**
**(a** and **b)** Fortuitous in vivo CT observations at two levels show multiple septa through the perirenal fat and contrast loculation (L) by a bridging dorsal renorenal septum. Note that the medial and lateral insertions of this septum vary somewhat at different levels. The fluid loculation may mimic a subcapsular collection. (Courtesy of Michiel Feldberg, MD, University of Utrecht, The Netherlands)

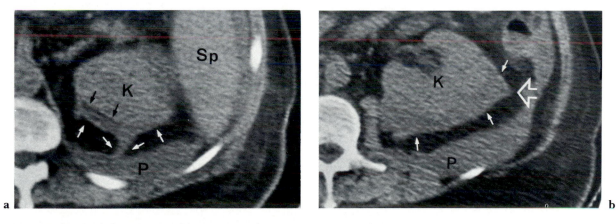

**Fig. 4–118. Bleeding deep to renorenal septum mimicking a subcapsular hematoma.**
**(a)** Small hematoma confined by the posterior renorenal bridging septum. Dark line (black arrows) between renal parenchyma (K) and hematoma (white arrows) is thought by some to represent swollen renal capsule and by others a CT artifact. The blood extends within another thickened septum to the posterior renal fascia which bounds a collection of blood within the posterior pararenal space (P). Sp = spleen.
**(b)** The hematoma extends external to the renal capsule from the posteromedial to the posterolateral aspect of the kidney. Laterally it becomes beak-shaped where it is tethered by another septum bridging to the renal fascia (open arrow). Tension within the hematoma deep to the renorenal septum displaces the kidney anteriorly.
  These findings were proven at autopsy.

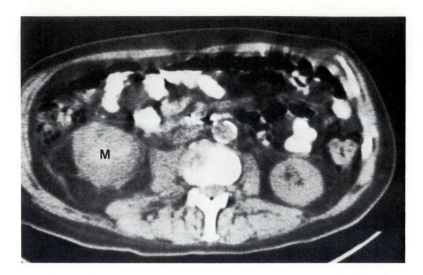

**Fig. 4–119. Stage II hypernephroma.**
CT scan shows the tumor mass (M) on the right has broken through the renal capsule and approaches the secondarily thickened Gerota's fascia. Increased reticular strands permeate the perirenal fat.

involved renal tissue may be preferable to nephrectomy.

## Staging of Renal Cell Carcinoma

Survival rates in patients with renal cell carcinoma have been correlated with the extent of tumor at the time of presentation.[106–108] Stage I denotes lesions entirely confined within the renal capsule. Stage II indicates extension through the capsule into the perirenal fat but not beyond the renal fascia. Stage III indicates involvement of the renal veins or lymph nodes, and Stage IV denotes either distant metastases or direct invasion of adjacent visceral structures. Five-year survival decreases with advancing stage, approximating 60% for Stage I lesions and decreasing to less than 10% with Stage IV tumors.

The prognosis in patients with vena cava extension depends on whether the tumors can be excised completely.[109,110] In patients who have renal vein or vena cava extension without extension outside the renal parenchyma itself and without nodal or distant metastases, the survival at 5 years is 50%. Nodal spread is a poor prognostic indicator, and only 5–10% of these patients survive 5 years.[111]

Computed tomography often readily provides helpful information in preoperative staging with an accuracy of over 90%[112] which may affect the therapeutic approach and aid the choice of the appropriate surgical procedure.[7,113] Extracapsular extension is shown by an indistinct tumor margin with strands of soft-tissue density extending into or obliterating the perirenal fat (Fig. 4–119). The relation of the tumor to Gerota's fascia can be evaluated (Fig. 4–120). The sensitivity of CT in detection of lymph node metastases provides valuable additional information for the surgeon planning lymphadenectomy, and CT is accurate in evaluating tumor extension into the main renal vein or inferior vena cava,[112–114] a finding that can also be demonstrated by ultrasonography[115,116] (Figs. 4–121 and 4–122). Contiguous invasion is also readily documented (Figs. 4–123 and 4–124).

Magnetic resonance imaging appears to be similar to CT in staging renal cell carcinoma.[117,118] These lesions have a varied MR signal with the most common appearance being a mass with an intensity intermediate between the renal cortex and the medulla on $T_1$-weighted images and hyperintense on $T_2$-weighted images. While CT and MRI are least reliable in differentiating Stage I from Stage II lesions, MRI appears superior in differentiating lymphadenopathy from small vascular structures.

Stage I and Stage II tumors can be approached by a retroperitoneal incision whereas Stage III and Stage IV tumors require an abdominal approach. If the vena cava is involved, a thoracoabdominal approach is required.

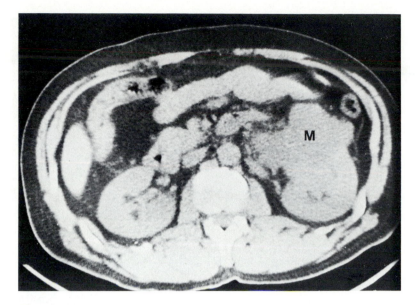

**Fig. 4–120. Stage III hypernephroma.**
CT scan demonstrates the faintly calcified tumor mass (M) on the left has extended anteriorly and medially beyond Gerota's fascia, with nodal involvement.

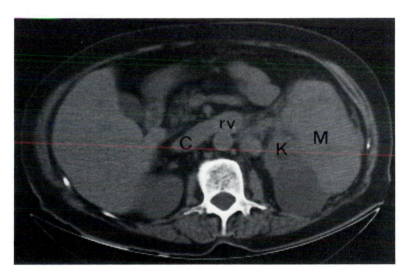

**Fig. 4–121. Stage III hypernephroma.**
CT shows the large tumor mass (M) on the left extending beyond the kidney (K). Tumor thrombus widens the left renal vein (rv) and inferior vena cava (C).

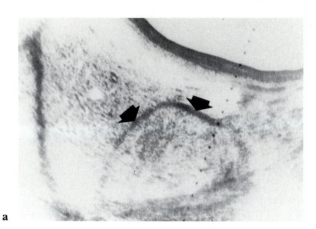

a

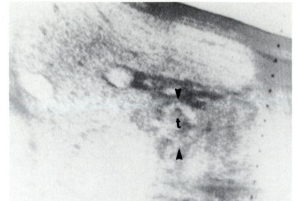

b

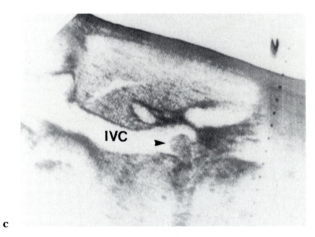

c

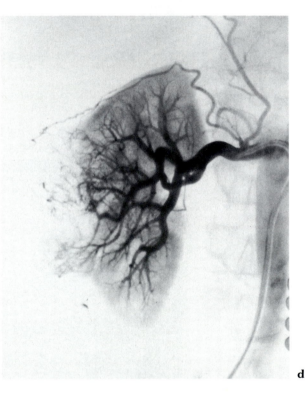

d

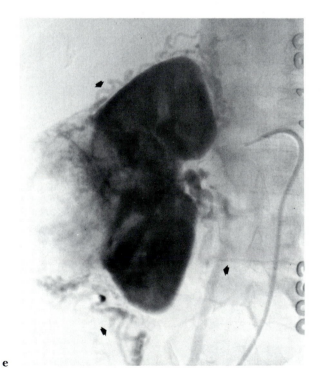

e

**Fig. 4–122. Stage III hypernephroma with extension into inferior vena cava.**

(a) Parasagittal ultrasonogram demonstrates the tumor mass (arrows) within the right kidney.

(b) More medially, tumor extension (t) within the right renal vein (arrowheads) is shown.

(c) Parasagittal ultrasonography at the level of the inferior vena cava (IVC) reveals it to contain tumor thrombus (arrowhead).

(d and e) Arterial and venous phases of selective right renal arteriogram demonstrate neovascularity of the tumor extending into the perirenal fat and nonopacification of the renal vein. Numerous venous collaterals (arrows) drain the kidney.

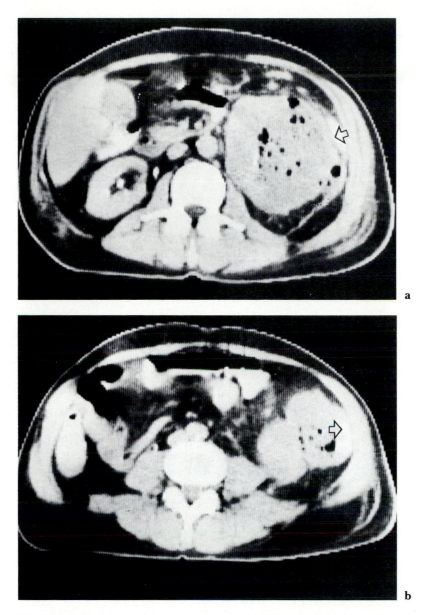

a

b

**Fig. 4–123. Stage IV infected hypernephroma invading perirenal and anterior pararenal spaces.**
**(a)** CT scan shows a huge gas-containing abscess, originating from the left kidney, which bulges throughout the perirenal space. The wall of the descending colon is thickened (arrow).
**(b)** At a lower level, the process has clearly extended into the anterior pararenal space and invaded the descending colon (arrow).

At surgery, a large necrotic and infected hypernephroma was found which involved the perirenal space and descending colon.
(From Love et al[7])

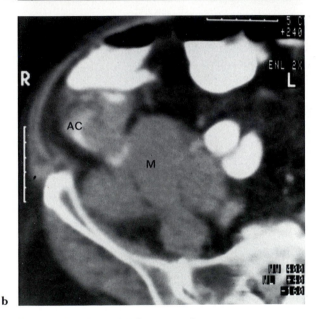

**Fig. 4–124. Stage IV hypernephroma.**
(**a** and **b**) CT shows the large lobulated tumor mass (M) extending posteriorly from the displaced right kidney (K) and inferiorly where it invades the ascending colon (AC).
(Courtesy of Michiel Feldberg, MD, University of Utrecht, The Netherlands)

# Posterior Pararenal Space

## Roentgen Anatomy of Distribution and Localization of Collections

Selective opacification of the posterior pararenal space in the cadaver permits identification of the preferential pathway of spread and the characteristic localizing features. This is shown in Figure 4–125. The natural spread is inferior and lateral because of gravity, lumbar lordosis, and the fact that this space is open toward the flanks. The fluid density thus assumes an axis paralleling that of the psoas muscle and tends to displace the lower pole of the kidney laterally as well as anteriorly and upward. The kidney outline and perirenal fat shadows tend to be preserved. These features further distinguish these collections from effusions within the perirenal space. The psoas muscle shadow is obliterated by fluid collections, although it may actually be highlighted by gas collections. Further progression is shown by anterior and medial displacement of the ascending or descending colon and then encroachment on, or obliteration of, the flank stripe (Fig. 4–126).

The significant criteria for the localization and distinction of collections within the posterior pararenal space are outlined in Table 4–1.

## Clinical Sources of Effusions

The posterior pararenal space is a common site of spontaneous retroperitoneal hemorrhage in conditions such as a bleeding diathesis or overanticoagulation. Hemorrhage from ruptured abdominal aneurysms also may typically localize within this compartment. Trauma (including stab wounds and rib fractures) and retroperitoneal lymphatic extravasation are other sources of effusions.

Infection limited solely to this compartment is rare. The posterior pararenal space itself does not include organs from which infection can arise directly. Except for the unusual case caused by bacteremia, infection here may develop as a complication of osteomyelitis of the vertebral column or 12th rib[3] or of an aortic graft. Abscess behind the transversalis fascia is not, strictly speaking, extraperitoneal, but retrofascial abscess (largely of osseous origin from infection in the spine or 12th rib, often from

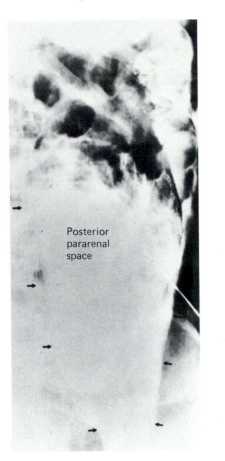

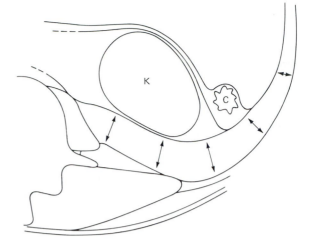

**Fig. 4–126. Fluid collection in the posterior pararenal compartment with viscus displacement and extension into the properitoneal fat.**
K = kidney, C = colon. (From Meyers[12])

**Fig. 4–125. Postmortem injection into the left posterior pararenal space.**
Medially the collection parallels the psoas muscle and obliterates its outline. Laterally there is direct extension into the flank fat. The axis of the collection is inferior and lateral. (From Meyers[12])

tuberculosis or actinomycosis) occasionally may transgress fascial planes to involve the posterior pararenal space. Fulminating perirenal infection rarely does this.

Extravasates originating in the pelvis, as in perforation of the rectum or sigmoid colon, may spread upward into this compartment.

## Hemorrhage

Retroperitoneal bleeding accompanying fractures of the spine (Fig. 4–127) or posterior ribs

**Fig. 4–127. Posterior pararenal hemorrhage.**
Following severe blunt trauma with fractures of both transverse processes (arrows), enhanced CT scan shows a large collection of blood in the posterior pararenal space on the left, displacing the kidney anteriorly and laterally. The blood extends into the flank to obliterate portions of the properitoneal fat (curved arrow). Associated hemorrhage into the psoas and paraspinal muscles contributes to displacement of the ureter. (Reproduced from Love et al[7])

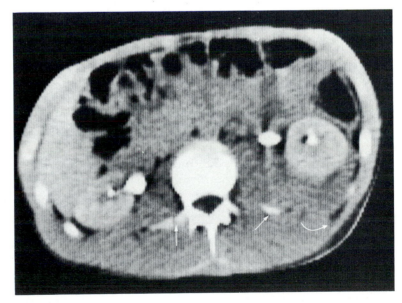

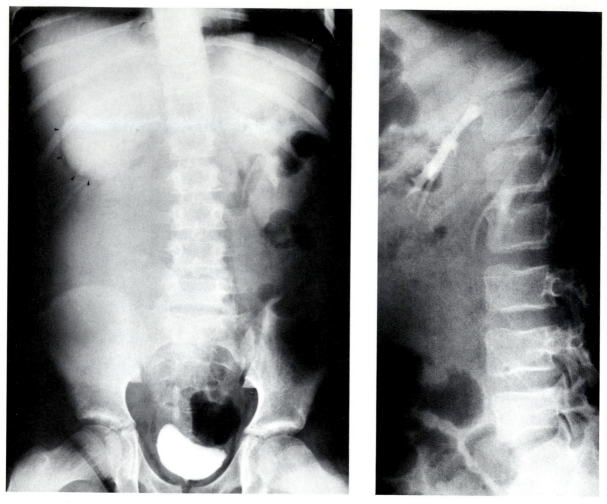

**Fig. 4–128. Posterior pararenal hemorrhage in a hemophiliac.**
**(a)** Intravenous urogram. The axis of the extraperitoneal density on the right is oriented inferolaterally. The psoas shadow is obliterated and the flank stripe obscured. The collection displaces the kidney laterally and superiorly. The obstructive nephrogram is outlined further by intact perirenal fat (arrowheads).
**(b)** Right lateral projection. The posterior collection displaces the kidney anteriorly.
(From Meyers et al[12])

may be identified as residing largely within this space.

Many cases of extraperitoneal hemorrhage due to bleeding dyscrasias (Fig. 4–128) or over-anticoagulation (Fig. 4–129) can be identified precisely as developing within the posterior pararenal compartment. The distinctive complex of findings is evaluated easily, and the radiologic evaluation may be crucial in uncovering the primary disorder. Figure 4–130 illustrates the case of a 58-year-old man with chronic bilateral hematomas identified within the posterior pararenal compartments; further investigation

then led to the diagnosis of a hemophiliac disorder.

Bleeding from a ruptured aortic aneurysm frequently extends to this compartment. Plain films may show a large extraperitoneal fluid collection with occasional findings localizing the process to the posterior pararenal space, such as alterations of the properitoneal flank stripe[119] or lucent streaks through the fat[120] (Fig. 4–131). In a low leak of an abdominal aortic aneurysm, CT often demonstrates that bleeding may preferentially rise upward within the posterior pararenal space (Fig. 4–132). Aneurysms may also rup-

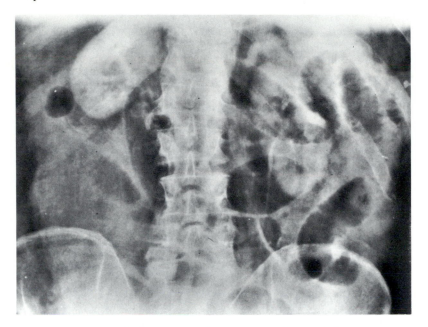

**Fig. 4–129. Posterior pararenal hemorrhage secondary to overanticoagulation.**
The partially obstructed kidney on the right is displaced superiorly and laterally by the collection of blood that extends in an inferolateral axis. The hemorrhage obscures the psoas muscle margin but has not yet extended into the flank fat. The perirenal fat is not involved.

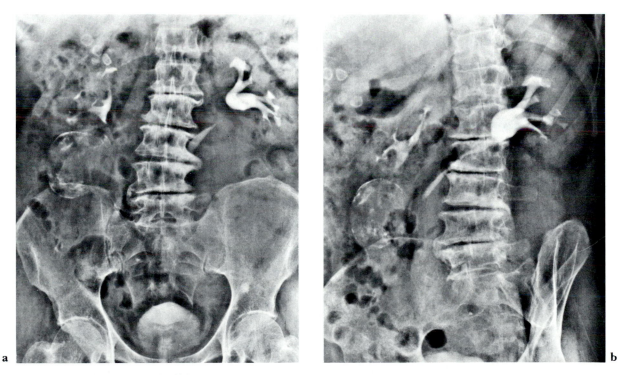

**Fig. 4–130. Chronic bilateral hematomas in the posterior pararenal spaces in an adult hemophiliac.**
**(a** and **b)** Intravenous urography demonstrates a calcified mass on the right and a soft-tissue density on the left. The lower segments of the psoas muscles are obliterated. The larger blood collection on the left displaces the lower pole of the kidney superiorly and laterally, and the ureter medially and anteriorly.

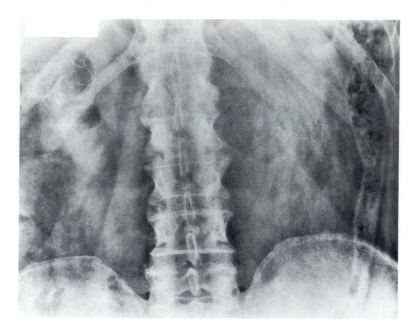

**Fig. 4–131. Posterior pararenal hemorrhage from ruptured aneurysm of the abdominal aorta.**
Plain film demonstrates streaky radiolucent lines on the left in an area of an ill-defined mass which also causes loss of visualization of the psoas muscle border. These changes are secondary to blood dissecting, often in sheets, through the posterior pararenal fat. (Courtesy of John Williams, MD, Geisinger Clinic, Danville, Pa.)

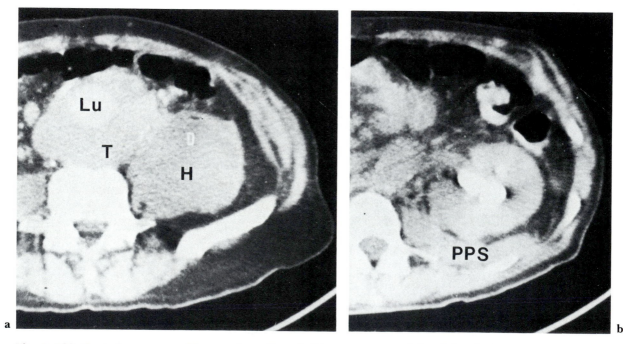

**Fig. 4–132. Posterior pararenal hemorrhage from leaking aneurysm of the abdominal aorta.**
**(a)** CT scan after intravenous contrast medium demonstrates a large aneurysm of the abdominal aorta containing thrombus (T) surrounding its residual opacified lumen (Lu). Hemorrhage (H) has extended from a site of rupture into the adjacent tissues on the left.
**(b)** At a higher level, the hemorrhage has risen into the posterior pararenal space (PPS), displacing the kidney anteriorly and laterally.

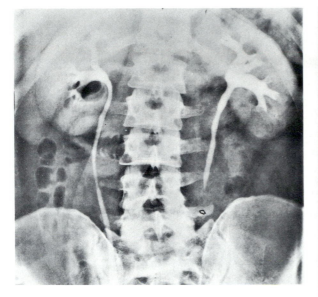

**Fig. 4–133. Posterior pararenal abscess secondary to spinal osteomyelitis.**
Staphylococcal osteomyelitis involves the left transverse process of L5 (arrow). Infection in the posterior pararenal space is revealed by the characteristic displacement of the lower pole of the left kidney upward and outward. Loss of visualization of the psoas margin may be due to the abscess as well, or it may be a consequence only of the scoliosis present.

ture first into the psoas muscle and then into the posterior pararenal space.[121]

## Abscess

Infection of this space consequent to osteomyelitis (Fig. 4–133) is now much less common than it has been in the past. Fascial transgression with infection may be seen as a complication of bowel surgery (Fig. 4–134) or severe renal disease (Fig. 4–135). Other sources include unusual extraperitoneal positions of the appendix (Fig. 4–136) and infections complicating aortic grafts[18,122,123] (Fig. 4–137).

## Lymphatic Extravasation

Extraperitoneal extravasation of lymph often selectively involves the posterior pararenal compartment (Figs. 4–138 and 4–139). Drainage laterally may coalesce into a flank lymphocyst (Fig. 4–140).

At times, circumscribed solid masses of extraperitoneal lymph node origin can be identified clearly as localized to the posterior pararenal

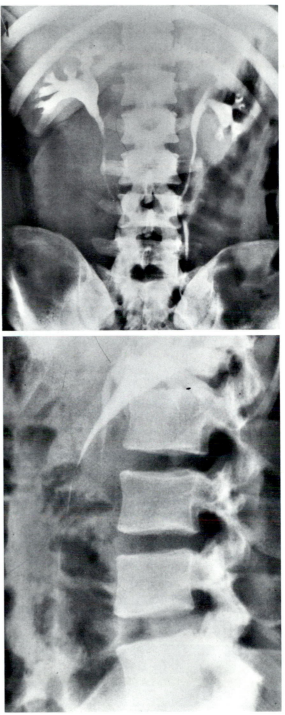

**Fig. 4–134. Posterior pararenal abscess following bowel resection for regional enteritis.**
**(a)** The density on the right is directed inferiorly and laterally, obscures the psoas margin, and displaces the lower pole of the kidney upward and outward.
**(b)** Right lateral view confirms the extreme posterior position of the abscess, which displaces the kidney and ureter forward.

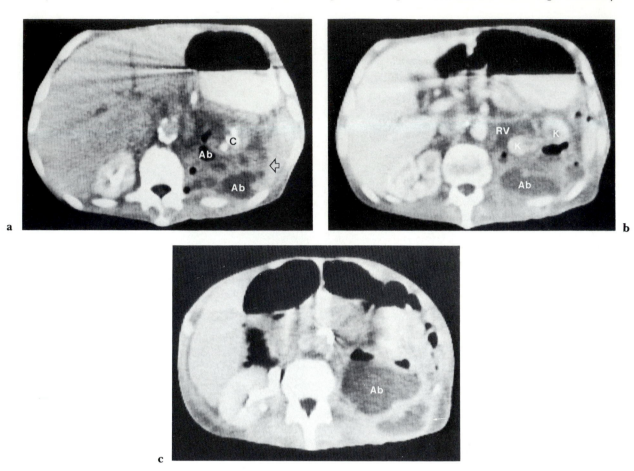

**Fig. 4–135. Calculus pyonephrosis with extension into the perirenal and posterior pararenal spaces.**
**(a–c)** There is a large left gas-containing extraperitoneal abscess (Ab) which involves the perirenal space with obliteration of its fat, renal contour, and splenic angle (arrow), and which causes anterior displacement of the atrophic kidney (K) containing calculi (C) and of the left renal vein (RV). There is also extension into the posterior pararenal space and into the subcutaneous tissues (white arrow).
(From Love et al[7])

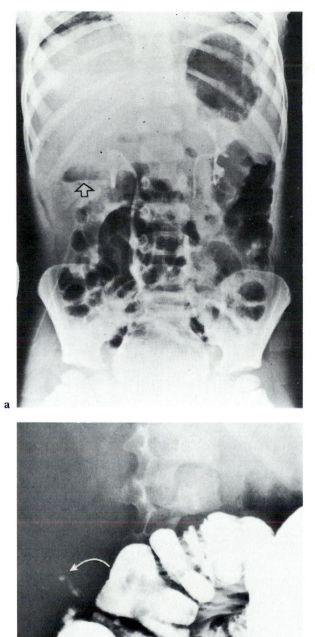

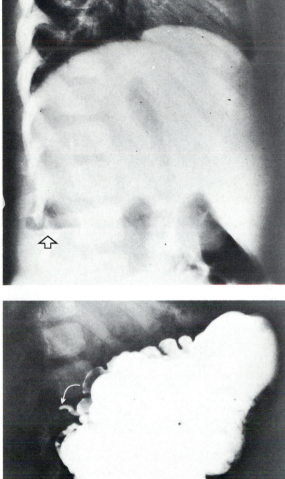

**Fig. 4–136. Posterior pararenal abscess secondary to extraperitoneal appendicitis.**

(a and b) Erect AP urogram and lateral plain film in a child demonstrate an air–fluid level in an abscess (arrows) behind and a little lateral to the right kidney.

(c and d) Frontal and lateral views of barium enema study demonstrate an undescended subhepatic cecum from which arises an ascending appendix (curved arrows). In this situation, the appendix is extraperitoneal in location and its perforation can then lead to infection in unusual sites.

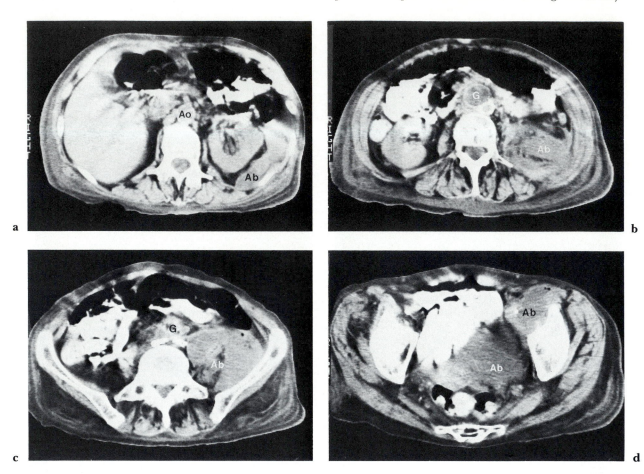

**Fig. 4–137. Posterior pararenal abscess with extension to the inguinal area secondary to an infected aorta graft.**

This patient developed sepsis and a fluctuant left inguinal mass following an aortofemoral prosthetic graft. The graft had been placed end-to-side on the abdominal aorta, passed beneath the inguinal ligament, and then anastomosed to the left common femoral artery.

**(a)** CT scan shows abscess (Ab) in the left posterior pararenal space extending into the flank. The perirenal fat is maintained. The abdominal aorta (Ao) is calcified.

**(b and c)** At and below the level of the proximal anastomosis, inflammatory reaction surrounds the graft (G) anterior to the heavily calcified aorta and its bifurcation. The abscess develops extension into the left pelvis along the plane of the iliopsoas muscle.

**(d)** The abscess extends from the pelvis to the left groin.

(Courtesy of Patrick Freeny, MD, Mason Clinic, Seattle, Wash.)

**Fig. 4–138. Posterior pararenal lympho-cyst after sympathectomy.**
A mass density on the right displaces the lower pole of the kidney superiorly and laterally and obscures the psoas margin.

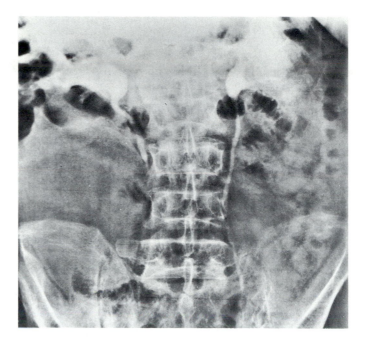

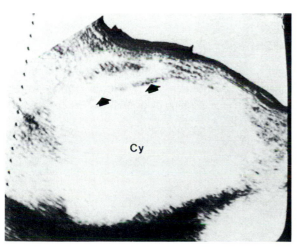

a

**Fig. 4–139. Posterior pararenal lymphocyst secondary to surgical node biopsies for staging purposes.**
(a) Left parasagittal ultrasonogram in supine position demonstrates large unilocular cyst (Cy) displacing the left kidney far anteriorly and flattening it against the anterior abdominal wall. Note posterior aspect of kidney and anterior margin of lymphocele (arrows).
(b) Percutaneous injection of cyst delineates its extent within the posterior pararenal space and its communication from the pelvis.

This abdominal lymphocyst originated from the pelvis at the site of extensive iliac node biopsies, presenting in the flank at a considerable distance from the site of the disrupted lymphatics. This case confirms that collections localized to the posterior pararenal compartment may be the result of cephalad spread from processes originating in the extraperitoneal pelvis.

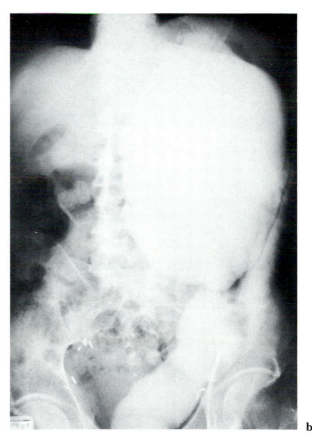

b

(Reproduced from Morin ME, Baker DA: Lymphocele: A complication of surgical staging of carcinoma of the prostate. Am J Roentgenol 129: 333–334, 1977)

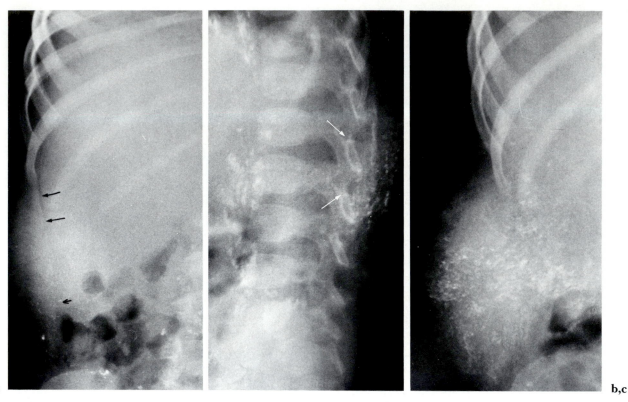

a                                                                                                                                    b,c

**Fig. 4–140. Posterior pararenal lymphatic extravasation** in a child presenting with a cystic flank mass.
**(a)** Lymphangiogram. Extravasated droplets of contrast material extend laterally toward flank mass. At this site, the flank-stripe fat is discretely lost and is maintained only in segments bordering the lymphocyst (arrows). The posterior collection also causes loss of visualization of the hepatic angle.
**(b)** Lateral projection documents the extreme posterior extravasation (arrows).
**(c)** Later film shows that with further extravasation into the enlarged mass all of the flank fat is effaced.
(From Meyers et al[12])

space. Figure 4–141 illustrates this in an instance of reticulum cell sarcoma.

## Diffuse Extraperitoneal Gas

Radiologic localization of diffuse extraperitoneal gas to a specific compartment is greatly advanced by anatomic knowledge gained from careful study of body sections, postmortem injections, and retroperitoneal pneumography. Fascial boundaries and tissue planes direct the spread and localization of extraperitoneal gas, depending on its source.

In presacral pneumography, if the needle is inserted in the midline behind the rectum, the gas ordinarily rises symmetrically up both sides.[13] While the kidneys and adrenal glands are shown with striking clarity, much of the ex-

traperitoneal gas is outside the perirenal space. A considerable part undoubtedly enters this compartment through its inferior communication with the iliac fossa, but there is also significant distribution into the posterior pararenal space in particular, outlining the contours of the liver, spleen, upper poles of the kidneys, medial crura of the diaphragm, and subphrenic extraperitoneal tissues (Fig. 4–142). Furthermore, because of the fusion of the renal fascial layers with the diaphragm superiorly, perirenal gas alone does not lead to pneumomediastinum and cervical emphysema, whereas gas in the posterior pararenal compartment frequently does.

It is also apparent that extraperitoneal gas is not truly fixed in position but retains some mobility through the tissues. This is demonstrable clinically by the changeable distribution between supine and erect films (Figs. 4–143 and 4–146).

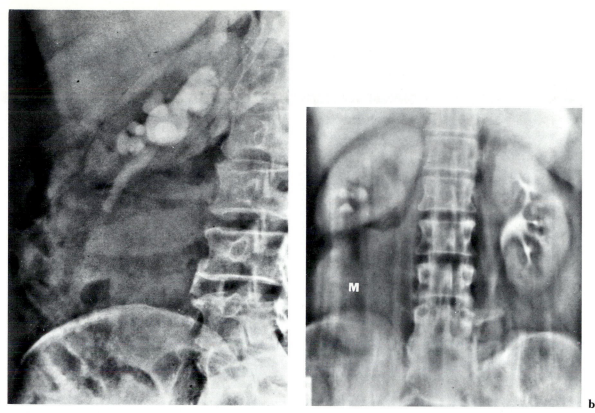

a                                                                                    b

**Fig. 4–141. Posterior pararenal development of reticulum cell sarcoma.**
**(a)** Excretory urogram, oblique projection. Large circumscribed mass displaces the right ureter and the lower pole of the right kidney anteriorly. Obstructive hydronephrosis is present.
**(b)** Nephrotomogram. The sarcomatous mass (M) results in loss of visualization of the lower psoas segment and lateral displacement of the lower renal pole. The perirenal fat and upper psoas segment are intact.
 These changes localize the lymphoma to the posterior pararenal space.

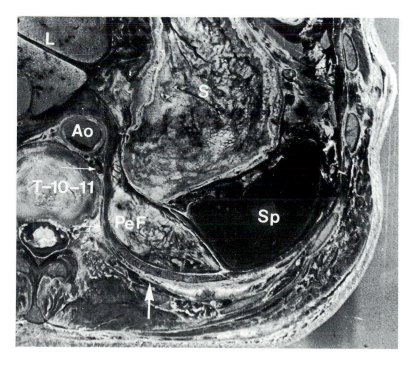

**Fig. 4–142. Posterior pararenal fat** (PeF).
This provides contrast to the medial crus (small arrows) and inferior margin (large arrow) of the diaphragm, and to the posteromedial border of the spleen (Sp). S = stomach, L = liver, Ao = aorta.

267

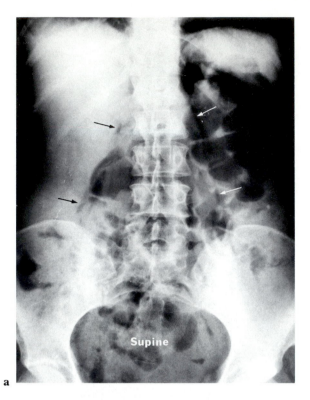

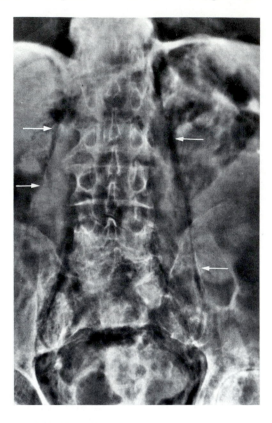

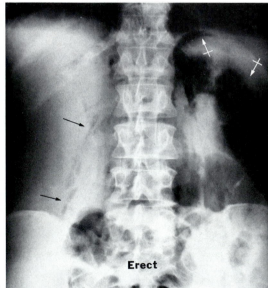

**Fig. 4–144. Rectal perforation.**
Bilateral gas in the posterior pararenal compartments outlines the complete lateral borders of the psoas muscles (arrows) and the upper poles of the kidneys and immediate subphrenic tissues.

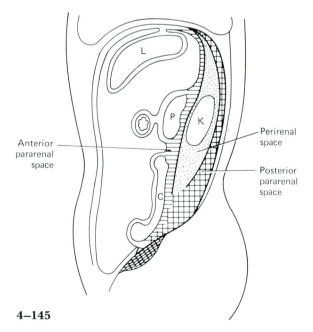

**Fig. 4–143. Rectal perforation.**
Supine and erect films demonstrate extraperitoneal gas paralleling the lateral borders of the psoas muscles (arrows). Cephalad extension on the left outlines the upper pole of the kidney, the adrenal gland, the medial border of the spleen, the medial crus of the diaphragm, and the immediate subphrenic tissues (crossed arrows). These findings localize the gas to the posterior pararenal compartments. The suprarenal and subphrenic gas collection increases in the erect position. (From Meyers[9])

4–145

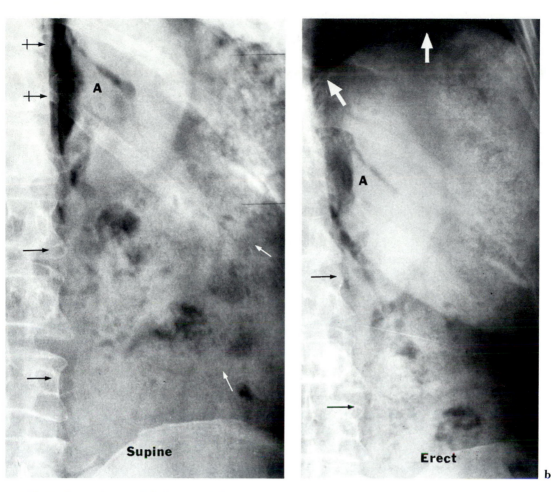

a    Supine

b    Erect

**Fig. 4–146. Perforated sigmoid diverticulitis.**
Extraperitoneal gas (arrows) extends anterior to the psoas muscle toward the spine within the anterior pararenal space.

Superiorly, the gas extends within the posterior pararenal space outlining the adrenal gland (A) and the posteromedial border of the spleen, the medial crus of the diaphragm (crossed arrows), and segments of the extraperitoneal subdiaphragmatic tissue (large white arrows). Note that the latter do not follow the highest plane of the diaphragm, in contradistinction to free intraperitoneal air. (From Meyers[9])

◁

**Fig. 4–145. Relationships and structures of the three extraperitoneal spaces on the left.**
The sigmoid colon is in continuity with the posterior and anterior pararenal compartments. L = liver, P = pancreas, K = kidney, C = colon. (From Meyers[8])

The general extraperitoneal region can be thought of as Y-shaped in the frontal and lateral planes of the body. In an anteroposterior plane, continuity from the pelvis extends to both sides. It consistently appears that extraperitoneal gaseous extravasation originating from disease processes in the pelvis or at the level of the iliac fossa does not enter the perirenal space; rather, it extends into the anterior and posterior pararenal spaces, presumably because the inferior apex of the cone of renal fascia is rapidly sealed off by associated inflammatory adhesions.

These considerations provide a rationale for the observation that bilateral spread of gas through the extraperitoneal tissue planes originates most often in the pelvic region. Extraperitoneal gas arising in the upper abdomen does not generally descend enough to cross over the midline to the opposite side at the level of the lumbosacral junction. An exception to unilateral confinement in the upper abdomen has been seen in gas-producing pancreatitis, presumably by virtue of the digestive enzymes involved. Extraperitoneal gas originating in and confined to the left upper quadrant is rare but may follow a perforated carcinoma or diverticulitis of the proximal descending colon or an abscess of the tail of the pancreas. If both intraperitoneal and extraperitoneal gas are present, it can be confidently assumed that the source is a perforation of an extraperitoneal structure that has broken through the posterior parietal peritoneum.

## Rectal Perforation

Since the rectum is subperitoneal and lies in the midline, gas that escapes from its lumen rises up both sides within the extraperitoneal tissues. Depending primarily on the exact site of perforation, the gas may predominate on one side, but bilateral spread remains evident. In my experience, spread has preferentially been to the posterior compartments. The gas may then parallel the lateral contour of the psoas muscles, outlining the suprarenal and subdiaphragmatic tissues (Figs. 4–143 and 4–144).

## Sigmoid Perforation

The sigmoid colon lies below the limits of the cone of renal fascia where it is in anatomic continuity with both the anterior and posterior pararenal spaces (Fig. 4–145). Gas from a sigmoid perforation may therefore enter either or both compartments.

Studies by Meyers et al[124,125] have confirmed that only one of the four rows of colonic diverticula faces the peritoneal cavity and that fully 75% of sigmoid diverticula are related to the extraperitoneal tissues. Extraperitoneal gas associated with perforated sigmoid diverticulitis typically progresses up the left side. The gas may extend medially over the psoas muscle in the form of mottled radiolucencies (Fig. 4–146), but extension into the posterior compartment often dominates the radiologic findings. The gas may enter the properitoneal flank fat directly, but superiorly is characterized by its outlining of the left adrenal gland and upper renal pole, the medial crus of the diaphragm, the medial contour of the posterior aspect of the spleen, and the extraperitoneal subdiaphragmatic plane (Fig. 4–146).

Only if the sigmoid perforation occurs between the leaves of the mesocolon does the extraperitoneal gas rise bilaterally within the anterior pararenal spaces.[9]

## Extraperitoneal Gas of Supradiaphragmatic Origin

Gas arising above the diaphragm may pass down the mediastinum through the diaphragmatic hiati and directly into the posterior pararenal space. If the gas gains entrance to structures of the chest wall, its extension to the extraperitoneal tissues of the abdomen may pursue a characteristic course. The endothoracic fascia of the chest is continuous with the transversalis fascia of the abdomen. Gas originating in the chest or even in the neck may pass deep to the endothoracic fascia, external to the parietal pleura, and continue directly into the abdominal wall. The lucencies may then extend preferentially within the flank fat (Fig. 4–147), although some gas may be seen in the deeper portions of the posterior pararenal compartment.

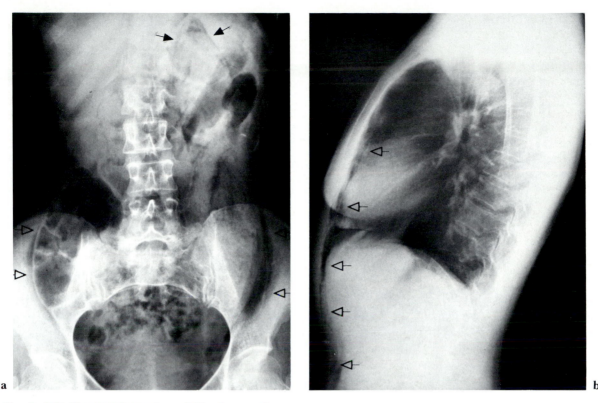

**Fig. 4–147. Extraperitoneal gas following tracheostomy.**
**(a)** Preferential spread into the flank fat (open arrows). A minimal amount outlines the left psoas muscle and suprarenal area (solid arrows).
**(b)** Lateral chest film demonstrates the continuous channel of gas from the chest to the abdomen deep to the endothoracic fascia and transversalis fascia (arrows).
(From Meyers[9])

## Differential Diagnosis of Small Amounts of Subdiaphragmatic Gas

The predominant extraperitoneal gas within the posterior pararenal fat may seek the immediate subdiaphragmatic tissue planes. While occasionally extraperitoneal air may be distinguished by its outlining of individual diaphragmatic muscle bundles,[125a] I have observed two further characteristics at this site on erect films which are particularly useful in differentiating even small amounts of extraperitoneal gas from free intraperitoneal air.

1. Free intraperitoneal air always conforms to the highest curvature of the dome of the diaphragm and may have a flat lower border. Gas in the subphrenic extraperitoneal tissues often parallels a lower plane of the diaphragmatic curvature, medial or lateral to its apex, and in-

variably demonstrates a crescentic outline (Figs. 4–143b and 4–146b).
2. The amount of free intraperitoneal subdiaphragmatic air increases on inspiration and decreases on expiration, presumably reflecting the influence of the greater negative intraabdominal pressure beneath the diaphragm during inspiration. In contrast, extraperitoneal subdiaphragmatic gas appears to increase on expiration and decrease on inspiration on erect frontal films (Fig. 4–148). The extraperitoneal tissues are not affected by respiratory variations in intraperitoneal pressure so that with descent of the diaphragm, extraperitoneal gas is simply compressed more diffusely, resulting in a thinner crescentic collection.

The anatomic boundaries of the three extraperitoneal spaces and the dynamics of the spread of extraperitoneal gas clearly explain its

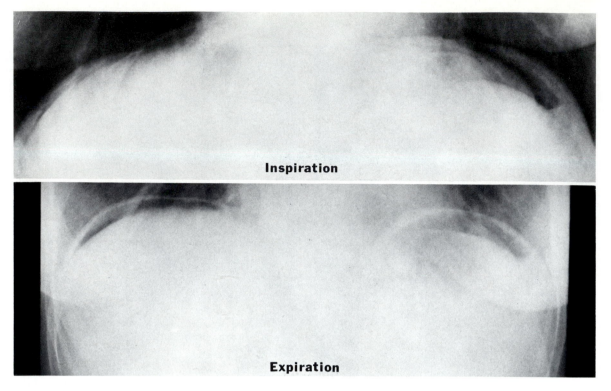

**Fig. 4–148.** Erect films demonstrate a greater accumulation of subdiaphragmatic extraperitoneal gas within the posterior pararenal spaces during expiration. (From Meyers[9])

**Table 4–2.** Spread and localization of extraperitoneal gas

| Extraperitoneal compartment | Localizing roentgen features | Side of abdomen | Most likely sources |
|---|---|---|---|
| Anterior pararenal | Medially: gas extends beyond the lateral border of the psoas muscle toward the spine; on oblique projections the outline of the muscle may be preserved. | Right | Perforation of the descending duodenum |
| | | Left | Perforated sigmoid diverticulitis |
| | Laterally: there is no extension into the flank stripe except possibly inferiorly, below the cone of renal fascia. | Bilateral | Sigmoid perforation into mesocolon; fulminating pancreatitis |
| | Superiorly: the renal outline may be preserved. | | |
| Perirenal | Gas collection presents an inferiorly convex border overlying the iliac crest. | Right | Renal infection |
| | | | Occasionally, perforation of the descending duodenum |
| | Most prominent within the rich fat posterior to the kidney. | Left | Renal infection |
| | Renal outline is enhanced. | | |
| | Inflammatory thickening and displacement of the renal fascia. | | |
| Posterior pararenal | Medially: gas is limited by and parallels the margin of the psoas muscle. | Left | Sigmoid diverticulitis |
| | Laterally: gas extends into the flank stripe. | Bilateral | Rectal perforation |
| | | | Supradiaphragmatic origin |
| | Superiorly: gas outlines the suprarenal area, diaphragm, and posterior aspects of the liver and spleen. | | |
| | Extension above the diaphragm leads to pneumomediastinum and cervical subcutaneous emphysema. | | |

distribution and localization. The radiologic criteria that allow identification of the likely primary source of extraperitoneal gas are summarized in Table 4–2.

# Psoas Abscess and Hematoma

Spontaneous dissection from a primary site in the retrofascial space deep to the transversalis fascia into the extraperitoneal compartments is rare.[3] Psoas abscesses generally do not originate within the psoas compartment but spread here from neighboring intraabdominal structures.[126]

Injection studies confirm clinical observations that the strong psoas fascia confines collections within it (Fig. 4–149). Indeed, this may provide

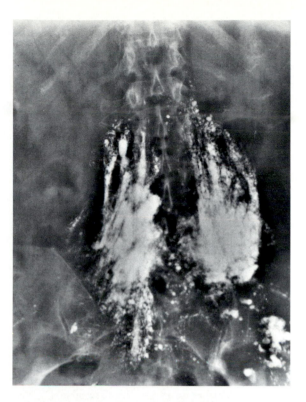

**Fig. 4–149. Contrast injection into the psoas muscles.**
The collections are restrained by the strong psoas fascia.

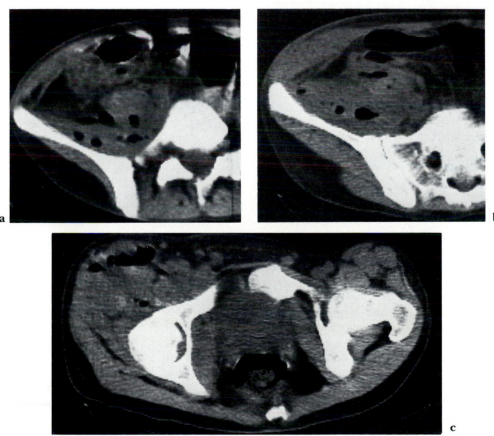

**Fig. 4–150. Iliopsoas abscess.**
**(a–c)** CT shows a gas-producing infection of the iliopsoas muscle tracking to a large abscess in the groin.

273

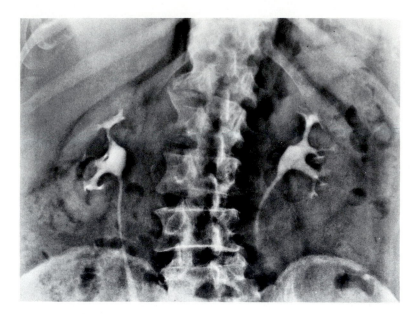

**Fig. 4–151. Right psoas abscess** secondary to osteomyelitis of L2.

Intravenous urogram demonstrates mass density displacing the right kidney laterally and effacing the upper segment of the psoas muscle.

a pathway for extension of the process to the hip and thigh (Fig. 4–150), as discussed in Chapter 11. More often, a psoas abscess is localized in a paraspinal location and is revealed by its efface-ment of the lateral border of the muscle and its lateral displacement of the kidney and ureter (Fig. 4–151). Psoas abscesses are shown by CT as enlargement of the muscle with low-density areas and perhaps gas.[126,127] The usefulness of magnetic resonance imaging in these conditions is under investigation.[128]

# References

1. Meyer HI: The reaction of retroperitoneal tis-sue to infection. Ann Surg 99: 246–250, 1934
2. Stevenson EO, Ozeran RS: Retroperitoneal space abscesses. Surg Gynecol Obstet 128: 1202–1208, 1969
3. Altemeier WA, Alexander JW: Retroperitoneal abscess. Arch Surg 83: 512–524, 1961
4. Elkin M, Cohen G: Diagnostic value of the psoas shadow. Clin Radiol 13: 210–217, 1962
5. Williams SM, Harned RK, Hultman SA, et al: The psoas sign: A reevaluation. Radiographic 5(4): 525–536, 1985
6. Editorial: Periureteric fibrosis. Lancet 2: 780–781, 1957
7. Love L, Meyers MA, Churchill RJ, et al: Com-puted tomography of extraperitoneal spaces. AJR 136: 781–789, 1981
8. Meyers MA: Acute extraperitoneal infection. Semin Roentgenol 8: 445–464, 1973
9. Meyers MA: Radiologic features of the spread and localization of extraperitoneal gas and their relationship to its source: An anatomical ap-proach. Radiology 111: 17–26, 1974
10. Meyers MA: Uriniferous perirenal pseudocyst: New observations. Radiology 117: 539–545, 1975
11. Meyers MA, Whalen JP, Evans JA: Diagnosis of perirenal and subcapsular masses: Anatomic-ra-diologic correlation. AJR Rad Ther Nucl Med 121: 523–538, 1974
12. Meyers MA, Whalen JP, Peelle K, et al: Radio-logic features of extraperitoneal effusions: An anatomic approach. Radiology 104: 249–257, 1972
13. Meyers MA: Diseases of the Adrenal Glands. Radiologic Diagnosis with Emphasis on the Use of Presacral Retroperitoneal Pneumography. CC Thomas, Springfield, Illinois, 1963, pp. 11–15, 20
14. Barbaric Z: Renal fascia in urinary tract diseases. Radiology 118: 561–565, 1976
15. Kochkodan EJ, Haggar AM: Visualization of the renal fascia: A normal finding in urography. AJR 140: 1243–1244, 1983
16. Whalen JP, Ziter FMH Jr: Visualization of the renal fascia: A new sign in localization of ab-dominal masses. Radiology 80: 861–863, 1967
17. Feldberg MAM: Computed Tomography of the Retroperitoneum: An Anatomical and Patholog-ical Atlas with Emphasis on the Fascial Planes. Martinus Nijhoff, Boston, 1983

18. Meyers MA: Dynamic Radiology of the Abdomen: Normal and Pathologic Anatomy, 2nd ed. Springer-Verlag, New York, 1982

19. Parienty RA, Pradel J, Picard J-D, et al: Visibility and thickening of the renal fascia on computed tomograms. Radiology 139: 119–124, 1981

20. Zuckerkandl E: Beitrage zur Anatomie des Menschlichen Korpers. Ueber den Fixationsapparat der Nieren. Med Jahr 13(2): 59–67, 1883

21. Gerota D: Beiträge zur Kenntnis des Befestigungsapparates der Niere. Arch Anat Entwicklungsgesch 265–286, 1895

22. Meyers MA, Oliphant M, Berne AS, et al: The peritoneal ligaments and mesenteries: Pathways of intra-abdominal spread of disease. Annual Oration. Radiology 163: 593–604, 1987

23. Congdon ED, Edson JN: The cone of renal fascia in the adult white male. Anat Rec 80: 289–313, 1941

24. Mitchell GAG: The renal fascia. Br J Surg 37: 257, 1950

24a. Kneeland JB, Auh YH, Rubenstein WA et al: Perirenal spaces: CT evidence for communication across the midline. Radiology 164: 657–664, 1987

25. Martin CP: Anatomical notes: A note on the renal fascia. J Anat 77: 101–103, 1942

26. Southam AH: Fixation of the kidney. Q J Med 16: 283–308, 1923

27. Parienty RA, Pradel J: Radiological evaluation of the peri- and pararenal spaces by computed tomography. Crit Rev Diagn Imaging 20: 1–26, 1983

28. Nicholson RL: Abnormalities of the perinephric fascia and fat in pancreatitis. Radiology 139: 125–127, 1981

29. Chintapalli K, Lawson TL, Foley WD, et al: Renal fascial thickening in pancreatitis. J Comp Assisted Tomogr 6(5): 983–986, 1982

30. Hadar H, Meiraz D: Thickened renal fascia: A sign of retroperitoneal pathology. J Comp Assist Tomogr 5: 193–198, 1981

31. Feldberg MAM, Hendriks MJ, van Waes P, et al: Pancreatic lesions and transfascial perirenal spread: Computed tomographic demonstration. Gastrointest Radiol 12: 121–127, 1987

32. Rubenstein WA, Auh YH, Zirinsky K, et al: Posterior peritoneal recesses: Assessment using CT. Radiology 156: 461–468, 1985

33. William PL, Warwick R (eds): Gray's Anatomy, 36th ed. Edinburgh, Churchill Livingstone, 1980

34. Raptopoulos V, Kleinman PK, Marks S Jr, et al: Renal fascial pathway: Posterior extension of pancreatic effusions within the anterior pararenal space. Radiology 158: 367–374, 1986

35. Hopper KD, Sherman JL, Juethke J, et al: The retrorenal colon in the supine and prone patient. Radiology 162: 443–446, 1987

36. Love L, Demos TC, Posniak H: CT of retrorenal fluid collections. AJR 145: 87–91, 1985

37. Sherman JL, Hopper KD, Greene AJ, et al: The retrorenal colon on computed tomography: A normal variant. J Comp Assist Tomogr 9: 339–341, 1985

38. Kunin M: Bridging septa of the perinephric space: Anatomic, pathologic, and diagnostic considerations. Radiology 158: 361–365, 1986

39. Feuerstein IM, Zeman RK, Jaffe MH, et al: Perirenal cobwebs: The expanding CT differential diagnosis. J Comp Assist Tomogr 8: 1128–1130, 1984

40. McLennan BL, Lee JKT, Peterson RR: Anatomy of the perirenal area. Radiology 158: 555–557, 1986

41. Winfield AC, Gerlock AJJL, Shaff MI: Perirenal cobwebs: A CT sign of renal vein thrombosis. J Comp Assist Tomogr 5: 705–708, 1981

42. Skarby HG: Beiträge zur Diagnostik der Paranephritiden mit besonderer Berucksichtigung des Röntgenverfahrens. Acta Radiol Suppl 62: 1–165, 1946

43. Whalen JP, Berne AS, Riemenschneider PA: The extraperitoneal perivisceral fat pad. I. Its role in the roentgenological visualization of abdominal organs. Radiology 92: 466–472, 1969

44. McCort J: Anterior pararenal-space infection. Mt Sinai J Med 51: 482–490, 1984

45. Feldberg MAM, Hendriks MJ, van Waes P: Role of CT in diagnosis and management of complications of diverticular disease. Gastrointest Radiol 10: 370–377, 1985

46. Meyers MA, Oliphant M: Ascending retrocecal appendicitis. Radiology 110: 295–299, 1974

47. Feldberg MAM, Hendriks MJ, van Waes P: Computed tomography in complicated acute appendicitis. Gastrointest Radiol 10: 289–295, 1985

48. Ginzburg L, Oppenheimer GD: Urological complications of regional ileitis. J Urol 59: 948–952, 1948

49. Roman E, Silva Y, Lucas C: Management of blunt duodenal injury. Surg Gynecol Obstet 132: 7–14, 1971

50. Glazer GM, Buy JN, Moss AA, et al: CT detection of duodenal perforation. AJR 137: 333–336, 1981

51. Sperling L, Rigler LG: Traumatic retroperitoneal rupture of duodenum: description of valuable roentgen observations in its recognition. Radiology 29: 521–524, 1937

52. Toxopeus MD, Lucas CE, Krabbenhoft KL: Roentgenographic diagnosis in blunt retroperitoneal duodenal rupture. AJR 115: 281–288, 1972

53. Sagel SS, Siegel MG, Stanley RJ, et al: Detection of retroperitoneal hemorrhage by computed tomography. AJR 129: 403–409, 1977

54. Dembner AG, Jaffe CC, Simeone J, et al: A new computed tomographic sign of pancreatitis. AJR 133: 477–479, 1979

55. Mendez G Jr, Isikoff MB, Hill MC: CT of acute pancreatitis: Interim assessment. AJR 135: 463–469, 1980

56. Meyers MA, Evans JA: Effects of pancreatitis on the small bowel and colon: Spread along mesenteric planes. AJR 119: 151–165, 1973

57. Myerson PJ, Berg GR, Spencer RP, et al: Gallium-67 spread to the anterior pararenal space in pancreatitis: Case report. J Nucl Med 18: 893–895, 1977

58. Siegelman SS, Copeland BE, Saba GP, et al: CT of fluid collections associated with pancreatitis. AJR 134: 1121–1132, 1980

59. Griffin JF, Sekiya T, Isherwood I: Computed tomography of pararenal fluid collections in acute pancreatitis. Clin Radiol 35: 181–184, 1984

60. Susman N, Hammerman AM, Cohen E: The renal halo sign in pancreatitis. Radiology 142: 323–327, 1982

61. Dickson AP, Imrie CW: The incidence and prognosis of body wall ecchymosis in acute pancreatitis. Surg Gynecol Obstet 159: 343–347, 1984

62. Grey Turner G: Local discoloration of the abdominal wall as a sign of acute pancreatitis. Br J Surg 7: 394–395, 1919

63. Wulsin JH: Peptic ulcer of the posterior wall of the stomach and duodenum with retroperitoneal leak. Surg Gynecol Obstet 134: 425–429, 1972

63a. Casolo F, Bianco R, Franceschelli N: Perirenal fluid collection complicating chronic pancreatitis: CT demonstration. Gastrointest Radiol 12: 117–120, 1987

63b. Weil F, Brun P, Rohmer P et al: Migrations of fluid of pancreatic origin: Ultrasonic and CT study of 28 cases. Ultrasound in Med & Biol 9(5): 485–496, 1983

64. Meyers MA: Roentgen significance of the phrenicocolic ligament. Radiology 95: 539–545, 1970

65. Polkey HJ, Vynalek WJ: Spontaneous nontraumatic perirenal and renal hematomas: Experimental and clinical study. Arch Surg 26: 196–218, 1933

66. Evans JA, Meyers MA, Bosniak MA: Acute renal and perirenal infections. Semin Roentgenol 6: 274–291, 1971

67. Bacon RD: Respiratory pyelography: A study of renal motion in health and disease. AJR 44: 71, 1940

68. Nesbit RM, Dick VS: Pulmonary complications of acute renal and perirenal suppuration. AJR 44: 161–169, 1940

68a. Vermooten V: The mechanism of perinephric and perinephritic abscesses: A clinical and pathological study. J Urol 30: 181–193, 1933

69. Friedenberg RM, Moorehouse H, Gade M: Urinomas secondary to pyelosinus backflow. Urol Radiol 5: 23–29, 1983

70. Morgan CL Jr, Grossman H: Posterior ureteral valves as a cause of neonatal uriniferous perirenal pseudocyst (urinoma). Pediatr Radiol 7: 29–32, 1978

71. Crabtree EG: Pararenal pseudo-hydronephrosis: With report of three cases. Trans Am Assoc Genitourinary Surg 28: 9–40, 1935

72. Razzaboni G: Richerche sperimentali sulla pseudoidronefrosi. Arch Ital Chir 6: 365–372, 1922

73. Hudson HG, Hundley RR: Pararenal pseudocyst. J Urol 97: 439–443, 1967

74. Weintrab HD, Rall KL, Thompson IM, et al: Pararenal pseudocysts: Report of three cases. AJR 92: 286–290, 1964

75. Sauls CL, Nesbit RM: Pararenal pseudocysts: a report of four cases. J Urol 87: 288–296, 1962

76. Johnson CM, Smith DR: Calcified perirenal pseudohydronephrosis: Hydronephrosis with communicating perirenal cyst with calcification. J Urol 45: 152–164, 1941

77. Pyrah LN, Smiddy FG: Pararenal pseudohydronephrosis: A report of two cases. Br J Urol 25: 239–246, 1953

78. Itoh S, Yoshioka H, Kaeriyama M, et al: Ultrasonographic diagnosis of uriniferous perirenal pseudocyst. Pediatr Radiol 12: 156–158, 1982

79. Macpherson RI, Gordon L, Bradford BF: Neonatal urinomas: Imaging considerations. Pediatr Radiol 14: 396–399, 1984

80. Suzuki Y, Sugihara M, Kuribayashi S, et al: Uriniferous perirenal pseudocyst detected by 99m-Tc-dimercaptosuccinic acid renal scan. AJR 133: 306–308, 1979

81. Healey ME, Teng SS, Moss AA: Uriniferous pseudocyst: Computed tomographic findings. Radiology 153: 757–762, 1984

82. Hurwitz SP, Weisenthal CL: Pararenal pseudocyst. J Urol 97: 8–15, 1967

83. Kark RM, Muehrcke RC, Pollack VE, et al: An analysis of 500 percutaneous renal biopsies. Arch Intern Med 101: 439–450, 1958

84. Mukamel E, Nissenkorn I, Avidor I, et al: Spon-

taneous rupture of renal and ureteral tumors presenting as acute abdominal condition. J Urol 122: 696–698, 1979

85. Pollack HJ, Popky G: Spontaneous subcapsular renal hemorrhage: Its significance and roentgenographic diagnosis. J Urol 108: 530–533, 1972

86. Watnick M, Spindola-Franco H, Abrams HL: Small hypernephroma with subcapsular hematoma and renal infarction. J Urol 108: 534–536, 1972

87. Sherman JL, Hartman DS, Friedman AC, et al: Angiomyolipoma: Computed tomography—pathologic correlation of 17 cases. AJR 137: 1221–1226, 1981

88. Mastrodomenico L, Korobkin M, Silverman PM, et al: Perinephric hemorrhage from metastatic carcinoma to the kidney. J Comp Assist Tomogr 7(4): 727–729, 1983

89. Choyke PL, White EM, Zeman RK, et al: Renal metastases: Clinicopathologic and radiologic correlation. Radiology 162: 359–363, 1987

90. Shirkhoda A: Computed tomography of perirenal metastases. J Comp Assist Tomogr 10(3): 435–438, 1986

91. Rosen A, Korobkin M, Silverman PM, et al: CT diagnosis of ruptured abdominal aortic aneurysm. AJR 143: 265–268, 1984

92. Sandler CM, Jackson H, Kaminsky RI: Case report: Right perirenal hematoma secondary to a leaking abdominal aortic aneurysm. J Comp Assist Tomogr 5(2): 264–266, 1981

93. Mackenzie AR: Spontaneous subcapsular renal hematoma: Report of case misdiagnosed as acute appendicitis. J Urol 84: 243–245, 1960

94. Engel WJ, Page IH: Hypertension due to renal compression resulting from subcapsular hematoma. J Urol 73: 735–739, 1955

95. Marshall WH Jr, Castellino RA: Hypertension produced by constricting capsular renal lesions ("Page" kidney). Radiology 101: 561–565, 1971

96. Takahashi M, Tamakawa Y, Shibata A, et al: Computed tomography of "Page" kidney. J Comp Assist Tomogr 1: 344–348, 1977

97. Page IH: Production of persistent arterial hypertension by cellophane and perinephritis. JAMA 113: 2046–2048, 1939

98. Frank IN, Wieche DR: Nephrotomographic appearance of spontaneous subcapsular hemorrhage. Radiology 89: 477–482, 1967

99. Pollack HM, Popky GL: Roentgenographic manifestations of spontaneous renal hemorrhage. Radiology 110: 1–6, 1974

100. Meyers MA, Friedenberg RM, King MC, et al: The significance of the renal capsular arteries. Br J Radiol 40: 949–956, 1967

101. Koehler PR, Talner LB, Friedenberg MJ, et al: Association of subcapsular hematomas with nonfunctioning kidney. Radiology 101: 537–542, 1973

102. Schaner EG, Barlow JE, Doppman JL: Computed tomography in the diagnosis of subcapsular and perirenal hematoma. AJR 129: 83–88, 1977

103. Federle MP, Kaiser JA, McAninch JW, et al: The role of computed tomography in renal trauma. Radiology 141: 455–460, 1981

104. Sandler CM, Toombs BD: Computed tomographic evaluation of blunt renal injuries. Radiology 141: 461–466, 1981

105. Presman D, Rolnick D, Portney F: Spontaneous perinephric hematoma secondary to renal tumor. Am J Surg 102: 586–593, 1961

106. Robson CJ, Churchill BM, Anderson W: The results of radical nephrectomy for renal cell carcinoma. J Urol 101: 297–301, 1969

107. Skinner DG, Colvin RB, Vermillion CD, et al: Diagnosis and management of renal cell carcinoma: A clinical and pathologic study of 309 cases. Cancer 28: 1165–1177, 1979

108. Waters WB, Richie JP: Aggressive surgical approach to renal cell carcinoma: Review of 130 cases. J Urol 122: 306–309, 1979

109. Cherrie RJ, Goldman DG, Lindner A, et al: Prognostic implications of vena cava extension of renal cell carcinoma. J Urol 128: 910–912, 1982

110. Sogani PC, Herr HW, Bains MS, et al: Renal cell carcinoma extending into inferior vena cava. J Urol 130: 660–663, 1983

111. DeKirnion JB, Berry D: The diagnosis and treatment of renal cell carcinoma. Cancer 45: 1947–1956, 1980

112. Johnson CD, Dunnick NR, Cohan RH, et al: Renal adenocarcinoma: CT staging of 100 tumors. AJR 148: 59–63, 1987

113. Weyman PJ, McClennan BL, Stanley RJ, et al: Comparison of computed tomography and angiography in the evaluation of renal cell carcinoma. Radiology 137: 417–424, 1980

114. Lang EK: Angio-computed tomography and dynamic computed tomography in staging of renal cell carcinoma. Radiology 151: 149–155, 1984

115. Thomas JL, Bernardino ME: Neoplastic-induced renal vein enlargement. Sonographic evaluation. AJR 136: 75–79, 1981

116. Didier D, Racle A, Etievent JP, et al: Tumor thrombus of the inferior vena cava secondary to malignant abdominal neoplasms: US and CT evaluation. Radiology 162: 83–89, 1987

117. Fein AB, Lee JKT, Balfe DM, et al: Diagnosis and staging of renal cell carcinoma: A comparison of MR imaging and CT. AJR 148: 749–753, 1987

118. Hricak H, Demas BE, Williams RD, et al: Magnetic resonance imaging in the diagnosis and staging of renal and perirenal neoplasms. Radiology 154: 709–715, 1985

119. Loughran CF: A review of the plain abdominal radiography in acute rupture of abdominal aortic aneurysms. Clin Radiol 37(4): 383–387, 1986

120. Nichols GB, Schilling PJ: Pseudo-retroperitoneal gas in rupture of aneurysm of abdominal aorta. AJR 125: 134–137, 1975

121. Hopper KD, Sherman JL, Ghaed N: Aortic rupture into retroperitoneum. Letter to the editor. AJR 145: 435–437, 1985

122. Kam J, Patel S, Ward RE: Computed tomography of aortic and aortoiliofemoral grafts. J Comp Assist Tomogr 6(2): 298–303, 1982

123. Mark A, Moss AA, Lusby R, et al: CT evaluation of complications of abdominal aortic surgery. Radiology 145: 409–414, 1982

124. Meyers MA, Volberg F, Katzen B, et al: Haustral anatomy and pathology: A new look. I. Roentgen identification of normal patterns and relationships. Radiology 108: 497–504, 1973

125. Meyers MA, Volberg F, Katzen B, et al: Haustral anatomy and pathology: A new look. II. Roentgen interpretation of pathologic alterations. Radiology 108: 505–512, 1973

125a. Christensen EE, Landay MJ: Visible muscle of the diaphragm: Sign of extraperitoneal air. AJR 135: 521–523, 1980

126. Feldberg MAM, Koehler PR, van Waes P: Psoas compartment disease studied by computed tomography: Analysis of 50 cases and subject review. Radiology 148: 505–512, 1983

127. Williams MP: Non-tuberculous psoas abscess. Clin Radiol 37: 253–256, 1986

128. Lee JKT, Glazer HS: Psoas muscle disorders: MR imaging. Radiology 160: 683–687, 1986

129. Gavant ML, Salazar JE, Ellis J: Intrarenal rupture of the abdominal aorta: CT features. J Comp Assist Tomogr 10(3): 516–518, 1986

# 5 The Renointestinal Relationships: Normal and Pathologic Anatomy

## General Introduction

Many patients with renal disease present with symptoms that seem to arise from the digestive tract. Practically every case of urinary tract disease is known to be accompanied by some gastrointestinal complaint of a transitory or permanent character, particularly nausea, vomiting, epigastric distress, constipation, or diarrhea.[1] Gastrointestinal symptoms alone have been noted in up to 43% of patients. Since clinical investigation of such patients is often started with barium contrast studies, it is important to recognize that characteristic effects on specific portions of the bowel may uncover the primary renal disease and redirect the course of evaluation.[2]

Basic to a radiologic appreciation of the characteristic bowel changes is an understanding of the renointestinal anatomic relationships.

## Anatomic Considerations

### The Right Kidney

The right kidney is in intimate relationship to two segments of the gastrointestinal tract: the descending duodenum and the hepatic flexure of the colon. Figures 5–1 and 5–2 illustrate these relationships and the reflections of the posterior parietal peritoneum in the right flank. Virtually all of the right kidney is invested anteriorly by peritoneum except at two sites constituting its "bare areas":

(1) Medially, the second portion of the duodenum descends immediately in front of the right kidney. Here the peritoneum reflects to continue anterior to the duodenum and pancreas.

(2) Inferiorly, the extraperitoneal colon courses obliquely over the lower pole of the kidney. This occurs precisely at its level between (a) the distal ascending colon and the posterior hepatic flexure, which is related superiorly to the deep inferior visceral surface of the liver; and (b) the anterior hepatic flexure as it crosses the descending duodenum; this segment marks the beginning of the transverse mesocolon and is related superiorly to the gallbladder.

A common variant exists in the extent of peritonealization of the second portion of the duodenum. Frequently, the postapical segment of the duodenum remains intraperitoneal for several centimeters, even as it courses inferiorly, suspended by the lesser omentum. The point at which it penetrates the posterior parietal peritoneum to descend extraperitoneally as a straight segment is marked characteristically by a mild junctional flexure. An exaggerated form of this is seen as the "hammock" duodenum.

Because of the oblique position of the kidney along the lateral edge of the psoas muscle, its medial surface projects somewhat anterior to its lateral border. Thus, it can be appreciated that both anterior and medial displacement of the descending duodenum, distal to its postapical segment, would result from a right renal mass.

While some variation occasionally exists, the descending duodenum usually lies on a more posterior plane than the duodenojejunal (DJ)

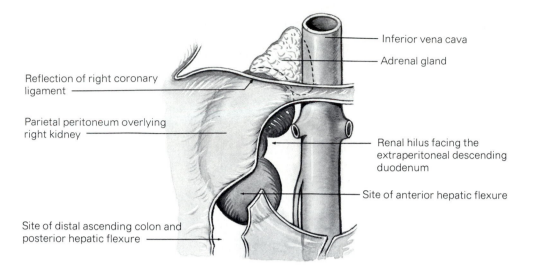

**Fig. 5–1. Frontal drawing emphasizing relationships of right kidney to descending duodenum and hepatic flexure of the colon by virtue of their peritoneal reflections.**

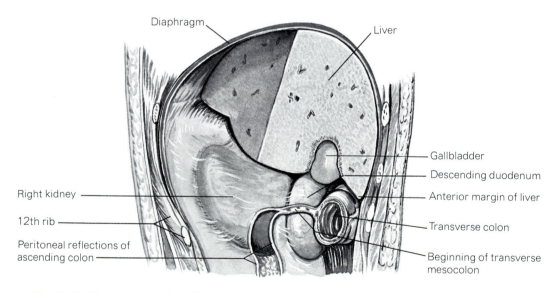

**Fig. 5–2. Right parasagittal drawing showing anatomic relationships to the right kidney.**

junction at the ligament of Treitz. In a standard right lateral projection of an upper GI series, therefore, projection of the second duodenum anterior to the fourth (ascending) duodenum and DJ junction should be viewed with suspicion of a right renal mass.

The upper two-thirds of the right kidney are related to the right colon between its two flexures, whereas the lower pole is inframesocolic and is related laterally and anteriorly to the distal ascending colon.

## The Left Kidney

The relationships of the left kidney to the bowel are most intimate to the distal transverse and proximal descending colon. Figure 5–3 illustrates these relationships and the complex peritoneal reflections in the left flank. The reflections of the transverse mesocolon cross the left kidney anteriorly along a narrow "bare area" at the junction of its middle and lower thirds to continue with the peritoneal reflections over the

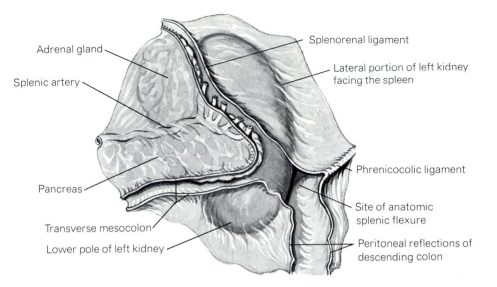

**Fig. 5–3. Frontal drawing emphasizing the relationship of the left kidney to the colon by virtue of their peritoneal reflections.**

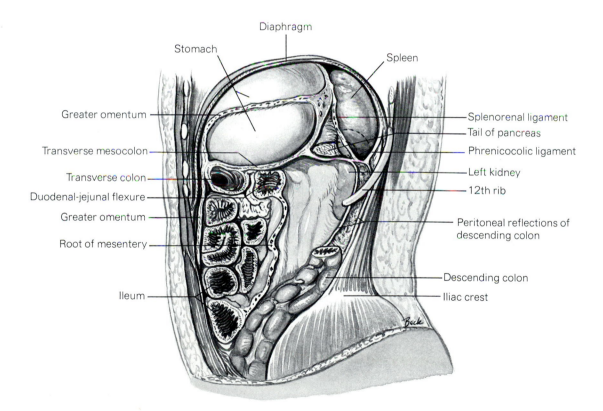

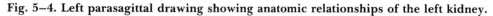

**Fig. 5–4. Left parasagittal drawing showing anatomic relationships of the left kidney.**

descending colon. At the junction of the transverse and the descending colon, the peritoneum reflects from the anatomic splenic flexure to form the phrenicocolic ligament that inserts on the left diaphragm at the level of the 10th and 11th ribs. The distal transverse colon is related to the anterior surface of the lower half of the left kidney, although at variable distances, depending upon the length of the transverse mesocolon. The lower pole is fully inframesocolic. The extraperitoneal descending colon passes downward along the lateral border of the left kidney, turning somewhat medially toward the lower border of the psoas muscle at the lower pole. Other peritoneal reflections account for the splenorenal ligament, within which the tail of the pancreas inserts and the splenic vessels course. More anterior to the medial surface of the left kidney lie the greater curvature of the stomach, and inferiorly, the duodenojejunal junction and jejunal loops. Figure 5–4 clarifies these relationships in a parasagittal dimension.

# Radiologic Observations

The intimate anatomic relationships of the kidneys to specific portions of the gastrointestinal tract precisely account for characteristic changes of deformity, displacement, or distortion.[2]

## *Characteristic Mass Displacements*

### The Right Kidney

*Duodenum.* Right renal masses typically cause medial and anterior displacement of the descending duodenum, while the immediate postapical segment tends to be unaffected. This produces a characteristic appearance on frontal and lateral projections. In anteroposterior or posteroanterior views, the immediately proximal second portion of the duodenum descends vertically, but the distal two-thirds is deflected medially (Figs. 5–5 through 5–8). In right lateral projections, correspondingly, the normal descent of the proximal segment is maintained but the distal portion is displaced anteriorly; this may result in a gentle axis inferiorly and anteriorly (Figs. 5–5b and 5–6b) or in a striking ven-

tral bowing (Figs. 5–7 and 5–8b). Extrinsic pressure on the mucosal folds themselves may be best appreciated in only one view. This may be shown as mass flattening of the normal mucosal contour, undulations, or gross mass distortion on the lateral or posterior wall.

These changes in the descending duodenum are usually easily distinguishable from other extrinsic masses. Right adrenal masses may attain a size to affect the postapical segment (Fig. 5–9). Enlargement of the right lobe of the liver typically produces a more uniform medial displacement (Fig. 5–10).

*Small Bowel.* Massive kidney enlargement displaces jejunal loops anteriorly and inferiorly. With progression, particularly if the process is bilateral as in polycystic renal disease, the small bowel may be crowded into the midline (Fig. 5–11).

*Colon.* In masses originating within the upper two-thirds of the right kidney, the right colon segment most typically involved is that extending between the posterior and anterior hepatic flexures. This demonstrates displacement inferiorly, medially, and anteriorly (Figs. 5–12 through 5–14). Extrinsic pressure may be further shown by flattening and compression of the superior and posterior haustral rows at this site. Dilatation of an extrarenal pelvis in some cases of obstructive hydronephrosis may produce a more generalized mass effect extending to the anterior hepatic flexure (Fig. 5–15).

Occasionally, similar changes may be produced by a liver mass projecting downward from the visceral surface of the right lobe of the liver (Fig. 5–16).

Extension of a renal mass laterally into the flank displaces the posterior hepatic flexure inferiorly (Figs. 5–12 through 5–14). Further progression may result in striking displacement of the ascending colon medially and anteriorly (Figs. 5–17 and 5–18). Maintenance of the lateral haustral contours with extrinsic flattening of the posterior haustral sacculations (Fig. 5–18b) characterize the mass effects as extraperitoneal in site, rather than those from a mass within the intraperitoneal lateral paracolic gutter.[3,4]

A mass originating in the lower pole of the right kidney characteristically elevates the colon

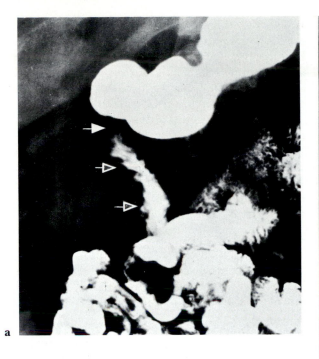

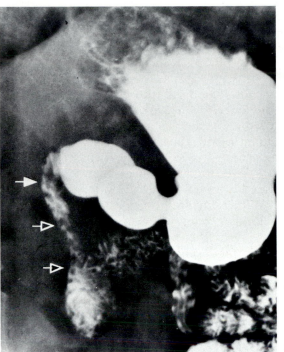

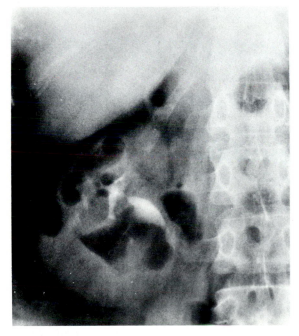

**Fig. 5–5. Displacement of descending duodenum by right renal cyst.**
(a) Frontal and (b) right lateral views. The proximal portion descends normally (closed arrow), but there is medial and anterior displacement of the distal two-thirds (open arrows).
(c) Intravenous urography demonstrates enlargement of lower pole of right kidney by a large cyst. (From Meyers[2])

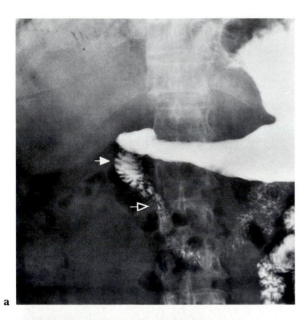

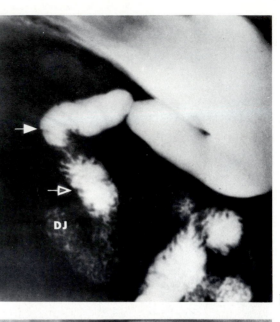

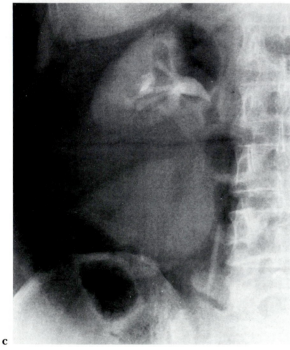

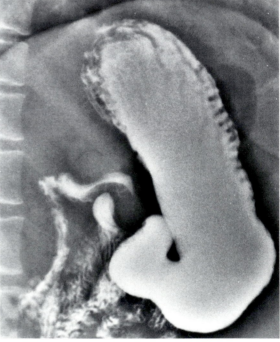

**Fig. 5–6. Displacement of descending duodenum by right renal cyst.**

(a) Frontal and (b) right lateral views. The postapical portion of the duodenum descends normally (closed arrow), but there is medial and anterior deflection of the distal two-thirds (open arrow). The descending duodenum projects anterior to the duodenojejunal junction (DJ). In (a) note the renal mass also causes elevation of the hepatic flexure of the colon.

(c) Intravenous urography demonstrates a huge cyst arising from the lower pole.

(From Meyers[2])

**Fig. 5–7. Displacement of descending duodenum by right renal cyst.**

Bowed anterior displacement of second portion of duodenum.

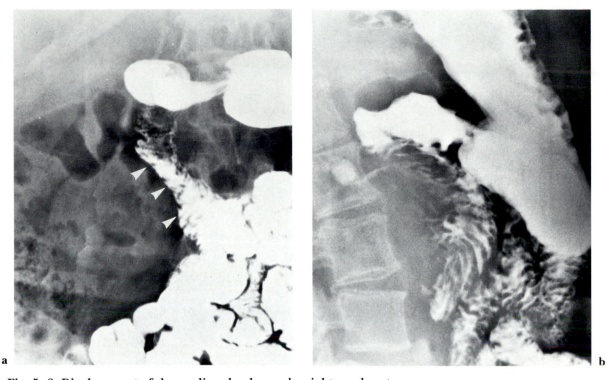

a                                                                          b

**Fig. 5–8. Displacement of descending duodenum by right renal cyst.**
The proximal second portion of the duodenum descends normally. While the frontal projection **(a)** shows only relatively mild medial displacement of the distal two-thirds with flattening of the mucosal folds laterally (arrowheads), the lateral view **(b)** demonstrates striking anterior bowing and extrinsic mucosal distortion. In **(a)** note that the renal mass also elevates the hepatic flexure of the colon.
(From Meyers[2])

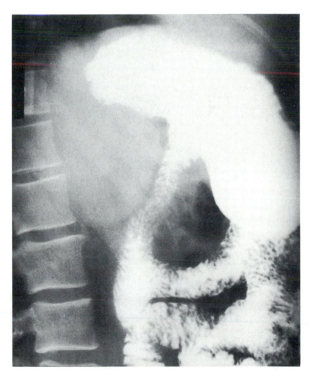

**Fig. 5–9. Displacement of descending duodenum by right adrenal mass.**
The proximal portion of the descending duodenum is displaced anteriorly by an adrenal mass. Its soft tissue outline distinctly conforms to its effect upon the duodenum.

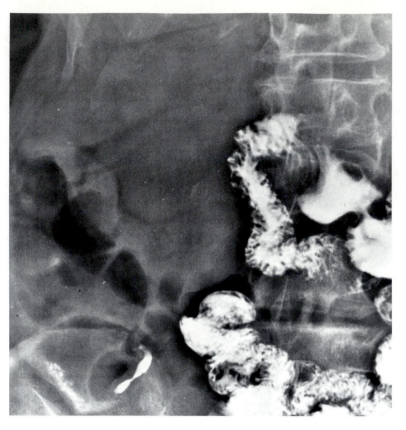

**Fig. 5–10. Displacement of descending duodenum by liver enlarged with metastases.**
There is mild medial displacement of the descending duodenum and compression upon the gas-filled hepatic flexure of the colon.

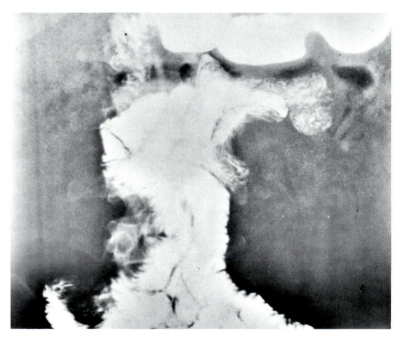

**Fig. 5–11. Displacement of small bowel by polycystic renal disease.**
Massive renal enlargement bilaterally crowds jejunal loops toward the midline. (From Meyers[2])

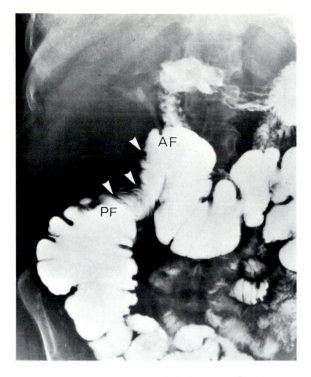

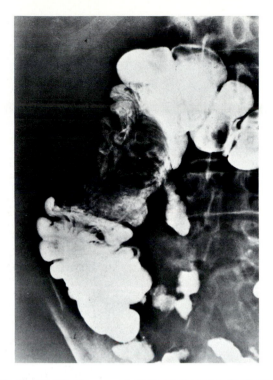

**Fig. 5–12. Displacement of right colon by right renal cyst.**
The large intestine between the posterior (PF) and anterior (AF) hepatic flexures is displaced inferiorly and medially, with extrinsic compression of its superior haustral row (arrowheads). The posterior flexure is mildly displaced downward as the mass, originating in the middle third of the kidney, extends laterally into the flank. Note that there is no displacement of the descending duodenum. (From Meyers[2])

**Fig. 5–13. Displacement of the right colon by hydronephrotic right kidney.**
The segment between the two hepatic flexures is displaced inferiorly and medially. There is extrinsic flattening of its superior haustral border and marked compression of the lumen by the hugely dilated renal pelvis. (From Meyers[2])

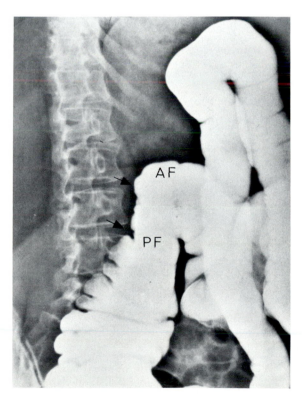

**Fig. 5–14. Displacement of right colon by right renal cyst.**
Oblique view shows the large intestine between the posterior (PF) and anterior (AF) hepatic flexures displaced anteriorly and medially, with extrisic flattening of its posterior haustral row (arrows). (From Meyers[2])

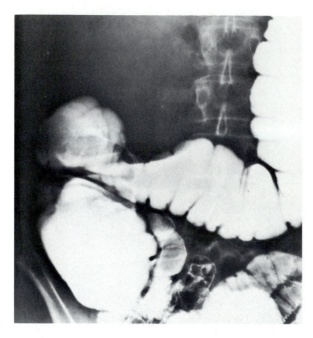

**Fig. 5-15. Displacement of right colon by dilated extrarenal pelvis.**
Marked pyelectasis from obstruction of the upper ureter results in mass pressure extending to the anterior hepatic flexure.

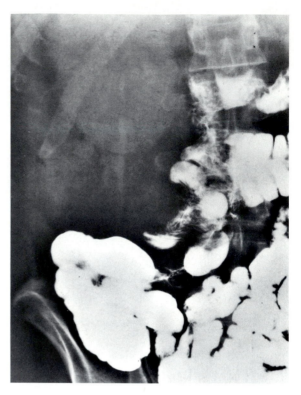

**Fig. 5-16. Displacement of right colon by liver mass.**
The segment between the two hepatic flexures is displaced inferiorly and medially by a large mass extending from the inferior surface of the liver anterior to the right kidney.

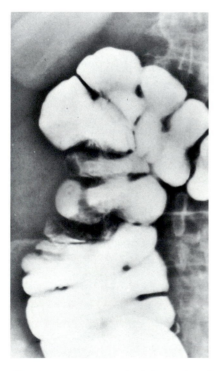

**Fig. 5-17. Displacement of right colon by right multicystic kidney.**
Medial displacement and mass effect on the distal ascending colon.

between the two hepatic flexures (Figs. 5-19 and 5-20). Extrinsic compression occurs on the inferior haustral rows at this site, and the process may affect adjacent segments of the transverse and ascending colon. Oblique projections document that the affected colon also is usually displaced anteriorly and medially. At times, very discrete pressure changes, selectively on the posterior haustra of this segment, may be recognizable, even on frontal projections (Fig. 5-20), an observation further indicating the extraperitoneal nature of the mass.[4]

## The Left Kidney

*Colon.* Left renal masses come into relationship to the colon usually before they attain a size that displaces the stomach, DJ junction, or small bowel. Masses arising in the upper half may displace the distal transverse colon inferiorly and anteriorly. Those originating in the lower half are often first revealed by typical effects on specific portions of the left colon. The descending

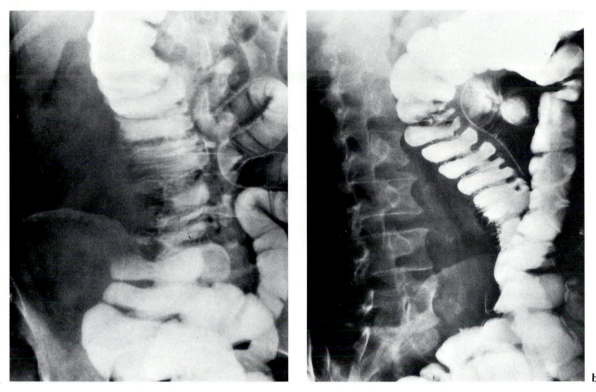

**Fig. 5–18. Displacement of right colon by right renal hypernephroma.**
(**a** and **b**) The mass extends deeply in the flank and markedly displaces the ascending colon medially and anteriorly. The oblique view shows that the posterior haustral contours are flattened by the mass.
(From Meyers[2])

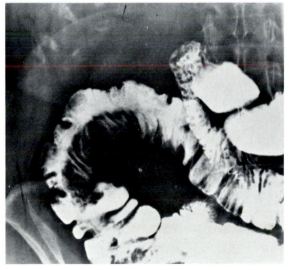

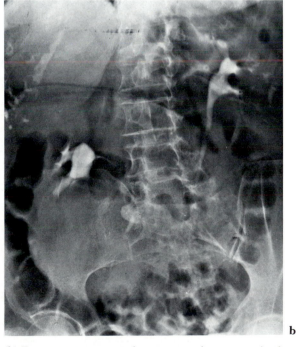

**Fig. 5–19. Displacement of right colon by right renal cyst.**
(**a**) Superior displacement of segment between the two hepatic flexures, with extrinsic compression of its inferior haustral row. The mass also affects the ascending colon. The descending duodenum is uninvolved.

(**b**) Excretory urogram documents a large mass in the lower renal pole with inframesocolic extension.
(From Meyers[2])

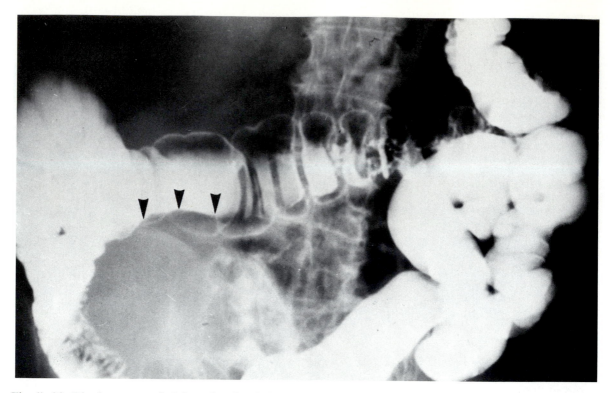

**Fig. 5–20. Displacement of right colon by right renal sarcoma.**
There is mild extrinsic pressure on the inferior border of the segment between the two hepatic flexures by the inframesocolic mass projecting from the lower renal pole. Note that the pressure effects can be localized particularly to the posterior haustral rows (arrowheads). (From Meyers[2])

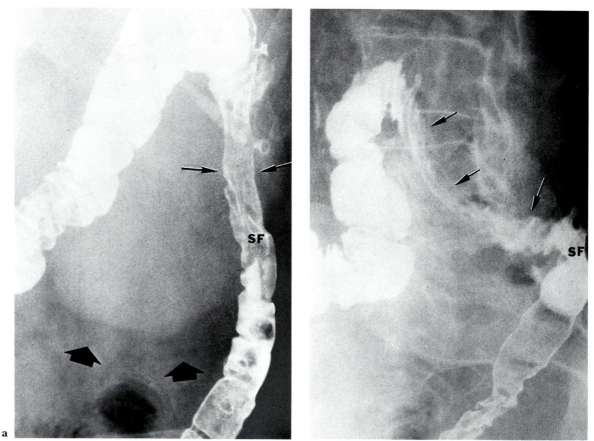

limb of the distal transverse colon appears compressed and displaced laterally and anteriorly (Figs. 5–21 and 5–22). Significantly, the landmark of the anatomic splenic flexure is preserved. Masses projecting from the lower pole displace the descending colon laterally and anteriorly (Fig. 5–23). Again, the anatomic splenic flexure is unaffected.

*Stomach and Small Bowel.* A left renal mass may bulge through into the peritoneal cavity, as shown in Figures 5–24 through 5–26, to displace the greater curvature of the stomach and jejunal loops.

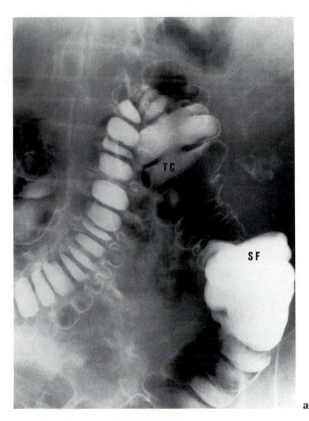

**Fig. 5–22. Displacement of the left colon by left renal carcinoma.**
(a and b) Barium enema and CT show calcified left renal mass (M) producing anterior displacement of distal mesenteric transverse colon (TC). The anatomic splenic flexure (SF) is maintained.

a

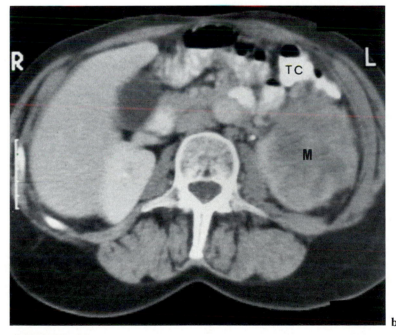

b

**Fig. 5–21. Displacement of the left colon by left renal cyst.**
(a and b) The anatomic splenic flexure (SF) is maintained, but there is lateral and anterior displacement of the descending limb of the distal transverse colon (arrows). The mass enlargement of the lower pole of the kidney is identifiable (large arrows).
(From Meyers[2])

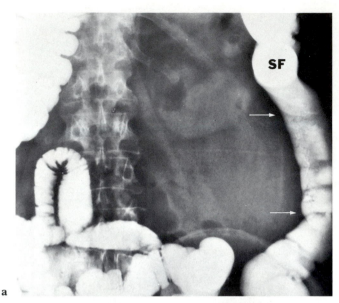

**Fig. 5–23. Displacement of left colon by left renal cyst.**

**(a** and **b)** The descending colon is displaced laterally and anteriorly (arrows) by a large cyst originating from the lower renal pole. The anatomic splenic flexure (SF) is unaffected.
**(c)** Intravenous urography confirms a huge cyst arising from the lower pole.
(From Meyers[2])

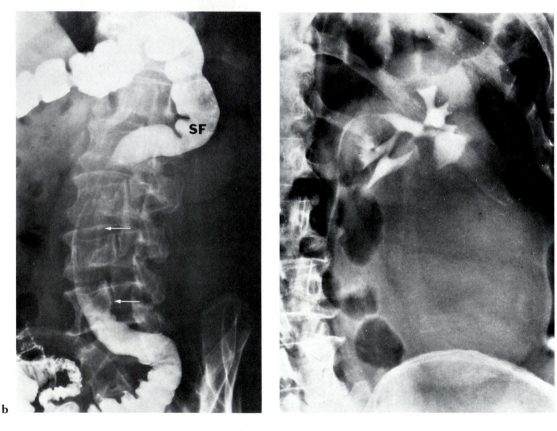

**Fig. 5–25. Displacement of stomach and small bowel by left renal cyst.**
**(a)** The round mass elevates the greater curvature of the stomach and displaces the duodenojejunal junction medially and small bowel loops inferiorly.
**(b)** Selective inferior mesenteric arteriogram shows arcuate displacement of the ascending left colic artery and its branches by the renal mass as it bulges through into the peritoneal cavity.
(From Meyers[2])

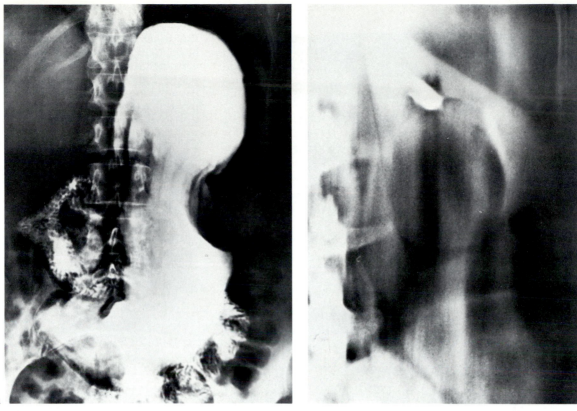

**Fig. 5–24. Displacement of stomach by left renal cyst.**
**(a)** Smooth extrinsic pressure upon the greater curvature of the stomach.
**(b)** Nephrotomogram documents a large cyst arising from the left kidney. It can be presumed to be spherical, with as great an AP dimension to bring it into relationship to the stomach as its coronal dimension.

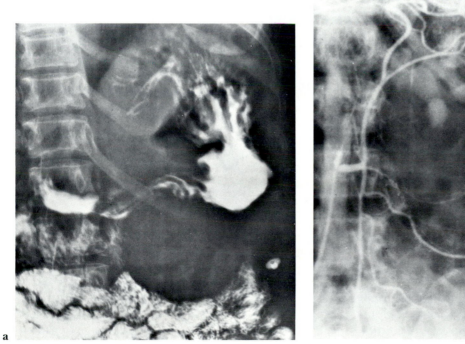
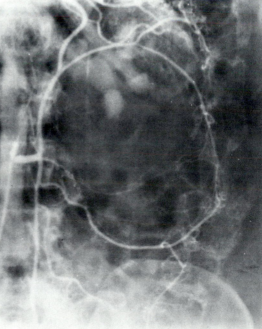

5–25

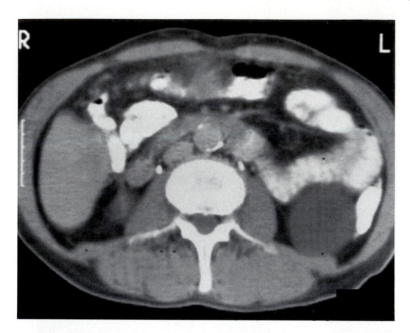

**Fig. 5–26. Displacement of small bowel by left renal cyst.**
CT demonstrates jejunal loops displaced anteriorly by cyst arising from the lower pole of the left kidney.

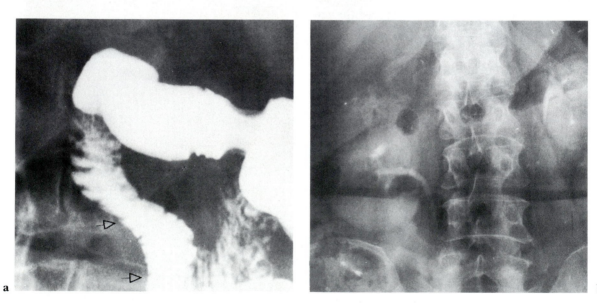

**Fig. 5–27. Displacement of the descending duodenum by a ptotic right kidney.**
**(a)** The distal segment of the descending duodenum is displaced anteriorly and medially (arrows).
**(b)** Intravenous urogram shows a ptotic right kidney with rotation about its vertical axis.
(From Meyers[2])

## Ptosis and Rotation

Ptotic descent of the kidney is frequently accompanied by rotation about its vertical axis. The condition is more common on the right where its effects on the bowel may be misleading unless the anatomic relationships are recognized.[2] The distal descending duodenum may be displaced medially and anteriorly in a manner indistinguishable from a true renal mass (Fig. 5–27). The ptotic kidney may further descend fully to the inframesocolic right lower quadrant so that with rotation it displaces primarily small bowel loops (Fig. 5–28).

## Invasive Hypernephroma

Renal neoplasms may directly invade adjacent segments of bowel, sometimes as recurrences many years after the primary tumor has been resected. On the right, the descending duodenum, and on the left, the distal transverse and proximal descending colon are typically involved. They tend to produce bulky intraluminal masses without significant obstruction, since they generally elicit no desmoplastic response (Fig. 5–29).[24a]

## Perinephritis and Renointestinal Fistulas

Advanced perirenal infection may break through fascial boundaries to involve overlying bowel.[5] The anatomic relationships of the kidneys, the enveloping fascial planes, and the colon are basic to an understanding of the spread of inflammation (Figs. 5–30 and 5–31). The distal transverse colon courses anterior to the lower half of the left kidney. The splenic flexure demarcates the transition between the mesenteric transverse colon and the extraperitoneal descending colon. It lies on a plane posterior to the hepatic flexure and is attached to the diaphragm, opposite the 10th and 11th ribs, by the phrenicocolic ligament, which helps support the lower end of the spleen. The descending colon passes downward along the lateral border of the left kidney, turning somewhat medially toward the lateral border of the psoas muscle at the lower pole. At this level the descending colon lies within areolar tissue in the anterior pararenal space behind the posterior parietal peritoneum. Normally, it is separated posteriorly from the kidney and perirenal fat by the anterior renal fascia; however, its medial and posterior walls face the left kidney and the richest deposit of perirenal fat, which resides behind and lateral to the lower renal pole.

The pathogenesis involves a site of renal infection that breaks through the capsule of the kidney to contaminate the perirenal space. The infection may spread through the perirenal fat as diffuse perinephritis, but coalescence into an abscess has a definite tendency to localize in the rich fat dorsolateral to the lower renal pole.[6,7] The inflammatory process is usually confined to

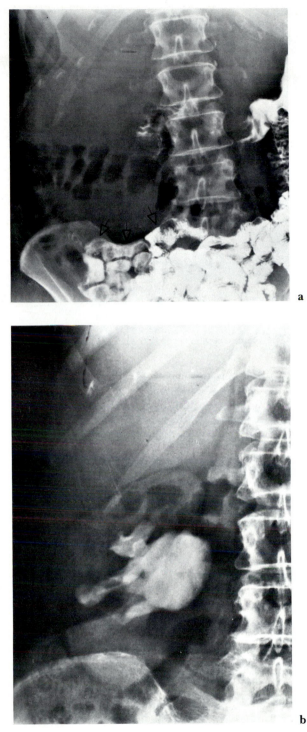

a

b

**Fig. 5–28. Displacement of small bowel by a ptotic right kidney.**
**(a)** There is gentle arcuate displacement of ileal loops (arrows) by a soft-tissue right lower quadrant mass. **(b)** Intravenous urogram shows a hydronephrotic, ptotic right kidney.
(From Meyers[2])

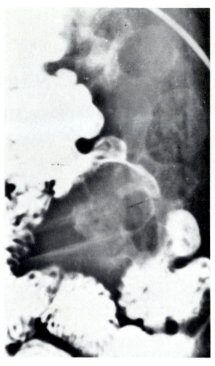

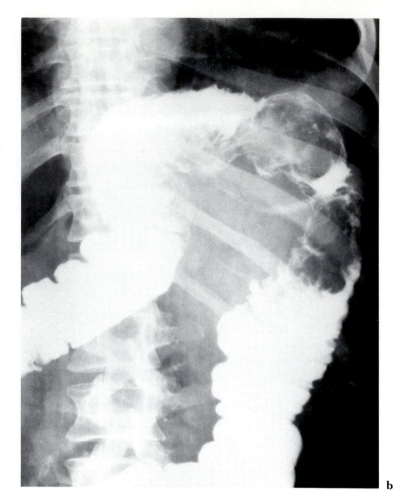

**Fig. 5–29. Direct invasion of the colon by left renal carcinoma.**
(a and b) Two different cases showing extrinsic and intramural masses of the distal transverse and proximal descending colon with bulky polypoid intraluminal extensions.
(b from Meyers[2])

the perirenal compartment by the renal fascia. More fulminating infections break through the fascial boundaries and spread to the overlying structures. On the left, the distal transverse colon and, particularly, the proximal or mid-descending colon and on the right, the ascending colon are involved.

Changes reflecting at least inflammatory adherence may affect principally the medial or posterior contour of the colon or be circumferential. They are manifested primarily by spastic narrowing, scalloped induration, and inflammatory mucosal thickening[5] (Figs. 5–32 through

5–35). In the descending colon, localization to the area distal to the splenic flexure overlaps the site involved in the extension of pancreatitis to the colon,[8] but lack of associated changes involving the flexure itself is a helpful differential point. Extravasated pancreatic enzymes passing along the transverse mesocolon into the phrenicocolic ligament result in inflammatory changes affecting, most characteristically, the splenic flexure. The defects do not closely simulate either the ulcerations and pseudosacculations of granulomatous colitis or the mucosal edema and thumbprinting of ischemic colitis.

⟶

**Fig. 5–32. Colonic changes secondary to left perinephritis.**
Lateral radiograph (a) and frontal spot film (b) demonstrate persistent irregular narrowing 5 cm in length (arrows) just distal to the splenic flexure. The mucosal folds are intact and there is no significant obstruction. Attention was then directed toward the left kidney, and a radiologic workup revealed three 5 × 4 cm perirenal abscesses. At nephrectomy, the lateral surfaces of the masses were adherent to the descending colon.
(From Meyers[5])

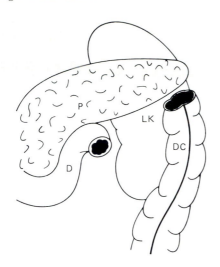

**Fig. 5–30. Frontal drawing illustrating the relationship of the descending colon (DC) to the left kidney (LK) distal to the splenic flexure.**
P = pancreas, D = duodenum. (From Meyers[5])

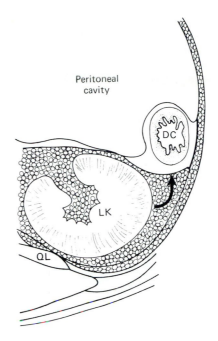

**Fig. 5–31. Horizontal cross-section through the left flank** demonstrating the anatomic relationships. The anterior renal fascia (arrow) demarcates the extraperitoneal descending colon (DC) from the left kidney (LK) and perirenal fat. QL = quadratus lumborum. (From Meyers[5])

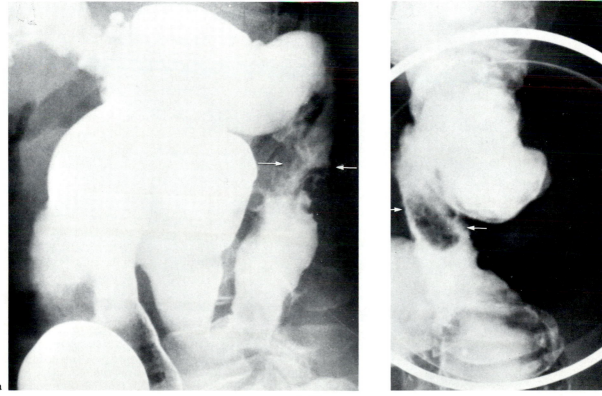

a                                                                                                                                          b

5–32

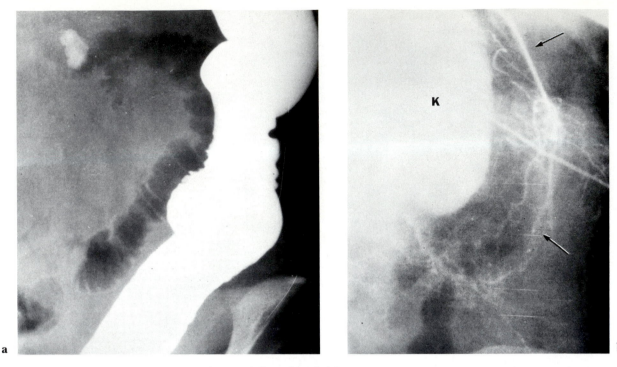

a

b

**Fig. 5–33. Colonic changes secondary to left perinephritis.**
**(a)** Barium enema study reveals localized rigidity and scalloping along the medial wall of the mid-descending colon. A left renal calculus is evident.
**(b)** Selective renal arteriography documented changes of xanthogranulomatous pyelonephritis. On nephrogram phase, wide displacement of the capsular artery (arrows) indicates a diffuse perirenal abscess. This was confirmed at nephrectomy, which also revealed the inflammatory process adhering to the medial wall of the descending colon. K = kidney.
(From Meyers[5])

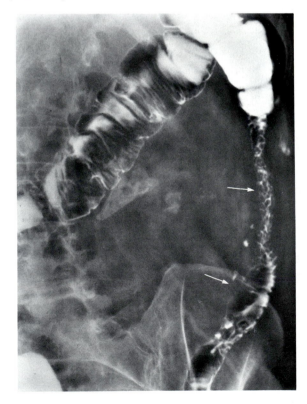

**Fig. 5–34. Colonic changes secondary to left perinephritis.**
Barium enema study shows displacement and mucosal fixation (arrows) along the medial wall of the descending colon. Staghorn calculi are evident in the left kidney. The colonic changes are secondary to a large peripheral abscess which required drainage.

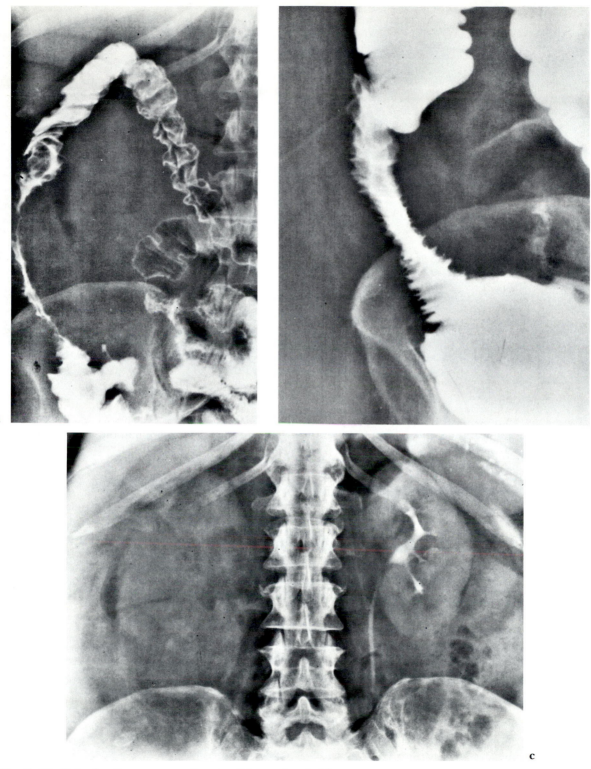

**Fig. 5–35. Colonic changes secondary to right perinephritis.**
(**a** and **b**) Barium enema study shows mass displacement and inflammatory mucosal thickening of the ascending colon.
(**c**) Intravenous urography demonstrates no function in an enlarged right kidney containing an opaque calculus.
    Nephrectomy confirmed the presence of xanthogranulomatous pyelonephritis with a perirenal abscess adherent to the ascending colon.

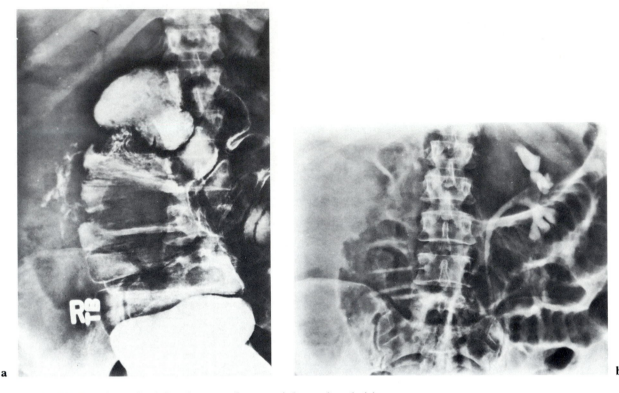

Fig. 5–36. Renointestinal fistula secondary to right perinephritis.
(a) Barium enema study shows loculated extravasation from the distal ascending colon which also presents a stricture with intact mucosal folds.
(b) Excretory urography demonstrates no function on the right. Distortion of the colonic gas shadow with faint extraluminal gas collections are apparent.
    A perirenal abscess secondary to xanthogranulomatous pyelonephritis had established a fistulous communication with the colon.

A gross extraperitoneal sinus communication represents advanced transmural erosion (Figs. 5–36 and 5–37). Most renointestinal fistulas are secondary to an underlying chronic kidney infection that establishes communication usually with the descending duodenum or left colon.[9] Traumatic fistulas are not common but their relative incidence appears to be increasing. Although they may be immediately obvious, they may also appear insidiously months later. Rarely is the communication caused by a primary process of the bowel[10] (Fig. 5–38).

Operative intervention is almost always indicated in renointestinal fistulas. In most cases, the affected kidneys have been the seat of parenchymal infection and stone disease for long periods before detection and have little if any remaining function. Most reported successes involve nephrectomy and bowel closure.[9]

Conservative methods are indicated for renointestinal fistulas detected before severe renal damage has occurred and in selected cases of fistulas.

## Renal Agenesis and Ectopia

Agenesis or ectopia of the kidney is frequently accompanied by characteristic malposition of specific portions of the bowel.[11] Particular segments of the intestine may occupy the area of the renal fossa on the side of agenesis or ectopia, or show characteristic displacement and extrinsic mass effect by an ectopic kidney in as high as 75% of the cases.[11,12]

The clinical value of these observations is twofold:

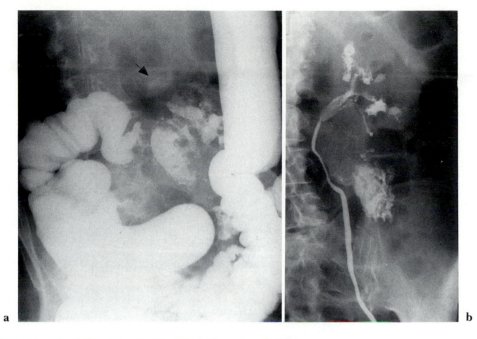

a                                                                                                             b

**Fig. 5–37. Renointestinal fistula secondary to left perinephritis.**
**(a)** Barium enema study demonstrates loculated extravasation from the distal transverse colon confined to the lower left perirenal space. A faintly opaque left renal calculus is evident (arrow).
**(b)** Excretory urography showed no function on the left. Left retrograde pyelography reveals a severely pyelonephritic kidney with a calculus in the renal pelvis. The extravasated barium is contained within an irregular loculated compartment external to the lower renal pole.

Nephrectomy was accomplished with some difficulty because of the marked inflammatory reaction and adherence of the distal transverse colon. The posterior wall of the defect was closed, and multiple large perirenal abscesses were drained.
(From Meyers[2])

1. Identification of the characteristic intestinal malposition or displacement on a barium contrast study uncovers the renal anomaly, which may have multiple clinical implications.

These observations not only allow one to suspect congenital renal anomalies during barium enema examinations, but help in assessment of the nature of the renal abnormality when excretory urography reveals an apparently solitary kidney. In the pediatric patient they may be particularly helpful in the differential diagnosis between renal agenesis and multicystic dysplastic kidney.[13] Although the ureter and trigone are absent in 80% of cases of agenesis,[14,17] one-third of cases of multicystic dysplastic kidney also have no demonstrable ureter or trigone at cystoscopy.[14] Several observers have concluded that nonvisualization of the kidney on excretory urography with normal position of the colon excludes agenesis or ectopia as diagnostic considerations.[13,16]

2. Such bowel changes should not be mistaken for a form of internal hernia, abnormality of rotation of the intestines, or displacement by a tumor mass or organomegaly.

*Embryologic Considerations.* Ashley and Mostofi[14] believe that the initiating factor in renal agenesis is in the metanephric blastema. Disturbances of embryologic growth from the fourth to the eighth week of fetal life may result in renal ectopia. Normally, the kidney reaches its mature level opposite the second lumbar vertebra at the end of the second month. During their migration, the kidneys also rotate 90° so that their convex borders, originally directed dorsally, become directed laterally.

The normal developmental ascent of the kid-

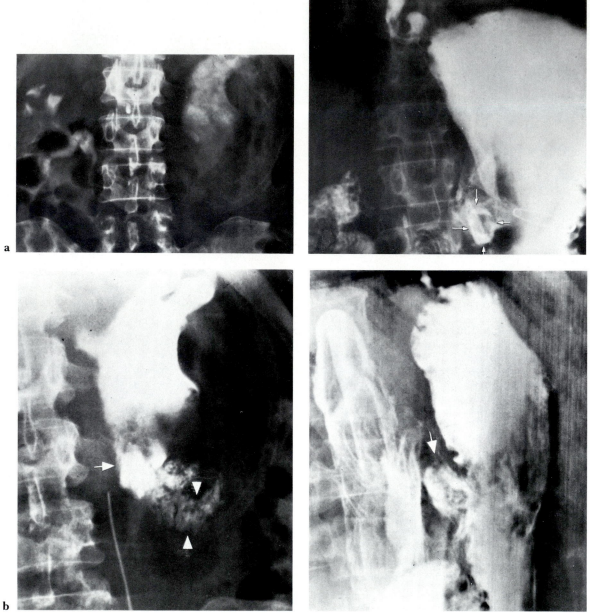

**Fig. 5–38. Renogastric fistula secondary to gastric ulcer.**
(a) Excretory urogram. Gross chronic inflammatory changes with distorted collecting system on the left.
(b) Retrograde pyelogram. Loculated extravasation (arrow) with opacification of gastric mucosa (arrowheads).
(c and d) Upper gastrointestinal series documents large ulcer on posterior wall of stomach (arrows) penetrating to the left kidney.
(From Meyers[2])

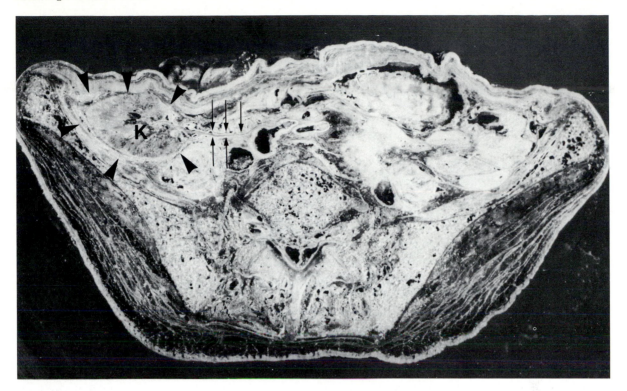

**Fig. 5–39. Anatomic cross-section through pelvis at the level of the iliac crest.**
An ectopic right kidney (K), deriving its blood supply (arrows) from the lower abdominal aorta, maintains its investment by well-defined extraperitoneal fascial planes (arrowheads). These layers of perirenal fascia are not developed cephalad to the ectopic kidney, where only pliable fat constitutes the extraperitoneal tissues. (From Meyers et al[11])

neys is necessary for the formation of the extraperitoneal perirenal fascial planes.[11,17,18] With either agenesis or ectopia of the kidney, extraperitoneal connective tissue in the flanks fails to condense into well-defined fascial layers. In contrast, the perirenal fascia is present in cases of ptotic kidney.

Figure 5–39 is an anatomic cross-section through an ectopic kidney in the pelvis. While the usual perirenal fascial layers immediately enveloping it are clearly demarcated, these could not be identified in the upper extraperitoneal space on the same side; they were present on the opposite side where the kidney was normally positioned. I have documented these associated features *in vivo* by computed tomography. Similarly, cases of renal agenesis and crossed fused ectopia studied by retroperitoneal pneumography document failure of the perirenal fascia to form on the side of the absent kidney (Figs. 5–40 and 5–41).

The lack of restraining fascia appears to contribute to the ease with which bowel malpositions itself into the pliable extraperitoneal fat in the "empty" renal fossa. The associated findings strongly suggest that development of not only the extraperitoneal perirenal fascia, but also portions of the intestinal mesenteric fixation, are embryologically dependent on normal ascent of the kidney.[11]

*Incidence.* These anomalies are not rare. Unilateral renal agenesis and renal ectopia have been found more frequently on roentgen examination (1 in 500) than in autopsy series (1 in 700 to 1500).[14,31a,35] The incidence of crossed fused ectopia is only 1 in 7500. An overrepresentation may be assumed in urologic cases because pathologic conditions, such as stone formation or hydronephrosis, are more common. There is a male to female preponderance in a ratio of 3 : 2 and the anomalies are more common on the left side.[14,17,20]

*Complications and Associated Anomalies.* While such renal anomalies may be compatible with a long life, the incidence of renal disease in a congenitally solitary kidney as a cause of death is high.[14] In unilateral agenesis, the opposite kidney has been found to be diseased in one-third[20] to almost two-thirds[21] of the cases, usually secondary to chronic pyelonephritis. Compensatory hypertrophy of the solitary kidney results in a palpable mass in the flank about 25% of the time.[21] Furthermore, because it projects below the rib cage, it is more susceptible to injury.

In an ectopic kidney or crossed renal ectopia with fusion, the incidence of complications such as lithiasis, infection, and hydronephrosis also approaches 50%.[22] Pain in the lower abdomen may lead to such erroneous diagnoses as appendicitis, diverticulitis, neoplasm of the colon, mesenteric cyst, and ovarian disease.

Pelvic ectopy is important in obstetrics because it may complicate delivery. In a review of the subject, Anderson and associates concluded that most women with pelvic kidney may be delivered vaginally, but if all of the renal tissue lies in the pelvis, as in bilateral ectopy or solitary fused pelvic kidney, cesarean section is the best method of delivery.[19]

Anomalies of structures arising from the urogenital ridge are associated with these renal conditions in as many as 18.5% of cases.[14,20,22-24] These include vaginal atresia, hypoplastic or unicornuate uterus, and the absence of an ovary; less often, monoorchidism and abnormality of the vas deferens are seen in males. The müllerian duct system develops at a later stage in embryogenesis than the wolffian duct and is therefore more likely to undergo malformation, which has been postulated to account for the higher incidence of associated genital anomalies in females than males.

The ipsilateral adrenal gland is often identified on CT as a disk-shaped organ with a parasagittal orientation that appears linear on cross-section.[12,25] Presumably this results from the absence of a normally located kidney which exerts a mass effect on the large, globular fetal adrenal before it shrinks.

Extragenitourinary tract anomalies are frequently associated with unilateral renal agenesis in children[20,26] (Fig. 5–42).

## The Right Side

On the right side, the descending duodenum may be abnormally positioned posteriorly. Normally, the second portion of the duodenum descends immediately anterior to the medial half of the right kidney. In the right lateral projection during an upper gastrointestinal series, the descending duodenum projects anterior to the lumbar spine. With congenital absence or failure of ascent of the right kidney, the descending duodenum may occupy the area of the renal bed and project well over the lumbar spine (Figs. 5–43 and 5–44). Its course on a frontal radiograph appears normal.

Proximal jejunal loops may also occupy a similar position, filling in the renal fossa and coursing abnormally posteriorly (Figs. 5–43 and 5–44).

In right renal agenesis or ectopia, the posterior position of jejunal loops within the renal bed might be most readily confused with a right paraduodenal hernia.[27] The loops, however, do not possess the characteristic circular grouping, stasis, and dilatation; the identifiable afferent and efferent limbs; or the fixation and nondisplacement within an encapsulated hernial sac, despite multiple positions. Distinction is further made by arteriography. In agenesis of the right kidney, jejunal loops and their mesentery and vessels are deflected *anterior* to the superior mesenteric artery into the right flank. In a right paraduodenal hernia, jejunal loops and their mesentery and vessels pass through the fossa of Waldeyer *posterior* to the superior mesenteric artery into a hernial sac of the ascending mesocolon. Frontal projections alone thus show similar findings, with the jejunal arteries arising normally from the left side of the superior mesenteric artery and then coursing abruptly to the right to supply a group of small bowel loops in the right abdomen. Lateral projections during aortography or, more clearly, during selective superior mesenteric arteriography readily differentiate between the two.

The posterior hepatic flexure of the colon may show characteristic posteromedial angulation, occupying the area of the right renal fossa[16] (Figs. 5–45 and 5–46).

## The Left Side

On the left side, there may be striking posteromedial malposition of the distal transverse co-

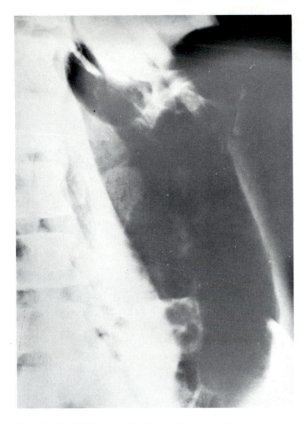

**Fig. 5–40. Unilateral left renal agenesis.**
Presacral retroperitoneal pneumography demonstrates that none of the perirenal fascial layers has developed on the affected side. (From Meyers et al[11])

**Fig. 5–41. Crossed renal ectopia with fusion.**
Presacral retroperitoneal pneumogram with excretory urography. While the adrenal glands (A) have developed normally, the extraperitoneal fat has failed to condense into well-defined connective tissue fascial layers on the left, opposite the fused kidneys (K). (From Meyers et al[11])

**Fig. 5–42. Renal agenesis in association with congenital scoliosis.**
This child presented with congenital scoliosis of the lumbar spine with anomalies including butterfly vertebrae. Intravenous urography demonstrates absence of the right kidney and compensatory hypertrophy on the left.

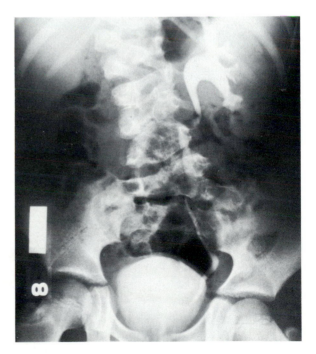

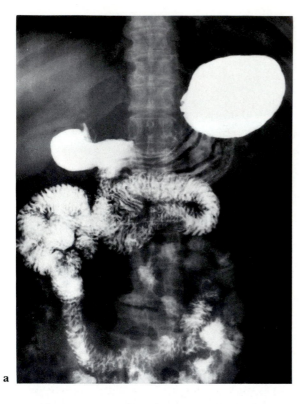

a

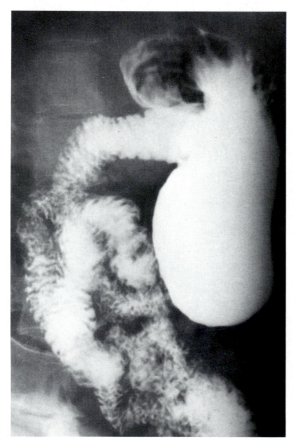

b

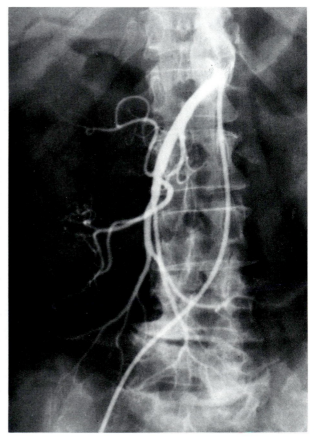

c

**Fig. 5–43. Right renal agenesis with intestinal malposition.**

(**a** and **b**) Upper gastrointestinal series demonstrates striking posterior malposition of the descending duodenum and proximal jejunal loops in the right flank region, simulating some of the features of a right paraduodenal hernia.

(**c** and **d**) Selective superior mesenteric arteriogram. The arterial phase demonstrates the jejunal arteries arising normally on the left, but then curving to the right midabdomen. The capillary blush of the jejunal loops assumes a general reniform contour.

(**e** and **f**) Flush aortogram and delayed film reveal absence of the right kidney and renal artery, with compensatory hypertrophy on the left.

(From Meyers et al[11])

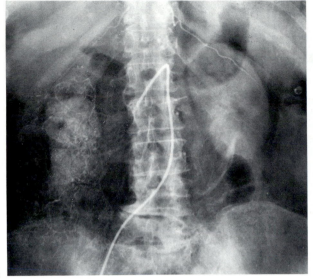

d

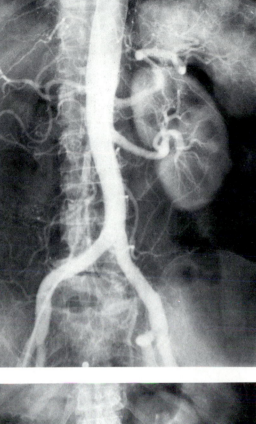

e

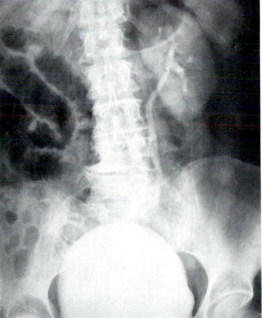

f

5–43

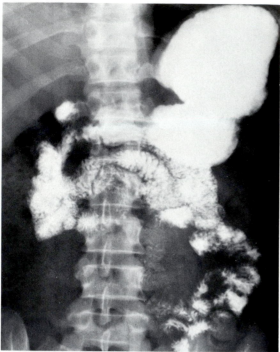

a

**Fig. 5—44. Crossed renal ectopia with intestinal malposition.**
(**a** and **b**) Upper GI series demonstrates posterior malposition of descending duodenum and abnormal location of jejunal loops in area of right renal bed. There is also a suggestion of separation of small bowel loops in the left lower quadrant.
(**c**) Intravenous urogram reveals crossed renal ectopia to the left side.
(From Meyers et al[11])

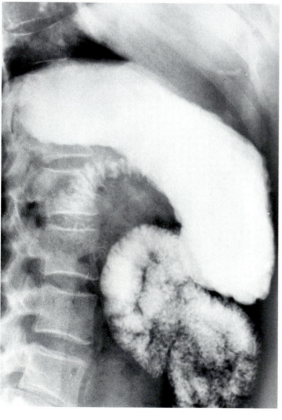

b

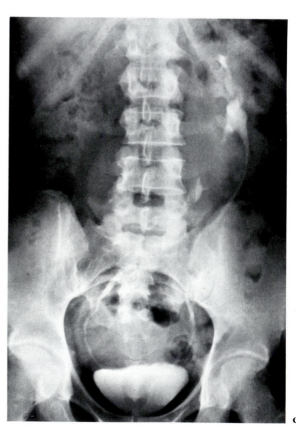

c

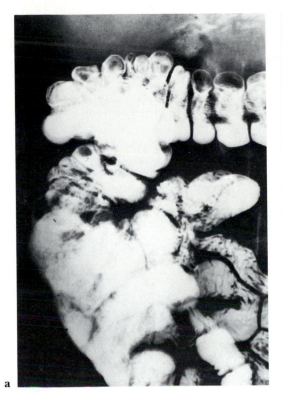

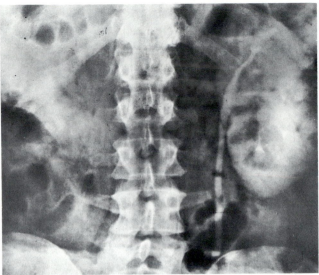

**Fig. 5–45. Colonic malposition in right renal agenesis.**
(a) Upper GI series, delayed film, demonstrates distal ascending colon and posterior hepatic flexure occupy area of right renal fossa.
(b) Excretory urography reveals absence of the right kidney and compensatory hypertrophy on the left.
(Part a reproduced from Curtis et al[16])

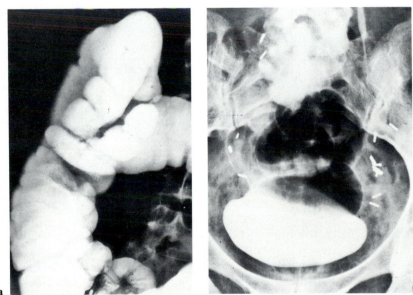

**Fig. 5–46. Colonic malposition in right renal ectopia.**
(a) Barium enema demonstrates angulated posteromedial deflection of posterior hepatic flexure.
(b) Intravenous urogram reveals right ectopic kidney overlying the lumbosacral junction. (Surgical clips are from a previous hysterectomy.)

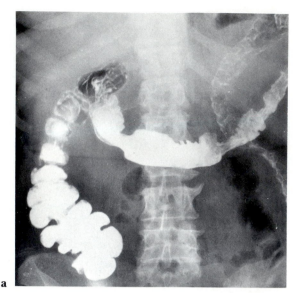

a

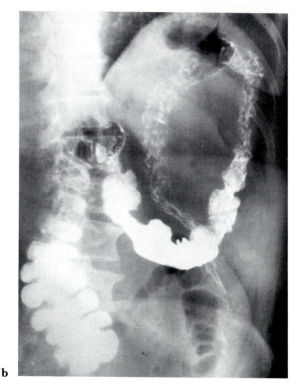

b

**Fig. 5–47. Colonic malposition in left renal agenesis.**
(a and b) Barium enema demonstrates marked medial and posterior malposition of the distal transverse colon and anatomic splenic flexure into the area of the left renal bed.
(c) Intravenous urogram reveals absence of the left kidney.
(From Meyers et al[11])

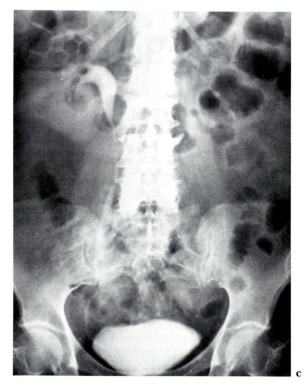

c

lon. Normally, the highest portion of the large intestine in the left upper quadrant ("roentgenographic" splenic flexure) retains the mesenteric attachment of the transverse colon. Distal to this, it courses inferiorly between the medial surface of the spleen and the anterolateral aspect of the left kidney to the anatomic splenic flexure in relation to the splenic angle. The anatomic splenic flexure is normally not only the most posterior but also the most fixed portion of the large intestine, being restrained by the phrenicocolic ligament.[28] Distal to this point, the colon continues as the extraperitoneal descending colon.

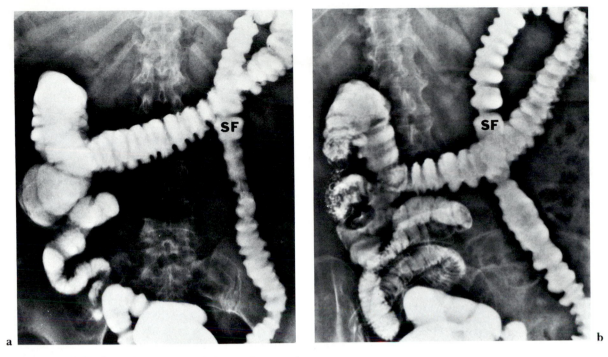

a                                                                                                                              b

**Fig. 5–48. Colonic malposition in left renal agenesis.**
(**a** and **b**) The anatomic splenic flexure (SF) is deflected medially and posteriorly, occupying the position of the "empty" renal fossa.
(From Meyers[2])

With agenesis or ectopia of the left kidney, the mesenteric distal transverse colon may be deflected posteriorly and medially into the "empty" renal fossa area. Similarly, the anatomic splenic flexure of the colon may be deflected toward the same site (Figs. 5–47 and 5–48). The colonic malposition may be evident as a finding on plain films (Fig. 5–49).

Figure 5–50 illustrates colonic herniation through a large foramen of Bochdalek. Associated left renal agenesis is indicated by the medial malposition of the subdiaphragmatic distal transverse colon and anatomic splenic flexure at the level of the phrenicocolic ligament.

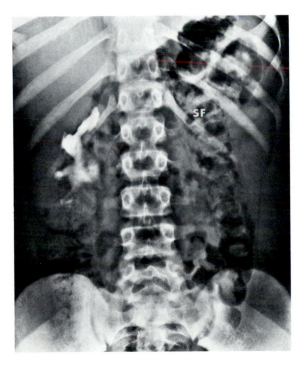

**Fig. 5–49. Colonic malposition in left renal agenesis.**
Excretory urogram. In this child, the anatomic splenic flexure (SF) occupies the "empty" renal fossa. There is compensatory hypertrophy of the right kidney. (From Meyers[2])

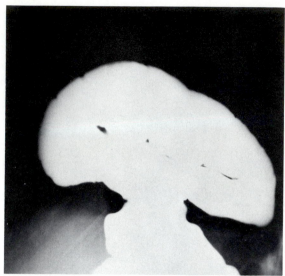

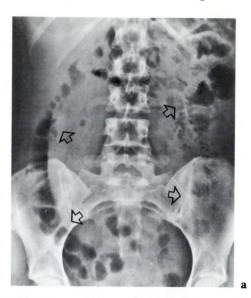

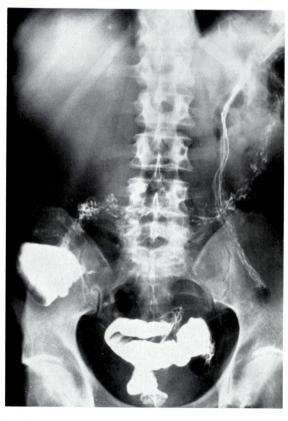

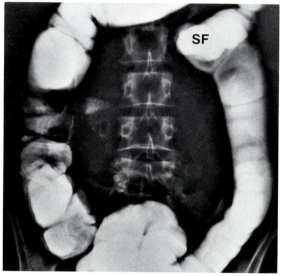

**Fig. 5–51. Torsion of wandering spleen.**
(a) Plain film shows a large central soft-tissue mass displacing bowel loops (arrows).
(b) Barium enema study demonstrates marked medial angulation and malposition of the anatomic splenic flexure (SF). This is produced by traction from the twisted splenic pedicle.

**Fig. 5–50. Intrathoracic colonic herniation.**
(a) Lateral view of barium enema study shows large intrathoracic herniation of the transverse colon through the foramen of Bochdalek.
(b) There is also marked medial malposition of the distal transverse colon and anatomic splenic flexure into the area of the left renal bed. These changes are secondary to associated agenesis of the left kidney.
(From Meyers et al[11])

The most common condition from which these characteristic changes must be distinguished is a congenital anomaly of fixation of the left colon.[15] Here, the splenic flexure may be medially situated, but it is in association with a freely mobile and medially located descending colon.

In left renal agenesis or ectopia, the posteromedial deflection of the distal transverse colon and anatomic splenic flexure into the renal bed should also not be confused for displacement by an enlarged spleen. Splenomegaly may depress the anatomic splenic flexure of the colon but does not displace it medially. In the entity known as wandering spleen,[29–31] laxity or absence of its supporting structures, including the phrenicocolic ligament, allows the organ to migrate from the left upper quadrant. The anatomic splenic flexure may then be sharply angulated medially (Figs. 5–51 and 5–52), a consequence of traction by the splenic pedicle.

These changes in intestinal position have not been seen with renal dysplasia, after flank nephrectomies, or with acquired atrophy of the kidney. In the latter, adipose replacement between the intact perirenal fascial layers contributes to this. However, colonic malposition may be noted after anterior nephrectomies (Figs. 5–53 through 5–56), because of the operative mobilization of the colon and violation of the anterior renal fascia. Occasionally, after left nephrectomy, the tail of the pancreas falls posteriorly and occupies the medial aspect of the renal bed, adjacent to the aorta and the left psoas muscle (Figs. 5–55 and 5–56).

Bowel may be a conspicuous component of lumbar hernias secondary to postoperative flank incisions[34] (Fig. 5–57).

## Direct Intestinal Effects Unique to Renal Ectopia

Ectopic kidneys may be located in the true pelvis (63%), in the iliac fossa or opposite the crest of the ilium (8%), or in the abdomen below the level of the second or third lumbar vertebra and

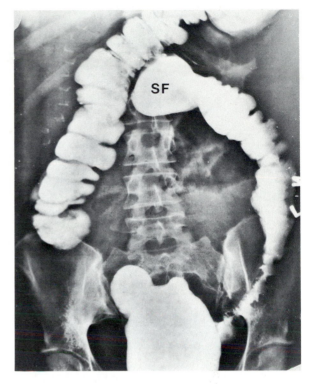

**Fig. 5–52. Torsion of wandering spleen.**
Barium enema study demonstrates sharply angulated medial malposition of the anatomic splenic flexure (SF), produced by traction from an elongated and twisted splenic pedicle. The enlarged congested spleen is indicated by the soft-tissue mass in the lower abdomen displacing the descending and sigmoid colon.

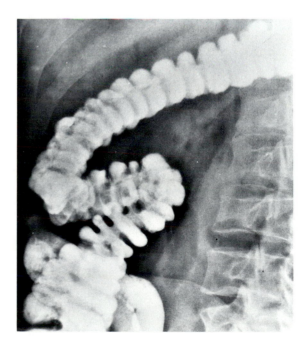

**Fig. 5–53. Malposition of the colon following right nephrectomy.**
The hepatic flexure is deviated into the "empty" renal fossa.

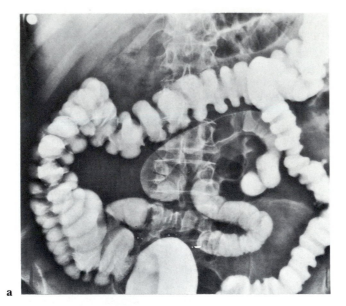

a

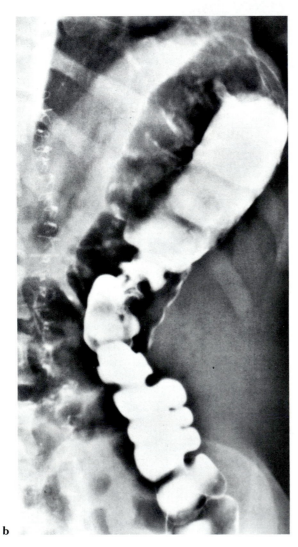

b

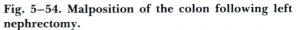

**Fig. 5–54. Malposition of the colon following left nephrectomy.**
In two different cases, the angulated splenic flexure occupies the area of the renal fossa.

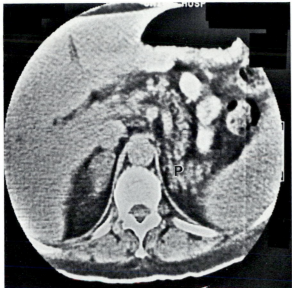

a

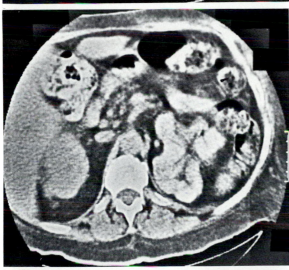

b

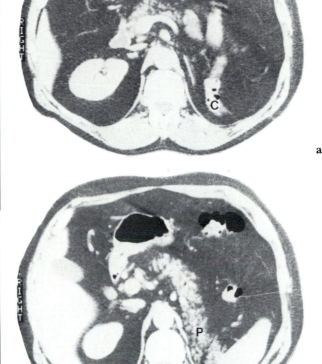

a

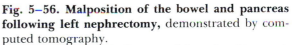

b

**Fig. 5–56. Malposition of the bowel and pancreas following left nephrectomy,** demonstrated by computed tomography.

(**a** and **b**) The splenic flexure of the colon (c), opacified by contrast medium, and the tail of the pancreas (P) are deviated into the renal bed.

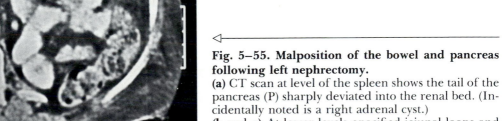

**Fig. 5–55. Malposition of the bowel and pancreas following left nephrectomy.**

(**a**) CT scan at level of the spleen shows the tail of the pancreas (P) sharply deviated into the renal bed. (Incidentally noted is a right adrenal cyst.)

(**b** and **c**) At lower levels opacified jejunal loops and feces-containing colon occupy the "empty" renal fossa.

c

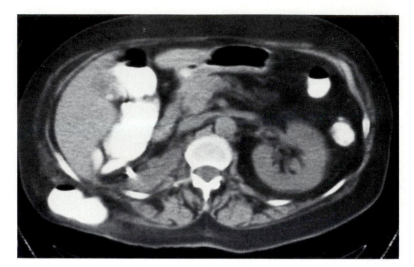

**Fig. 5–57. Herniation of the colon following right nephrectomy.**
CT demonstrates incisional herniation of the posterior hepatic flexure into the flank.

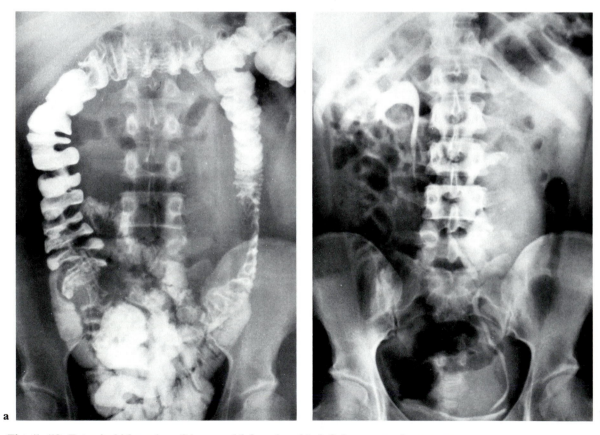

a                                                                                                                                          b

**Fig. 5–58. Ectopic kidney in a 24-year-old female with left lower quadrant mass.**
**(a)** Barium enema examination demonstrates extrinsic mass impression on medial aspect of lower descending colon. In addition, the splenic flexure is sharply angulated posteromedially, indicating an empty renal fossa.
**(b)** Intravenous urogram documents a left ectopic kidney with marked anterior malrotation in relationship laterally to the descending colon.
(From Meyers et al[11])

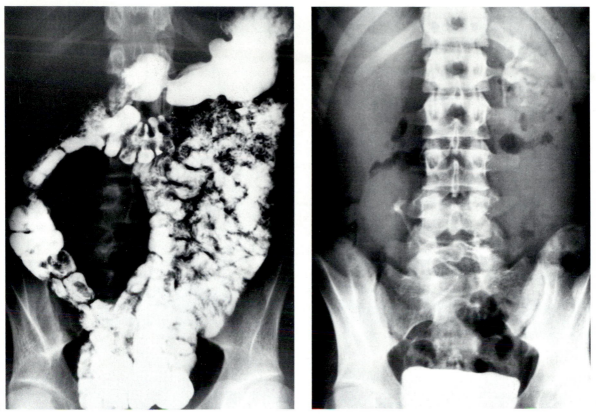

a b

**Fig. 5–59. Ectopic kidney.**
**(a)** Small bowel series. Inframesocolic mass displacement of the small bowel and colon in the right lower quadrant. Note reniform contour of mass displacement.
**(b)** Intravenous urogram reveals an ectopic right kidney with characteristic anterior malrotation.
(From Meyers et al[11])

above the crest of the ilium (29%).[35] In cases of ectopic kidney in the true pelvis, there is usually no definite pressure effect upon the sigmoid colon, presumably because the kidney within the sacral hollow does not come into relationship with the anteriorly directed sigmoid loops.[11]

However, renal ectopia in the iliac fossa or lower abdomen may result in a characteristic mass effect on or displacement of the ascending or descending colon.[11]

On plain films or barium contrast studies, the contour of the density that may be seen in ectopic kidneys usually is not clearly outlined. Two factors appear to account for this: (a) the relative lack of contrasting extraperitoneal fat in the lower abdomen and upper pelvis, and (b) the common marked anterior malrotation of the ectopic kidney. The latter feature also brings the ectopic kidney in the iliac or lower abdomi-

nal area into close relationship with the medial borders of the ascending and descending colon and small bowel loops (Fig. 5–58). Failure to recognize the characteristic mass effects and displacements as secondary to renal ectopia may lead to unnecessary surgery.

If displacement of small bowel loops toward the midline can also be demonstrated, the reniform contour of the "mass" may be shown more clearly (Fig. 5–59).

## References

1. Katz AB: Gastrointestinal manifestations of urinary tract disease. J Urol 69: 726–733, 1953
2. Meyers MA: The reno-alimentary relationships: Anatomic-roentgen study of their clinical significance. AJR Rad Ther Nucl Med 123: 386–400, 1975

3. Meyers MA, Volberg F, Katzen B, et al: Haustral anatomy and pathology: A new look. I. Roentgen identification of normal pattern and relationships. Radiology 108: 497–504, 1973

4. Meyers MA, Volberg F, Katzen B, et al: Haustral anatomy and pathology: A new look. II. Roentgen interpretation of pathologic alterations. Radiology 108: 505–512, 1973

5. Meyers MA: Colonic changes secondary to left perinephritis: New observations. Radiology 111: 525–528, 1974

6. Meyers MA: Acute extraperitoneal infection. Semin Roentgenol 8: 445–464, 1973

7. Meyers MA, Whalen JP, Peelle K, et al: Radiologic features of extraperitoneal effusions. An anatomic approach. Radiology 104: 249–257, 1972

8. Meyers MA, Evans JA: Effects of pancreatitis on the small bowel and colon: Spread along mesenteric planes. AJR 119: 151–165, 1973

9. Bissada NK, Cole AT, Fried FA: Renoalimentary fistula: Unusual urological problem. J Urol 110: 273–276, 1973

10. Dunn M, Kirk D: Renogastric fistula: Case report and review of the literature. J Urol 109: 785–787, 1973

11. Meyers MA, Whalen JP, Evans JA, et al: Malposition and displacement of bowel in renal agenesis and ectopia: New observations. AJR Rad Ther Nucl Med 117: 323–333, 1973

12. Hadar H, Gadoth N, Gillon G: Computed tomography of renal agenesis and ectopy. J Comp Assist Tomogr 8: 137–143, 1984

13. Mascatello V, Lebowitz RL: Malposition of the colon in left renal agenesis and ectopia. Radiology 120: 371–376, 1976

14. Ashley DJ, Mostofi FK: Renal agenesis and dysgenesis. J Urol 83: 211–230, 1960

15. Balthazar EJ: Congenital positional anomalies of the colon: Radiographic diagnosis and clinical implications. II. Abnormalities of fixation. Gastrointest Radiol 2: 49–56, 1977

16. Curtis JA, Sadhu V, Steiner RM: Malposition of the colon in right renal agenesis, ectopia, and anterior nephrectomy. AJR 129: 845–850, 1977

17. Benjamin JA, Tobin CE: Abnormalities of kidneys, ureters, and perinephric fascia: Anatomic and clinical study. J Urol 65: 715–731, 1951

18. Meyers MA: Diseases of the Adrenal Glands. Radiologic Diagnosis with Emphasis on the Use of Presacral Retroperitoneal Pneumography. Charles C Thomas, Springfield, Illinois, 1963

19. Anderson GW, Rice GG, Harris BA: Pregnancy and labor complicated by pelvic ectopic kidney. J Urol 65: 760–776, 1951

20. Doroshow L, Abeshouse BS: Congenital unilateral solitary kidney: Report of 37 cases and review of the literature. Urol Surv 11: 219–229, 1961

21. Braasch WF, Merricks JW: Clinical and radiological data associated with congenital and acquired single kidney. Surg Gynecol Obstet 67: 281–286, 1938

22. Farman F: Anomalies of the kidneys. Handbuch der Urologie, Vol 7. Malformations. Springer-Verlag, Berlin, 1968

23. Fried AM, Oliff M, Wilson EA, et al: Uterine anomalies associated with renal agenesis: Role of gray scale ultrasonography. AJR 131: 973–975, 1978

24. Wiersma AF, Peterson LF, Justema EJ: Uterine anomalies associated with unilateral renal agenesis. Obstet Gynecol 47: 654–657, 1976

24a. Meyers MA, McSweeney J: Secondary neoplasms of bowel. Radiology 105: 1–11, 1972

25. Kenney PJ, Robbins GL, Ellis DA, et al: Adrenal glands in patients with congenital renal anomalies: CT appearance. Radiology 155: 181–182, 1985

26. Macewen GD, Winter RB, Hardy JH: Evaluation of kidney anomalies in congenital scoliosis. J Bone J Surg 54A: 1451–1454, 1972

27. Meyers MA: Paraduodenal hernias: Radiologic and arteriographic diagnosis. Radiology 95: 29–37, 1970

28. Meyers MA: Roentgen significance of the phrenicocolic ligament. Radiology 95: 547–554, 1970

29. Gordon DH, Burrell MI, Levin DC, et al: Wandering spleen—The radiological and clinical spectrum. Radiology 125: 39–46, 1977

30. Smulewicz JJ, Clemett AR: Torsion of the wandering spleen. Am J Dig Dis 20: 274–279, 1975

31. Parker LA, Mittelstaedt CA, Mauro MA, et al: Torsion of a wandering spleen: CT appearance. J Comp Assist Tomogr 8(6): 1201–1204, 1984

31a. Thompson GJ: Incidence of congenital solitary kidney. J Urol 59: 119–128, 1948

32. Alter AJ, Uehling DT, Zwiebel WJ: Computed tomography of the retroperitoneum following nephrectomy. Radiology 133: 663–668, 1979

33. Neumann CH, Hessel SJ: CT of the pancreatic tail. AJR 135: 741–745, 1980

34. Baker ME, Weinerth JL, Andrian RT, et al: Lumbar hernia: Diagnosis by CT. AJR 148: 565–567, 1987

35. Thompson GJ, Pace JM: Ectopic kidney: Review of 97 cases. Surg Gynecol Obstet 64: 935–943, 1937

# 6 The Duodenocolic Relationships: Normal and Pathologic Anatomy

## General Introduction

The precise anatomic relationships between the duodenal loop and the transverse colon are often of critical importance in the radiologic interpretation of upper abdominal pathology. Their points of most intimate relationship represent anatomic crossroads between intraperitoneal and extraperitoneal structures and thus permit specific localization and diagnosis of a disease process.[1] Because of this relationship, a lesion originating in one may exert its major effects on the other. Particularly if radiologic investigation is initiated by a study that manifests the striking secondary effects, the presentation of findings may then be very misleading until the nature of the relationship and the primary site are appreciated.

Detailed knowledge of the intimate anatomic relationships is essential in the radiologic interpretation of a variety of diseases. These include defects of the mesocolon with internal herniation into the lesser sac, masses developing within the mesocolic leaves, extension of neoplasms, duodenocolic fistulas, gallbladder disease, renal masses, pancreatitis, abdominal aneurysm, and distinction between an abscess of Morison's pouch and an inframesocolic abscess.

## Anatomic and Normal Radiologic Features

The key to understanding the significance of the duodenocolic relationships is the insertion of the root of the transverse mesocolon and its planes of reflection (Fig. 6–1).

The hepatic flexure of the colon is characteristically composed of two curvatures.[2] The proximal, more posterior one continues from the fixed extraperitoneal ascending colon and is related to the inferior and lateral edge of the right kidney and the posterolateral tip of the liver. The colon then passes immediately anteromedially over the descending duodenum to the second curve of the hepatic flexure, which is more anterior and is related above to the gallbladder.

At a point between the two curvatures of the hepatic flexure, as the colon is in intimate relationship to the descending duodenum (Fig. 6–2), it begins to pick up the peritoneal sling of the transverse mesocolon. The colon in this area is then in virtual contiguity with the second portion of the duodenum, with the very short edge of the beginning reflection of the transverse mesocolon providing a mesenteric plane (Figs. 6–3 and 6–4).

The root of the transverse mesocolon broadly intersects the inframampullary portion of the descending duodenum and then continues along the anterior surface of the pancreas. Here it is attached to the midportion of the head and the inferior surface of the body and tail. The non-peritonealized bare area, wide on the right and progressively thinner toward the left, thus provides a shared anatomic plane, between the pancreas and descending duodenum behind and the transverse colon in front, along the leaves of the transverse mesocolon.

The transverse mesocolon itself is a fan-shaped structure in the horizontal plane of the body. Short at its beginning, it is longest in the

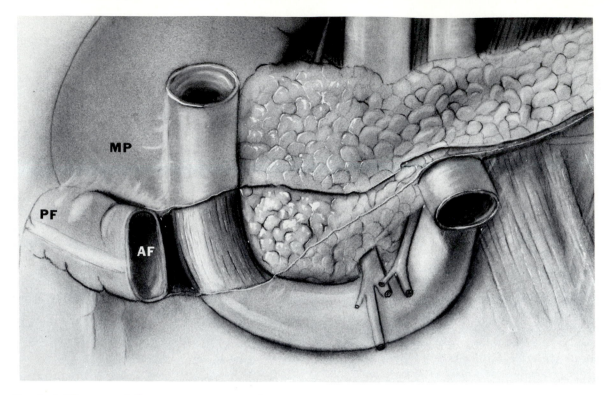

**Fig. 6–1. The root of the transverse mesocolon.**
It extends across the infraampullary portion of the duodenum and lower border of the pancreas. Note the relationships of the anterior hepatic flexure of the colon (AF) and of the duodenojejunal junction. **PF** = posterior hepatic flexure. **MP** marks the location of Morison's pouch, the intraperitoneal posterior extension of the right subhepatic space anterior to the right kidney. (From Meyers and Whalen[1])

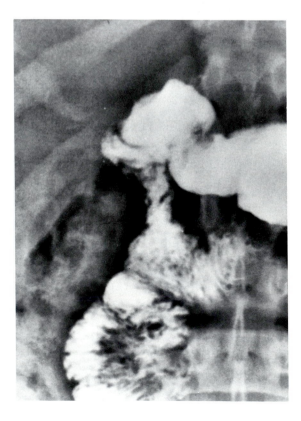

midsagittal plane, becoming abbreviated laterally once again as the colon comes into relationship to the left kidney and the spleen. The length of the transverse mesocolon varies. It tends to be short in stocky individuals and long in tall, thin patients.

The retroperitoneal duodenum bends forward after its ascending portion at the level of the ligament of Treitz to penetrate the posterior parietal peritoneum and continue as the intraperitoneal jejunum.

The duodenojejunal junction is then in intimate relationship to the inferior reflection of the transverse mesocolon (Figs. 6–1 and 6–5). It also serves as a useful landmark for dividing the body and tail of the pancreas.

The duodenojejunal junction, fixed by the ligament of Treitz, generally maintains its posi-

⊲ ————————————————

**Fig. 6–2. A normal upper GI series** frequently shows lateral pressure on the descending duodenum from a feces-distended anterior hepatic flexure of the colon. This reflects their contiguous anatomic relationship.

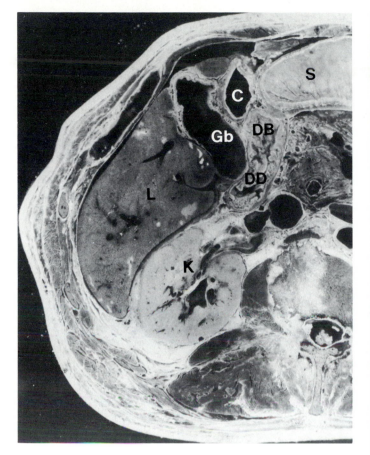

**Fig. 6–3. Transverse section through the right abdomen at the level of the duodenal bulb (DB) and the proximal descending duodenum (DD).**
Note the intimate relationship of the hepatic flexure of the colon (C) at the beginning reflection of the transverse mesocolon. S = stomach, Gb = gallbladder, L = liver, K = kidney. (From Meyers and Whalen[1])

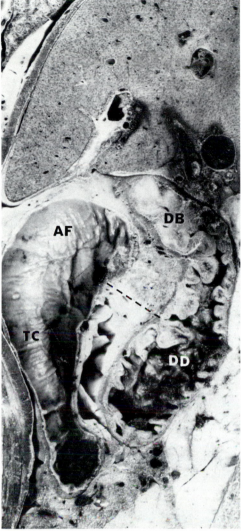

**Fig. 6–4. Right parasagittal section at the level of the duodenal bulb (DB) and the descending duodenum (DD),** showing their relationship to the anterior hepatic flexure (AF) of the colon before it continues ventrally as the transverse colon (TC). The dashed line indicates the transverse mesocolon. (From Meyers and Whalen[1])

tion throughout life at the approximate level of the lower border of L1. The duodenal bulb and proximal portion of the second duodenum, however, tend to descend with age, with progressive laxity of support, a change most marked in the fifth and sixth decades.[3] Nevertheless, the position of the root of the transverse mesocolon, which separates the peritoneal cavity from the lesser sac, can be constantly indicated on an upper GI series by a line drawn from the infraampullary segment of the descending duodenum to a point immediately above the duodenojejunal junction. This delimits the most superior ascent of small bowel loops posterior to the transverse colon normally possible (Fig. 6–6).

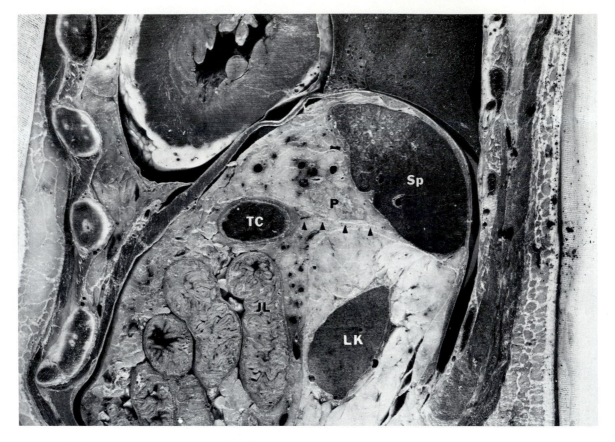

**Fig. 6–5. Left parasagittal section at a level lateral to the duodenojejunal junction.**
Shown are the relationships of the proximal jejunal loops (JL) to the transverse colon (TC) and its mesocolon
(arrowheads), coursing along the inferior aspect of the tail of the pancreas (P). The section is also through the
spleen (Sp) and the left kidney (LK). (From Meyers and Whalen[1])

On the right, the colon inferiorly and the descending duodenum medially provide two of the boundaries of the posterior extension of the subhepatic space (Morison's pouch) anterior to the kidney (Fig. 6–1).

## Abnormal Radiologic Features

### Defect of Mesocolon with Internal Herniation into Lesser Sac

Occasionally, jejunal loops may normally present within the upper abdomen anterior to the transverse colon and, perhaps, the stomach. Cephalad extension of small bowel loops posterior to the transverse colon above the line of the root of the transverse mesocolon in relationship to the descending duodenum and duodenojejunal junction indicates a defect of that mesentery with internal herniation into the lesser sac[1] (Fig. 6–7).

### Masses Within the Mesocolic Leaves

Pathologic alteration in the contour of the duodenum by a localized abnormality arising in the origin of the reflections of the transverse mesocolon is shown in Figure 6–8. The bare area is widest at this site so that symmetric growths developing within the leaves may impress upon the duodenum over a considerable length. The typical points of pressure then are at the immediate infraampullary and the genu locations.

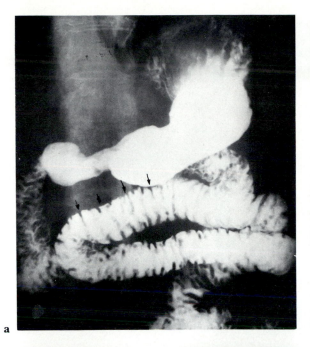

a

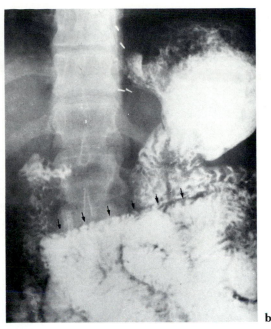

b

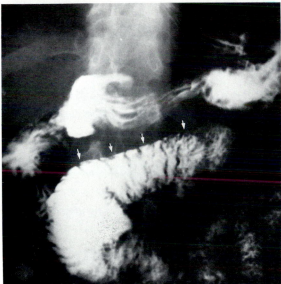

c

Fig. 6–6. The transverse mesocolon (arrows) is outlined by the limitation of cephalad extension of jejunal loops posterior to the transverse colon, resulting in flattening of their superior contour. It corresponds to a line drawn from the mid-descending duodenum to the duodenojejunal junction.
(a) Normal gastrointestinal series.
(b) Post-Billroth II antecolic gastrojejunostomy.
(c) Postduodenojejunostomy.
(From Meyers and Whalen[1])

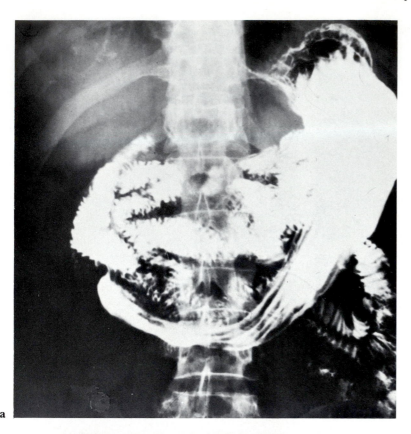

a

**Fig. 6–7. Internal hernia into the lesser sac through a large defect in the transverse mesocolon.**
This is indicated by the high position of the loops of small bowel above the normal insertion of the transverse mesocolon, which no longer determines their contour.
(**a**) Frontal.
(**b**) Prone oblique. Note that the herniated loops present posterior to the transverse colon and stomach.
(From Meyers and Whalen[1])

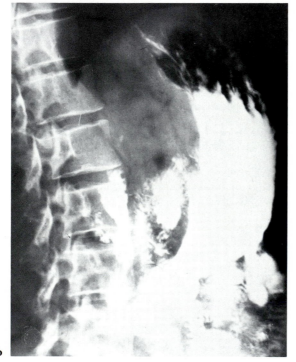

b

## Effect of the Descending Duodenum by Carcinoma of the Hepatic Flexure

The virtual contiguity of the hepatic flexure to the descending duodenum allows ready spread of a neoplasm.[1,4] Figures 6–9 and 6–10 illustrate early stages of this process. The occult nature of carcinoma of the right colon is well known and the presence of fever, abdominal distress, and a palpable epigastric mass may lead to radiologic investigation being initiated with an upper gastrointestinal series. In such cases, striking changes involving the descending duodenum may include extrinsic pressure defects and, occasionally, gas-containing cavities (Fig. 6–11a). These may be very misleading unless a barium enema study is done and the primary site in the hepatic flexure of the colon is revealed (Fig. 6–11b).

## Duodenocolic Fistulas

Although most duodenocolic fistulas result from an infiltrating adenocarcinoma of the hepatic flexure,[5] the communication may be estab-

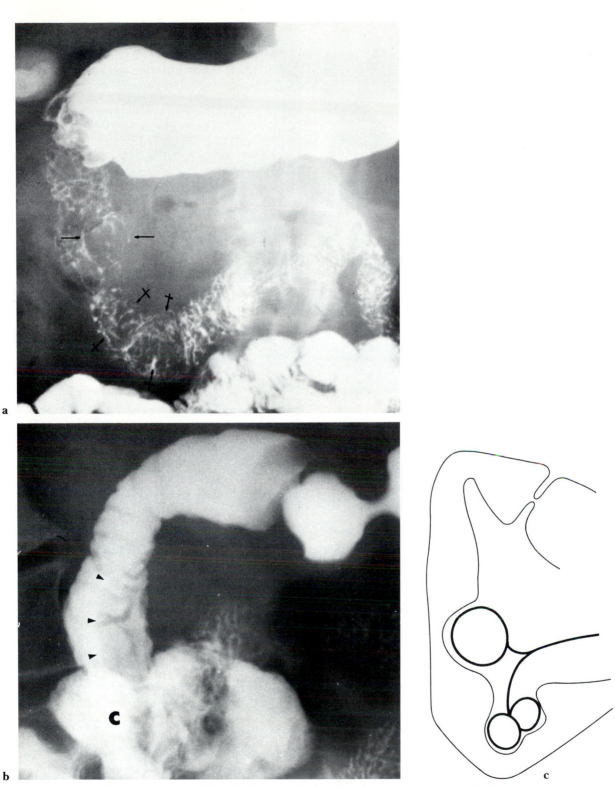

**Fig. 6–8. Lymphangitic cysts within the leaves of the transverse mesocolon** producing extrinsic nodular indentations on the descending duodenum.

(**a**) Prone. Three discrete mass impressions are shown (arrows).

(**b**) Right lateral projection. The larger, more proximal indentation presents on the anterior aspect of the descending duodenum (arrowheads). Note its relationship to the hepatic flexure of the colon (**C**).

(**c**) Cysts within the mesocolon leaves bridging the bare area of the descending duodenum.

(From Meyers and Whalen[1])

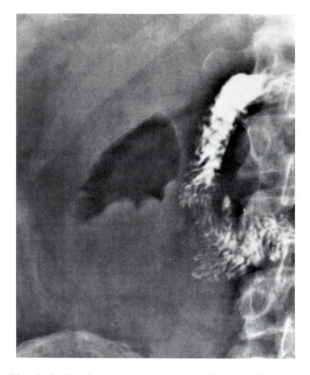

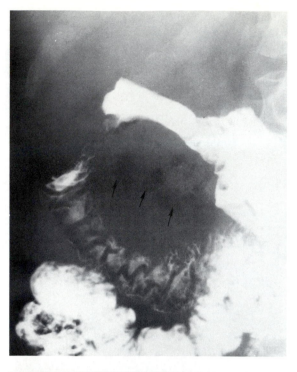

a

## Fig. 6–9. Carcinoma of the hepatic flexure adherent to the descending duodenum.

Upper GI series shows pressure effects on the duodenum by a nodular malignancy within the hepatic flexure outlined by gas. At surgery, this required careful dissection.

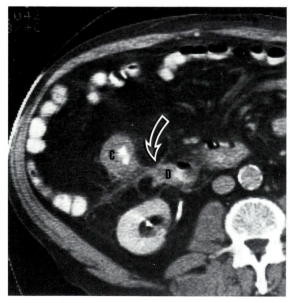

## Fig. 6–10. Adherence of colonic carcinoma to duodenum.

Computed tomography shows early adhesive contiguity (arrow) to the inferior genu of the duodenum (**D**) of a carcinoma which thickens the wall of the hepatic flexure of the colon (**C**). Thickening of the anterior renal fascia and increased reticulation through the perirenal fat are noted.

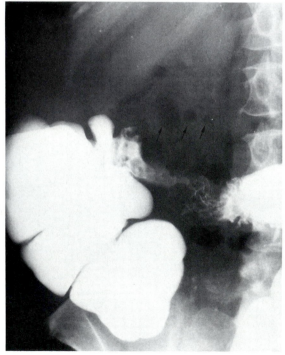

b

## Fig. 6–11. Extension of colonic carcinoma across the mesocolon to the paraduodenal area.

(**a**) Upper gastrointestinal series reveals numerous gas-containing abscess cavities (arrows) within a mass in the area of the head of the pancreas. There are edema and distortion of the mucosal folds of the descending duodenum.

(**b**) A subsequent barium enema shows a primary infiltrating carcinoma of the anterior hepatic flexure with a pericolonic–paraduodenal abscess.

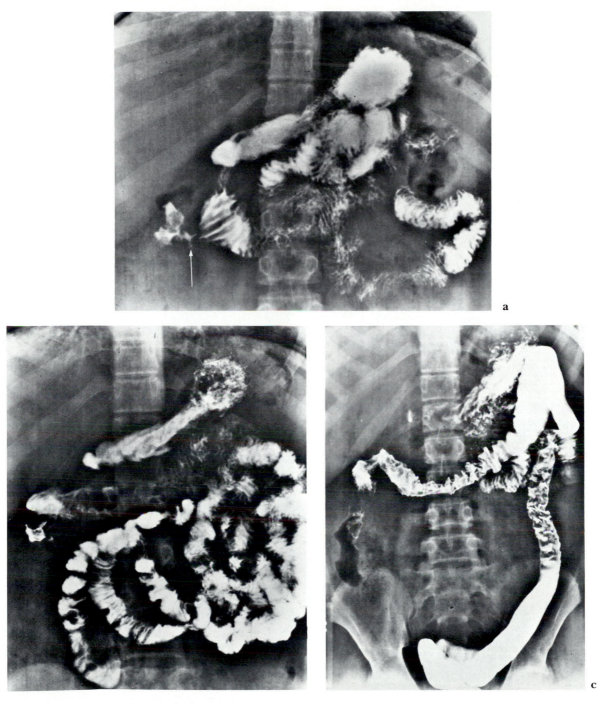

**Fig. 6–12. Duodenocolic fistula secondary to granulomatous colitis.**
Upper GI series demonstrates fistulous communication (arrow) from the intraampullary portion of the descending duodenum to the hepatic flexure, with premature opacification of the transverse colon. Crohn's disease of the large intestine is apparent.

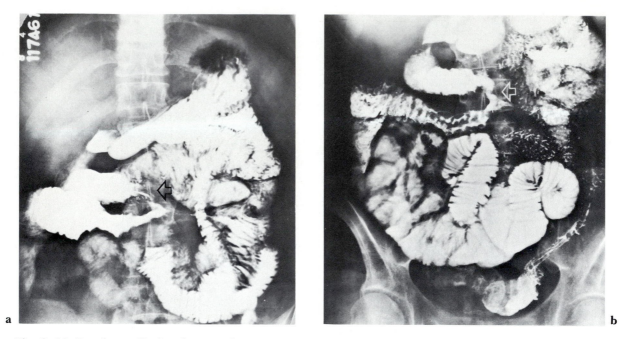

**Fig. 6–13. Duodenocolic fistula secondary to granulomatous colitis.**
(**a** and **b**) Upper GI series demonstrates wide communication (arrows) between the third portion of the duodenum and the transverse colon which is involved by Crohn's disease. The partially bypassed small intestinal loops show changes of malabsorption.

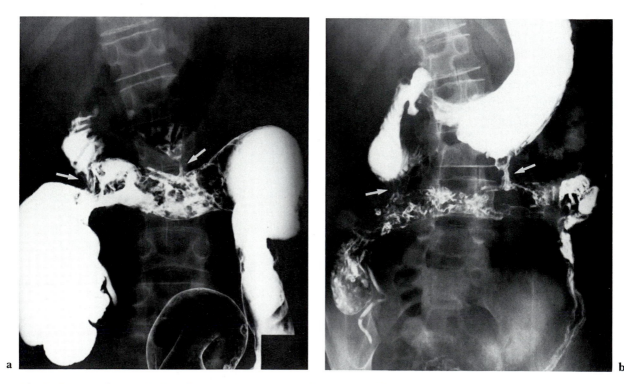

**Fig. 6–14. Duodenocolic fistula secondary to granulomatous colitis.**
Barium enema (**a**) and upper GI series (**b**) demonstrate fistulas between the hepatic flexure of the colon and the duodenum and between the transverse colon and the greater curvature of the stomach (arrows). Extensive Crohn's disease of the large intestine is evident.

**Fig. 6–15. Duodenocolic fistula from chronic "blow-out" of duodenal bulb.**
Following a Billroth II gastrojejunostomy, a fistulous communication (arrow) has developed between the sewn-over duodenal bulb and the hepatic flexure of the colon.

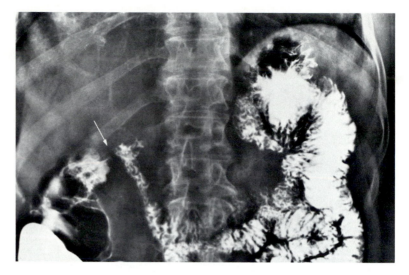

lished by ulcerative or inflammatory disease. Granulomatous colitis is being increasingly recognized as an underlying cause.[6,7] With the right-sided colonic involvement of this transmural inflammatory and ulcerating condition, fistulization may develop between the hepatic flexure particularly or the transverse colon and the duodenum (Figs. 6–12 through 6–14). Malabsorption may result if the small bowel is bypassed significantly, but the fistula need not be a serious complication of Crohn's disease and should not serve as an indication for surgical correction for its own sake.[6–8] A similar duodenocolic fistula may be seen as a postoperative complication (Fig. 6–15).

Examples have been described of fistulous communication between the third part of the duodenum and the transverse colon, which contained a well-marked muscular layer and an intact epithelium. This rare variety is presumably on an embryologic basis.[9]

## Effect of Gallbladder Disease on the Duodenocolic Relationships

The nonspecificity of signs and symptoms of diseases of the gallbladder often makes a clinical diagnosis difficult. At times, it is the striking manifestation of the secondary effects on the neighboring bowel that first brings the patient to medical attention.

Inflammatory adhesions may develop between the gallbladder and the postapical duodenum permitting the development of fistulous communication (Fig. 6–16).

The gallbladder is closely applied to the superior aspect of the anterior hepatic flexure in most individuals[10] (Fig. 6–17). The distance between the inner walls of the gallbladder and the adjacent colon is normally less than 1.5 cm.

When the gallbladder enlarges, as in acute cholecystitis, hydrops, empyema, or Courvoisier's sign of pancreaticoduodenal malignancy, plain films or barium enema study may reveal smooth extrinsic compression of the hepatic flexure (Figs. 6–18 and 6–19). Accompanying pericholecystitis or marked fibrous adhesions may result in mucosal edema or fixation. The postapical duodenum is characteristically displaced medially and may show features of spasm, luminal narrowing, and mucosal irregularities. Carcinoma of the gallbladder commonly infiltrates all layers of its wall and rapidly extends into the surrounding structures. As many as 15% show evidence of colonic invasion on barium enema studies (Fig. 6–20). Fistulous communication between the duodenum and colon may occur from acute cholecystitis or carcinoma of the gallbladder (Figs. 6–21 through 6–24).

## Duodenocolic Displacements from Right Renal Masses

The right kidney bears intimate relationships to both the descending duodenum and the region

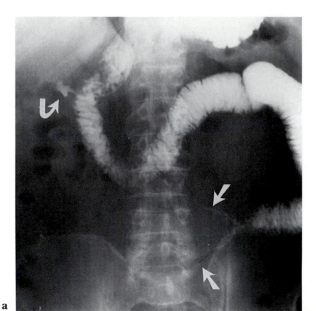

**Fig. 6–16. Cholecystoduodenal fistula with gall-stone ileus.**
(**a**) Upper GI series demonstrates tract (curved arrow) between the duodenum and gallbladder. A large gallstone is impacted in a proximal jejunal loop (arrows).
(**b**) CT shows inflammatory changes (arrow) between the duodenum (**D**) and the shrunken gallbladder (**GB**) which contains air. A dilated loop of jejunum (**J**) is evident. P = pancreas.
(**c**) At a lower level, the partially calcified cholesterol gallstone within the obstructed loop is documented (arrow).

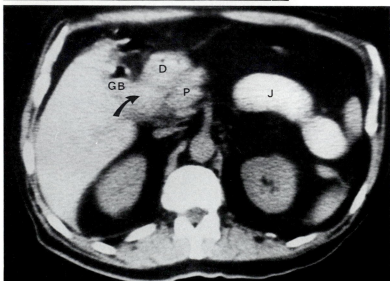

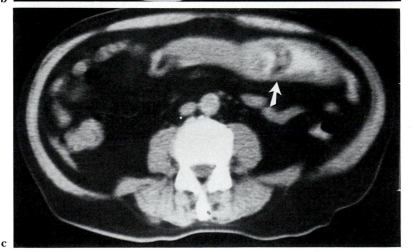

**Fig. 6–17. Right parasagittal section,** showing the close relationship of the gallbladder (GB) to the anterior hepatic flexure of the colon (**C**). **L** = liver, **RK** = right kidney.

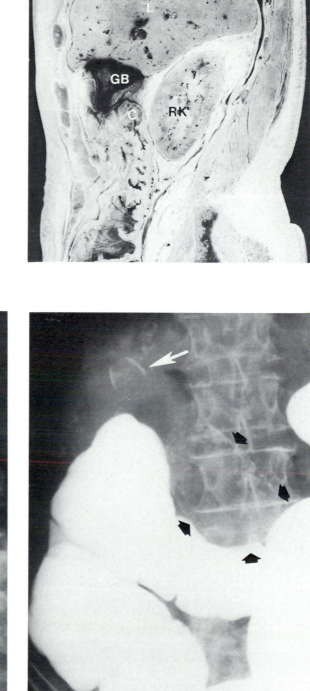

a

b

**Fig. 6–18. Impression of adherent "porcelain" gallbladder.**
(**a**) Plain film shows large calcified gallbladder with impacted stone in its neck (arrow).
(**b**) Barium enema study demonstrates displacement of gallbladder (black arrows) and impression upon anterior hepatic flexure to which it is adherent. White arrow shows impacted stone.
(From Ghahremani and Meyers[10])

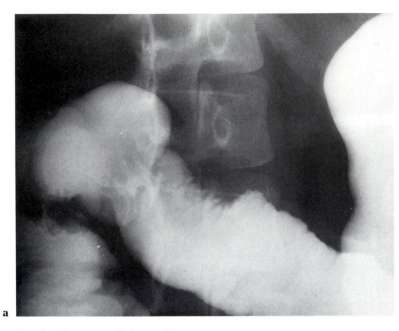
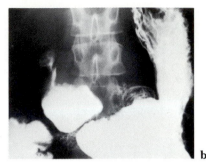

**Fig. 6–19. Acute cholecystitis.**
(a) Mass impression on superior aspect of anterior hepatic flexure, with mucosal irregularities.
(b) Medial displacement and spasm of proximal descending duodenum.
(From Ghahremani and Meyers[10])

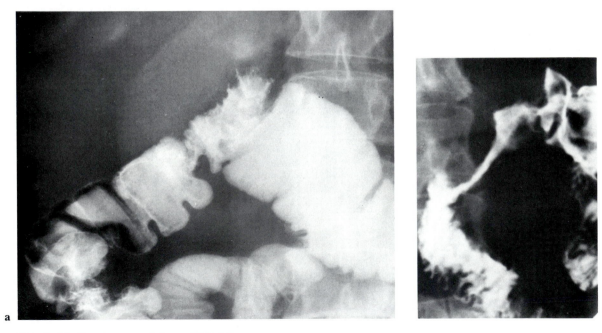

**Fig. 6–20. Carcinoma of the gallbladder.**
(a) Fixation of mucosal folds of anterior hepatic flexure.
(b) Marked compression, narrowing, and medial displacement of the proximal descending duodenum.
(From Ghahremani and Meyers[10])

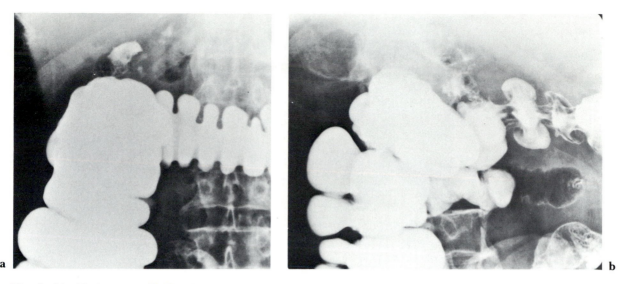

**Fig. 6–21. Cholecystocolic fistula secondary to chronic cholecystitis.**
(**a** and **b**) Frontal and oblique views during a barium enema study demonstrate communication between the anterior hepatic flexure and a small deformed gallbladder.

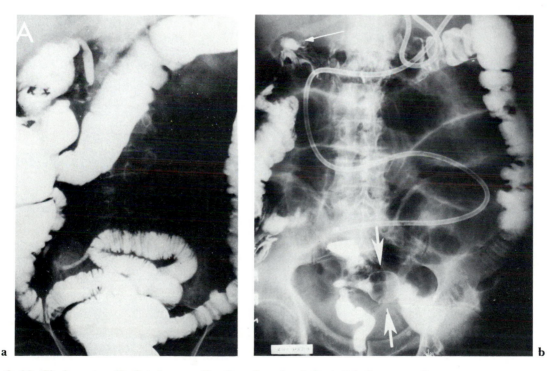

**Fig. 6–22. Cholecystocolic fistula complicating chronic cholecystitis in two patients.**
(**a**) Barium enema study demonstrates a wide communication between the fundus of the gallbladder containing stones and the adherent hepatic flexure.
(**b**) Gallstone ileus due to impaction of large nonopaque gallstones (large arrows) in the sigmoid colon with distended intestinal loops proximally. The cholecystocolic fistula and the shrunken gallbladder (small arrow) are partially opacified with barium.
(From Ghahremani and Meyers[10])

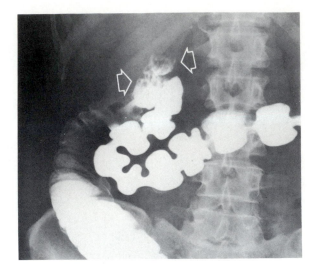

**Fig. 6–23. Cholecystocolic fistula secondary to carcinoma of the gallbladder.**
Barium enema study demonstrates the malignancy infiltrating the anterior hepatic flexure and projecting within the partially opacified gallbladder lumen (arrows).

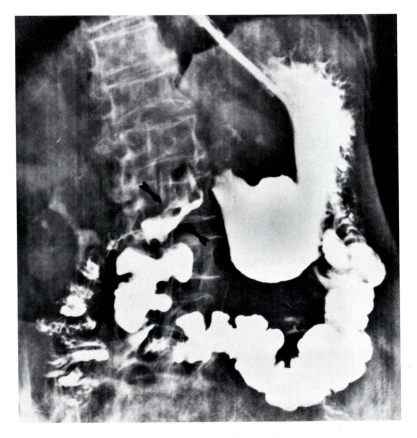

**Fig. 6–24. Carcinoma of the gallbladder with duodenocolic fistula.**
Upper GI series demonstrates the communication to the hepatic flexure of the colon across the malignant bed of the gallbladder (arrows). (From Ghahremani and Meyers[10])

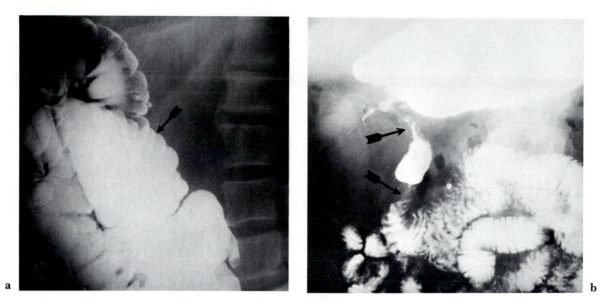

**Fig. 6–25. Leiomyosarcoma of second portion of duodenum with large extramural component.**
(**a**) Right lateral barium enema view shows anterior displacement of the distal hepatic flexure of the colon (arrow).
(**b**) Upper GI series then reveals narrowing, large ulceration, and mass effect on the descending duodenum (arrows).
(From Ghahremani and Meyers[10])

of the hepatic flexures of the colon. Renal masses may thus be revealed by their characteristic effects on the bowel. This is discussed in chapter 5.

## Effect on Colon of Mass Arising in Descending Duodenum

It has been shown that the distal hepatic flexure is in intimate relationship posteriorly to the descending duodenum. Localized anterior displacement of this portion of the colon then indicates a mass arising not in the nearby right kidney or gallbladder but specifically in the second portion of the duodenum (Fig. 6–25). Following identification of the displacement on an initial barium enema study, radiologic investigation can then be immediately directed to the primary site.

## Inframesocolic Extension of Neoplasm of Third Duodenum

The third portion of the duodenum lies retroperitoneally below the root of the transverse mesocolon. Extension of a mass arising in this structure is then revealed on barium enema examination by a characteristic elevation of the proximal transverse colon (Fig. 6–26a). While this type of displacement may occur secondary to such conditions as mesenteric cysts or primary retroperitoneal tumors, initial identification of this inframesocolic component should lead to careful investigation of the transverse duodenum (Fig. 6–26b).

## Acute Pancreatitis

Several of the plain film changes associated with acute pancreatitis, while strongly suggestive of the diagnosis, are by no means pathognomonic. Ileus of the transverse colon in a pattern approaching the "colon cut-off" sign may be seen in a variety of conditions.[1] "Sentinel-loop" dilatation of the descending duodenum may occur secondary to acute cholecystitis or acute right perinephritis. However, simultaneous paralytic dilatation of both, secondary to the effects of the extravasated enzymes along the shared anatomic planes, is diagnostic of acute pancreatitis (Fig. 6–27).

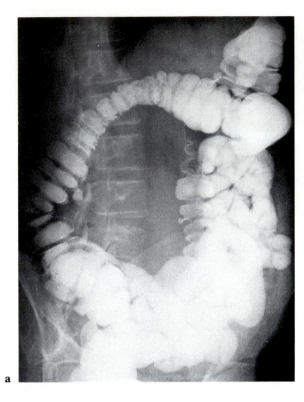

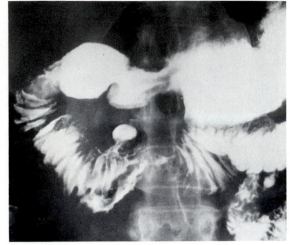

a

b

**Fig. 6–26. Leiomyosarcoma of third portion of the duodenum with large extramural component.**
(**a**) There is gross elevation and displacement of the proximal transverse colon by a huge mass.
(**b**) Upper GI series documents the changes of leiomyosarcoma arising in the transverse duodenum, characterized by irregular ulcerations and sinus tracts within a lobulated and serpiginous submucosal tumor.
(From Meyers[12])

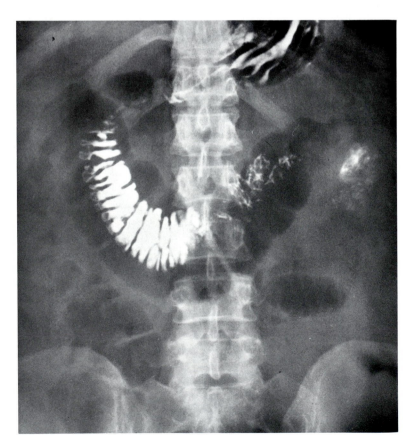

**Fig. 6–27. Acute pancreatitis.**
The radiologic finding of associated ileus of the transverse colon and of the descending duodenum (shown by stasis of barium within the dilated loop) is diagnostic of this condition.

**Fig. 6–28. Abscess of Morison's pouch.**
Right lateral decubitus projection. Margination by the descending duodenum (**DD**) medially and the hepatic flexure of the colon (**C**) inferiorly and laterally localizes the gas- and fluid-containing abscess specifically to the posterosuperior recess of the subhepatic space (Morison's pouch). (From Meyers and Whalen[1])

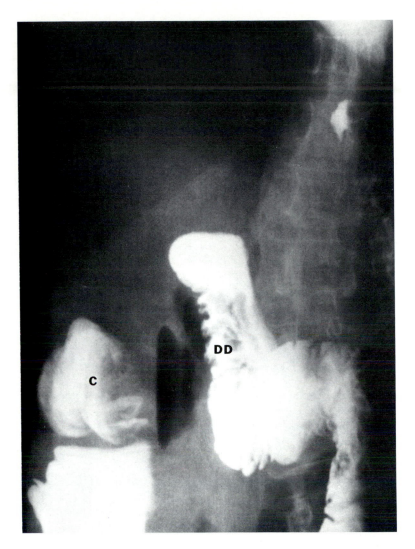

## Abscess of Morison's Pouch versus Inframesocolic Abscess

Two of the anatomic boundaries of Morison's pouch are provided by the point of juncture between the hepatic flexure and its mesocolon inferiorly and the descending duodenum medially. This peritoneal recess is the posterior extension of the right subhepatic space. It is one of the most common sites of an intraabdominal abscess, secondary to the pathways of spread and localization of acute intraperitoneal exudates.[11] Distinction of a gas-containing abscess of Morison's pouch from such conditions in the right upper quadrant as emphysematous cholecystitis, renal or perirenal abscess, liver abscess, and an anterior abdominal wall abscess can be made easily by recognizing its precise duodenocolic boundaries[1] (Fig. 6–28).

The duodenocolic relationships are of further significance in localizing an abscess to the infracolic space, observations that may lead to the identification of its site of origin. Figure 6–29 illustrates an abscess also relating to the duodenum and colon in a patient with an automobile lap-belt deceleration injury. While it lies anterior and primarily lateral to the descending duodenum in the plane of Morison's pouch (Fig. 6–29a), it is not until its inframesocolic position is documented that its source from a ruptured jejunal loop is ascertained (Fig. 6–29b).

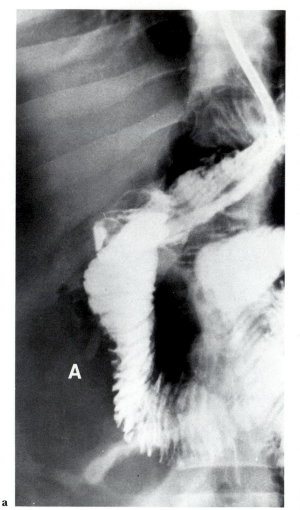

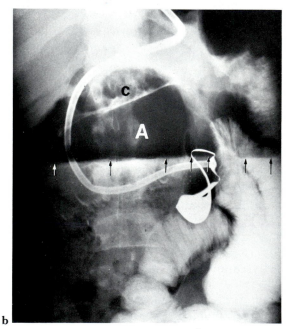

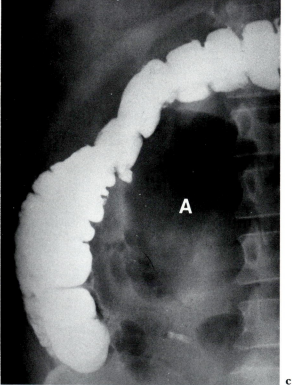

**Fig. 6–29. Rupture of mid-small bowel loop with intraperitoneal inframesocolic abscess.**
(**a**) Large gas-containing abscess (A) lateral and anterior to the descending duodenum. Its position could be misinterpreted as Morison's pouch.
(**b**) Erect. Inframesocolic position of abscess (A) is established by its elevation of the transverse colon (c). Note that its superior margination is provided by the root of the transverse mesocolon, which can be inferred from the landmarks provided by the Cantor tube within the descending duodenum. Communication of the abscess with an adjacent mid-small bowel loop is revealed by the identical planes of their air–fluid levels (arrows).
(**c**) A later barium enema study documents the position of the abscess within the right infracolic space.
(From Meyers and Whalen[1])

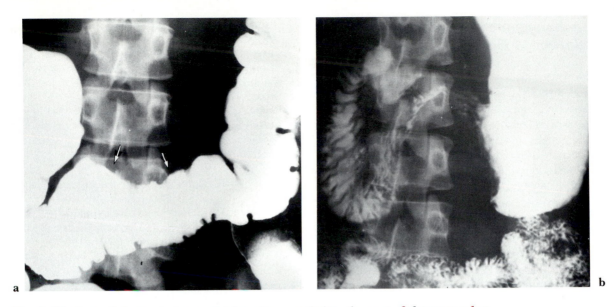

**Fig. 6–30. Cyst of the posterior parietal peritoneum below the root of the mesocolon.**
(**a**) Mild extrinsic pressure effect on the superior contour of the transverse colon (arrows).
(**b**) Gross medial displacement of the fourth portion of the duodenum and duodenojejunal junction, with pressure on the greater curvature of the gastric antrum.
(From Meyers and Whalen[1])

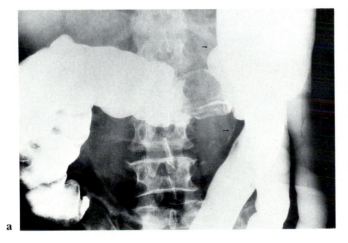

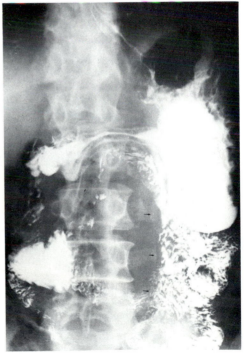

**Fig. 6–31. Large calcified aneurysm of the abdominal aorta** (arrows).
(**a**) There is mild pressure on the transverse colon, but (**b**) marked medial displacement of the ascending duodenum and superior displacement of the duodenojejunal junction. (From Meyers and Whalen[1])

## *Duodenojejunal Junction: Relation to Colon*

The intimate relationship of the duodenojejunal junction superiorly to the root of the transverse mesocolon as it extends across the pancreas is of importance in the identification of both locally arising processes and remote colonic pathology.

At this level, the mesocolon is generally long enough so that the transverse colon is considerably anterior. It is then apparent that minor effects on the distal transverse colon on an initial barium enema study may be shown to reflect a process that predominantly involves the ascending duodenum or duodenojejunal junction (Figs. 6–30 and 6–31).

## References

1. Meyers MA, Whalen JP: Roentgen significance of the duodenocolic relationships: An anatomic approach. AJR 117: 263–274, 1973
2. Whalen JP, Riemenschneider PA: Analysis of normal anatomic relationships of colon as applied to roentgenographic observations. AJR Rad Ther Nucl Med 99: 55–61, 1967
3. Friedman SM: Position and mobility of duodenum in living subject. Am J Anat 79: 147–165, 1946
4. Treitel H, Meyers MA, Maza V: Changes in the duodenal loop secondary to carcinoma of the hepatic flexure of the colon. Br J Radiol 43: 209–213, 1970
5. Vieta JO, Blanco R, Valentini GR: Malignant duodenocolic fistula: Report of two cases, each with one or more other synchronous gastrointestinal cancers. Dis Colon Rectum 19: 542–552, 1976
6. Korelitz BI: Colonic-duodenal fistula in Crohn's disease. Digest Dis 22: 1040–1048, 1977
7. Jacobson IM, Schapiro RH, Warshaw AL: Gastric and duodenal fistulas in Crohn's disease. Gastroenterology 89: 1347–1352, 1985
8. Herlinger H, O'Riordan D, Saul S, et al: Nonspecific involvement of bowel adjoining Crohn disease. Radiology 159: 47–51, 1986
9. Torrance B, Jones C: Three cases of spontaneous duodenocolic fistula. Gut 13: 627–630, 1972
10. Ghahremani GG, Meyers MA: The cholecystocolic relationships: A roentgen-anatomic study of the colonic manifestations of gallbladder disorders. AJR 125: 21–34, 1975
11. Meyers MA: Spread and localization of acute intraperitoneal effusions. Radiology 95: 547–554, 1970
12. Meyers MA: Leiomyosarcoma of the duodenum: Radiographic and arteriographic features. Clin Radiol 22: 257–260, 1971

# 7 Intestinal Effects of Pancreatitis: Spread Along Mesenteric Planes

## General Introduction

Acute inflammation of the pancreas may be classified into four groups:

1. *Acute edematous pancreatitis* is the most common form; there is localized or diffuse swelling of the organ.
2. *Acute hemorrhagic pancreatitis* is caused by the digestive effects of liberated trypsin and elastase on pancreatic vessels. The first changes caused by this vascular necrosis are found in the outer layer but the damage usually progresses rapidly to involve the entire thickness of the vessel wall, with disruption of the intima.[1]
3. *Acute gangrenous pancreatitis* is rare because of the rich vascularization of the pancreas.
4. *Acute suppurative pancreatitis* secondary to superimposed infection may range from a localized pancreatic abscess to diffuse involvement, perhaps as a gas-producing process.

Localized changes on characteristic portions of the small intestine and colon are produced by the extravasated enzymes of pancreatitis, which follow definite anatomic planes.[2] The lesions range from transient spasm to ischemic atrophy and the development of obstructive strictures as well as remote exudative abscesses. Extension of the effects of pancreatitis may occur through the loose retroperitoneal tissue planes of the anterior pararenal spaces. Notably, however, the mesenteric pathways most often involved and which direct the spread of pancreatic enzymes to remote sites in the intestinal tract are the transverse mesocolon and the small bowel mesentery. These observations have been confirmed by computed tomography.[3–5] Fat necrosis is most common in these two sites and in the omentum.[6]

## Anatomic Considerations

Virtually all of the pancreas is an extraperitoneal organ. However, a nonperitonealized bare area results from the reflections of the posterior parietal peritoneum to form the two leaves of the transverse mesocolon.[7] This extends across the lower border of the organ anteriorly (Fig. 7–1). On the right, the transverse mesocolon begins at the point where the anterior hepatic flexure of the colon immediately crosses ventral to the second portion of the duodenum. The bare area then extends as a broad strip across the infraampullary portion of the descending duodenum and continues across the head, body, and tail of the pancreas. The ascending colon and the proximal, more posterior hepatic flexure are completely extraperitoneal.

Significantly, the tail of the pancreas, after extending across the left kidney, is actually intraperitoneal in that it is incorporated or ensheathed within the leaves of the splenorenal ligament. By definition, any structure within a mesenteric attachment is intraperitoneal. Anatomic continuity is established by the peritoneal reflections constituting the supporting ligaments of the left upper quadrant. Figures 7–2 and 7–3 show the relationships of the tail of the pancreas within the splenorenal ligament to the transverse mesocolon, phrenicocolic ligament, and the peritoneal reflections of the descending

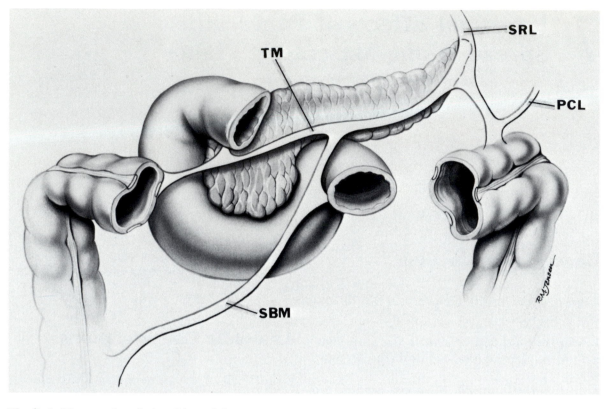

**Fig. 7–1. Mesenteric relationships of the pancreas.**
Frontal drawing shows the relationships of the transverse mesocolon (TM) and its continuity with the small bowel mesentery (SBM), splenorenal ligament (SRL), and phrenicocolic ligament (PCL). (Redrawn from Meyers and Evans[2])

colon. The phrenicocolic ligament[8] is attached to the anatomic splenic flexure of the colon and represents the most lateral continuity of the transverse mesocolon and splenorenal ligament. It thereby marks the site of transition from the intraperitoneal transverse colon to the extraperitoneal descending colon.

Of further clinical significance is the fact that the root of the small bowel mesentery, at its origin near the inferior portion of the pancreas, is anatomically continuous with that of the transverse mesocolon (Fig. 7–1). At this point it is in relationship to the midportion of the transverse duodenum. It then extends obliquely toward the right lower quadrant to insert, most often, at the cecocolic junction. Thus, anatomic continuity is established along the root of the mesentery from the pancreas to the third portion of the duodenum, jejunal loops, ileal loops, and cecum.

In this way, mesenteric planes are provided

for the direct spread of extravasated pancreatic enzymes (Figs. 7–4 and 7–5):

1. Along the mesocolon to the transverse colon. Extension along its planes to its lateral limits proceeds (a) on the right, to the hepatic flexure and perhaps the distal ascending colon, and (b) on the left, to the anatomic splenic flexure just below the tip of the spleen.
2. Along the small bowel mesentery to jejunal loops and the ileocecal region.

# Effects of Pancreatitis on the Colon: Spread Along the Transverse Mesocolon

The segment of large intestine involved by pancreatitis reflects the pathophysiology of the disease and the anatomic relationships of the pan-

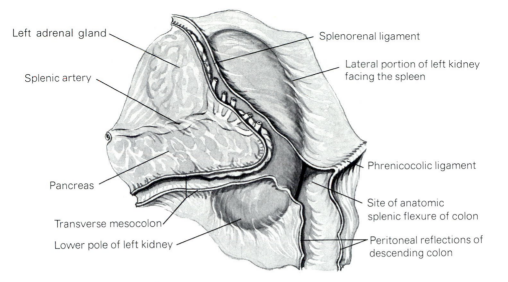

**Fig. 7–2. Posterior peritoneal reflections of the left upper quadrant,** demonstrating continuity of the transverse mesocolon and splenorenal ligament with the phrenicocolic ligament and the peritoneal reflections of the descending colon. The tail of the pancreas resides within the splenorenal ligament.

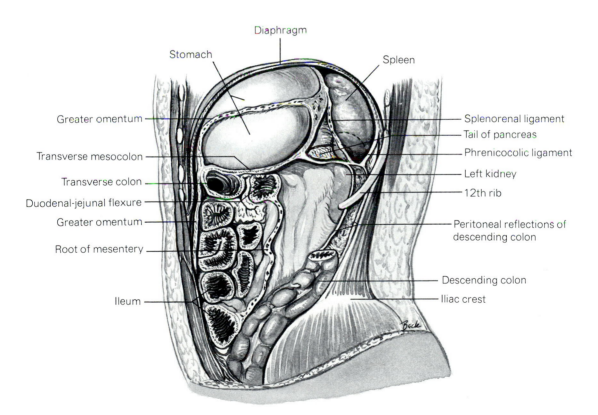

**Fig. 7–3. Left parasagittal drawing, emphasizing peritoneal reflections.**
Note the tail of the pancreas within the splenorenal ligament and its continuity with the transverse mesocolon and phrenicocolic ligament.

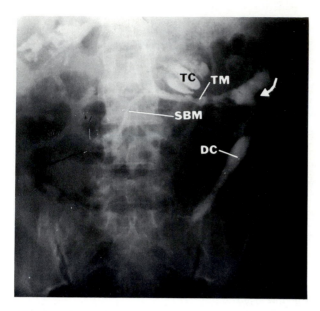

**Fig. 7–4. Opacification in vivo of continuity of mesenteric roots and bare areas in relationship to the pancreas.**
In this patient who has had a right hemicolectomy and ileotransverse colostomy, fistulography strikingly illustrates communication between the root of the transverse mesocolon (TM), root of the small bowel mesentery (SBM), and the bare area of the descending colon (DC). At the site of the phrenicocolic ligament (arrow), there is communication with the transverse colon (TC) and a left cutaneous fistula.

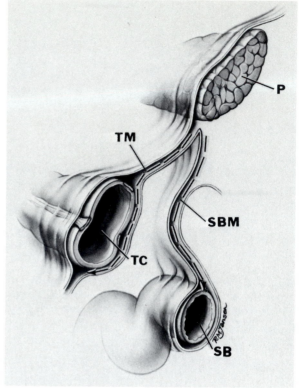

**Fig. 7–5. Anatomic pathways of spread from the pancreas.**
Lateral drawing. The arrowed-dashed lines show the planes of spread from the pancreas (P) to the transverse colon (TC), characteristically toward its lower border, and to the small bowel (SB). TM = transverse mesocolon, SMB = small bowel mesentery. (Redrawn from Meyers and Evans[2])

creas to the mesenteric planes of the transverse mesocolon. Inflammation localized to the head of the organ may extend to the hepatic flexure and perhaps the distal ascending colon. Diffuse pancreatitis may spread to involve the entire transverse colon, with a definite tendency to exert its major effects on the splenic flexure.

## Hepatic Flexure

With spread of liberated enzymes from the head of the pancreas into the right anterior pararenal space across the beginning of the transverse mesocolon, the hepatic flexure may show localized or diffuse inflammatory changes (Fig. 7–6). Occasionally, the "cut-off" process of a stricture resulting from pericolic fat necrosis may closely simulate an annular carcinoma[2,9] (Fig. 7–7).

In 1956 Price[10] coined the term "colon cut-off" sign in acute pancreatitis for isolated gaseous distention of the ascending colon and he-

patic flexure with sharp delimitation of the gas shadow just to the left of the flexure. In two patients he noted a similar cellulitis-like process spreading from the edematous head of the pancreas between the two layers of the transverse mesocolon to the mesocolic border of the colon just to the left of the hepatic flexure.

## Transverse Colon and Splenic Flexure

Since Price's report, however, the term "colon cut-off" sign has lost its original definition and has been applied to multiple sites of spasm and narrowing of the colon secondary to pancreatitis. Stuart[11] employed it to designate collapse with absence of gas in the midportion of the

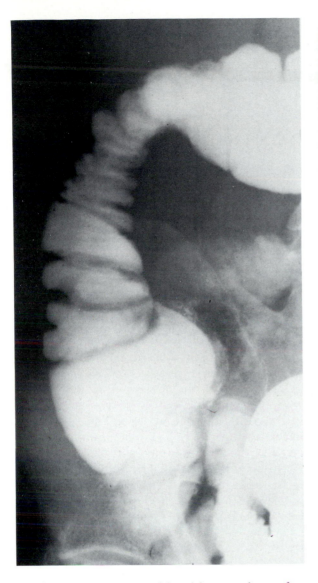

**Fig. 7–6. Acute pancreatitis with extension to hepatic flexure.**
Barium enema shows diffuse mild spasm and edematous mucosal changes of the hepatic flexure and distal ascending colon from extension of extravasated pancreatic enzymes via the right anterior pararenal compartment.

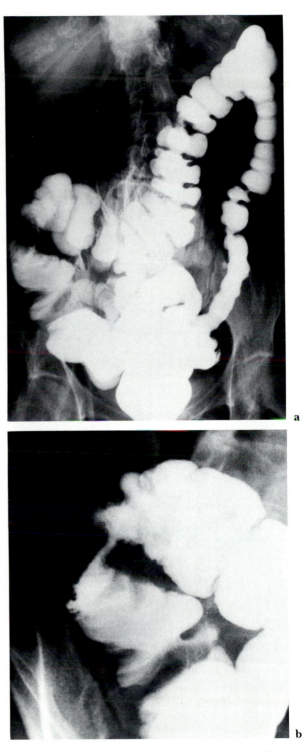

**Fig. 7–7. Acute suppurative pancreatitis with extension to hepatic flexure.**
(a and b) Barium enema and spot film demonstrate an annular constricting lesion of the distal ascending colon. The constant narrowing and overhanging shelflike margin mimic an "apple-core" carcinoma.

Exploratory laparotomy disclosed a large peripancreatic abscess with retroperitoneal extension down to and involving the hepatic flexure and distal ascending colon, where an extramural inflammatory stricture was encountered. Areas of fat necrosis were present in the transverse mesocolon, pericolonic tissue, and greater omentum.
(From Meyers and Evans[2])

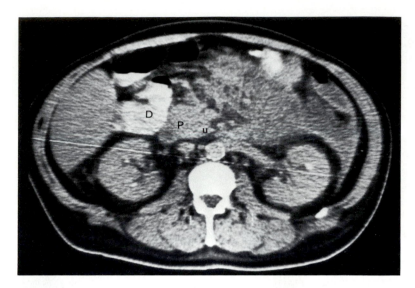

**Fig. 7–8. Pancreatitis extending through the transverse mesocolon.** CT demonstrates the inflammatory reaction accompanying the extravasated enzymes of acute pancreatitis spreading through the transverse mesocolon toward the transverse colon and splenic flexure. The process extends into the anterior pararenal space on the left. D = duodenum, P = head of pancreas, u = uncinate process. (From Meyers et al[5])

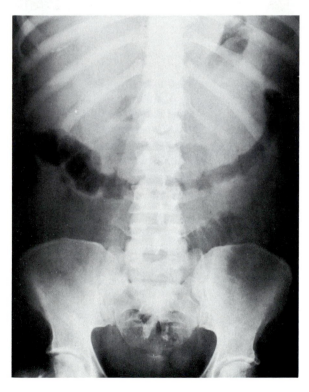

**Fig. 7–9. Acute pancreatitis.**
Plain film shows diffuse spasm and edema of the transverse colon due to extensive inflammatory exudate which also displaces the stomach superiorly and the transverse colon inferiorly.

transverse colon which appeared to be cut off from the gas-containing hepatic and splenic flexures. This was a constant finding in both supine and erect plain films of the abdomen in six patients with acute pancreatitis. Brascho and co-authors[12] found the gaseous dilatation to involve the ascending and entire transverse colon, with the cut-off point at the splenic flexure. In my experience,[2] as well as that of others,[13–16] this is by far the most common single site involved.

On plain films, the most common abnormality in the large intestine in cases of acute pancreatitis is gaseous distention of the transverse colon. This often represents a paralytic ileus secondary to the extravasated enzymes within the transverse mesocolon (Fig. 7–8). More directly irritative effects may be manifested by spasm and edema[17] (Figs. 7–9 through 7–11).

The natural extension of the inflammatory process into the phrenicocolic ligament may result in severe spasm or an incomplete mechanical obstruction at the level of the anatomic splenic flexure immediately inferior to the tip of the spleen.[8] The obstruction need not be permanent and may resolve as the pancreatitis subsides (Figs. 7–12 and 7–13). However, if the inflammation is more severe and particularly if accompanied by fat necrosis, barium enema study shows narrowing of the splenic flexure with irregular nodular or serrated margins and distorted mucosal folds secondary to the extramural inflammatory infiltrate. Occasionally a significant degree of retrograde obstruction may be met and the changes may simulate carcinoma.[18] A granulomatous and fibrotic reaction may then result in a stricture of the splenic flexure. It is for these reasons that most colon strictures secondary to pancreatitis occur in the splenic flexure.[2,14–16,19]

This is illustrated in Figure 7–14 in a case of traumatic pancreatitis. Barium enema examination discloses irregular flattening of the lower border of the transverse colon along its length, ending abruptly at the level of the anatomic splenic flexure (Fig. 7–14a). Distal to this site, the extraperitoneal descending colon resumes a normal haustral pattern. This pattern of asymmetric involvement of the lower contour of the mesenteric transverse colon is characteristic of extension of disease from the pancreas along the transverse mesocolon and phrenicocolic ligament.[20] The narrowing with irregular nodular defects demonstrated in the splenic flexure (Fig. 7–14b and c) are obviously organic and not functional in nature and thus indicate direct

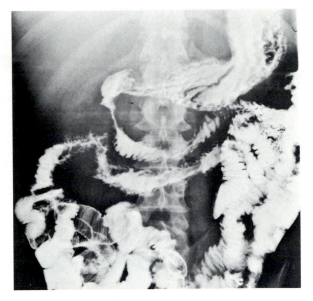

**Fig. 7–10. Acute pancreatitis.**
Diffuse inflammation of transverse colon, shown by spastic narrowing and gross mucosal irregularities on delayed film of upper GI series.

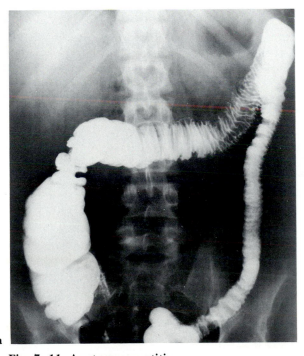

a

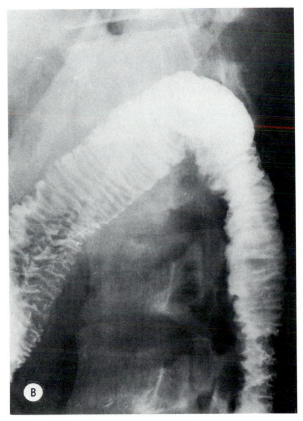

B

b

**Fig. 7–11. Acute pancreatitis.**
Diffuse inflammation of transverse colon. Frontal (a) and oblique (b) views of barium enema study demonstrate mucosal edema.
(Reproduced from Thompson et al[17])

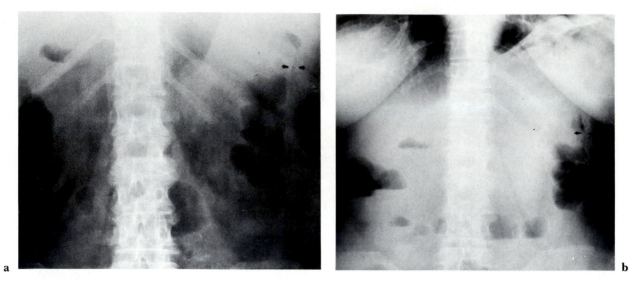

**Fig. 7–12. Acute pancreatitis.**
(a) Supine and (b) erect. Dilatation and air–fluid levels of the transverse colon extend to a narrowed segment of the splenic flexure (arrows).

Barium enema study 1 week after conservative therapy showed no abnormalities, indicating that these changes were due to spasm secondary to the irritating effects of enzymes within the phrenicocolic ligament. (From Meyers and Evans[2])

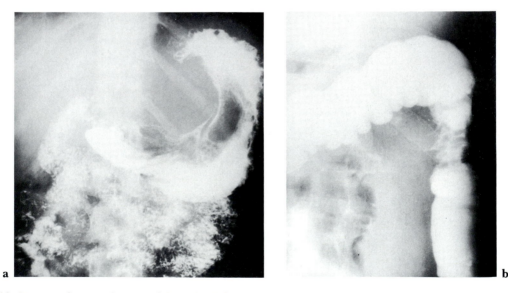

**Fig. 7–13. Pancreatic pseudocyst with pericolitis.**
While the upper gastrointestinal series (a) demonstrates the pressure effect on the stomach produced by a large organizing pancreatic pseudocyst, the barium enema study (b) shows localized narrowing and spiculation of the mucosal pattern of the anatomic splenic flexure from extravasated pancreatic enzymes.

passage of considerable pancreatic enzymes into the phrenicocolic ligament. From the severe changes in the splenic flexure, the probable development of a fibrotic stricture (Fig. 7–14d) should be anticipated and serial evaluations by barium enema studies obtained.

If the inflammatory process erodes through the wall of the colon at this site, extraperitoneal sinus tracts or fistulas to adherent small bowel loops may be demonstrated (Figs. 7–15 through 7–17).

Pancreatic pseudocysts may spontaneously

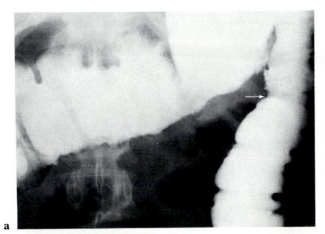

a

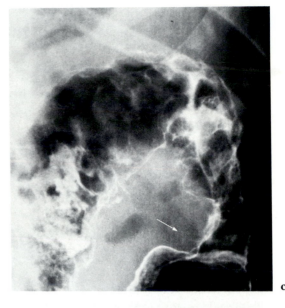

c

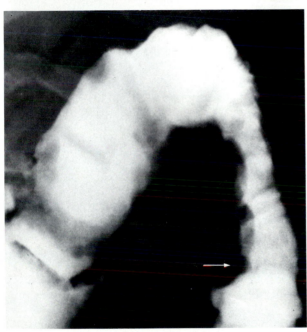

b

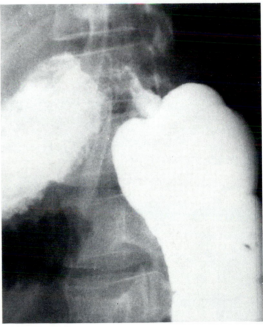

d

**Fig. 7–14. Traumatic pancreatitis, with development of stricture of splenic flexure.**
(a) Flattening of the inferior haustral contour of the transverse colon. Pseudosacculations result on the uninvolved superior border. The process ends at the level of the phrenicocolic ligament at the anatomic splenic flexure of the colon (arrow).
(b and c) Scalloped narrowing of the splenic flexure on filled and air studies. The intramural lesions end precisely at the level of the phrenicocolic ligament (arrows).

(d) Three months later there is a marked fibrotic stenosis of the splenic flexure, reducing its lumen to a diameter of less than 3 mm. Surgical resection of the stricture, induced by fat necrosis, was required.
(From Meyers and Evans[2])

rupture into an adjacent hollow viscus, the colon and particularly the splenic flexure being the most common site[21–23] (Figs. 7–18 through 7–20). Fistulization does not occur in the initial acute phase of pancreatitis, but rather as a consequence of pancreatic suppuration or pseudocyst. Pancreatic gas may be the consequence of fistulization, rather than secondary to pancreatic abscess alone.[24] The mechanism involves enzymatic digestion of the cyst wall or vascular in-

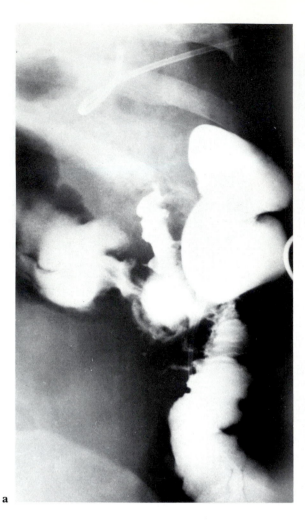
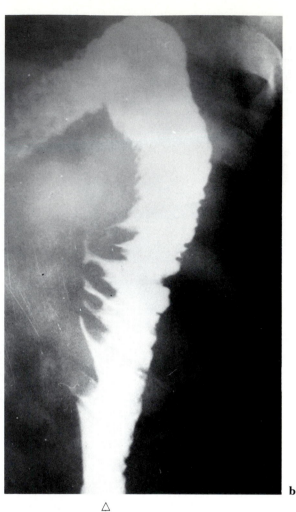

a

b

△

**Fig. 7–15. Gas-producing abscess of pancreas.**
(a) Multiple gaseous lucenies of tail of pancreas at site of draining catheter. Barium enema demonstrates extension via the phrenicocolic ligament to anatomic splenic flexure with multiple sinus tracts of varying size.
(b) Four months later, multiple residual sinus tracts are present. (From Meyers and Evans[2])

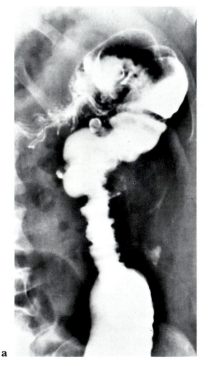
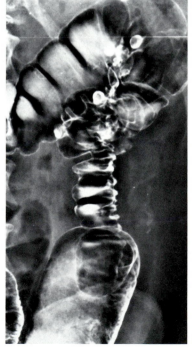

a

b

**Fig. 7–16. Acute pancreatitis with transmural erosion.**
(a and b) Severe spread of enzymes into the phrenicocolic ligament produces a fixed and irregular narrowing of the anatomic splenic flexure of the colon. Transmural erosion is shown by faint barium extravasation laterally.

**Fig. 7–17. Acute suppurative pancreatitis with transmural erosion.** Extravasated enzymes within the phrenicocolic ligament have resulted in incomplete obstruction of the splenic flexure (arrows) and transmural digestion with fistulization to a small bowel loop and a long extraperitoneal sinus tract from the narrowed splenic flexure. (From Meyers and Evans[2])

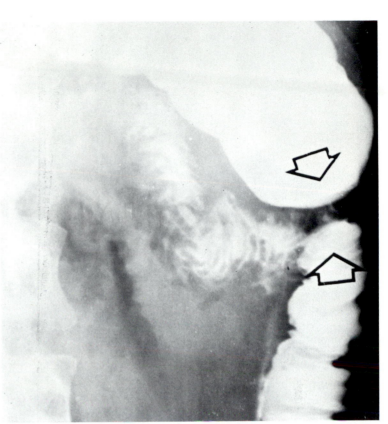

sult that produces progressive necrosis and rupture. While temporary or even permanent remission may result from this spontaneous decompression,[23] major gastrointestinal bleeding is seen in about 30% because of erosion of large arteries,[21,23] and sepsis with conversion of the pseudocyst into an abscess is frequent. The recommended operative procedure is proximal diverting colostomy and debridement with external drainage of the peripancreatic collection.[21]

Extraperitoneal dissection inferiorly may result in pseudocyst formation within the anterior pararenal space (Figs. 7–21 through 7–25) with effects on the long limbs of the colon, sigmoid colon, and rectum, and rarely may progress as far as the groin.[25–27] Fat necrosis at this site may mimic many other disease processes. The patient illustrated in Figure 7–26 presented with an acute abdomen and an inflamed scrotum which drained "beef-broth" material with a high amylase content secondary to fat necrosis. The barium enema study indicates the pathway of the pancreatic enzymes into the phrenicocolic ligament and inferiorly beyond the sigmoid colon to the inguinal region.

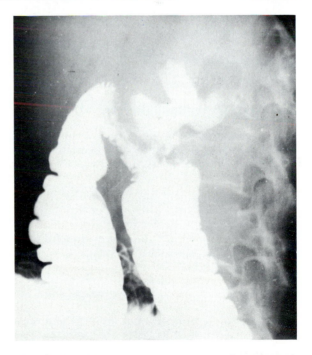

**Fig. 7–18. Spontaneous rupture of pancreatic pseudocyst into colon.** Barium enema study demonstrates communication at anatomic splenic flexure into pseudocyst cavity of tail of pancreas.

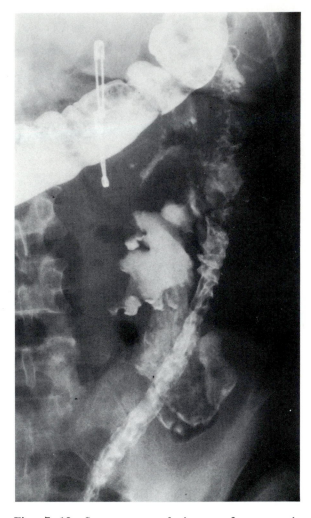

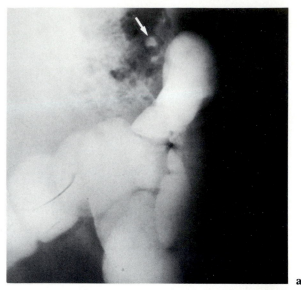

a

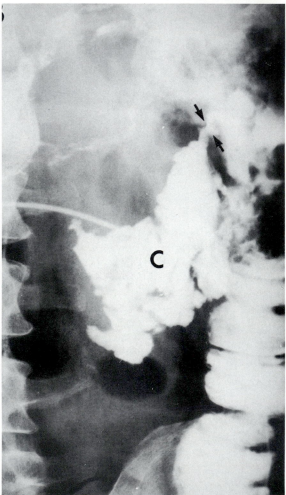

b

**Fig. 7–19. Spontaneous drainage of pancreatic pseudocyst into colon.**
Barium enema study reveals that a fistulous communication has been established between the region of the anatomic splenic flexure and an irregular pseudocyst extending retroperitoneally from the tail of the pancreas.

**Fig. 7–20. Spontaneous fistula formation from infected pancreatic pseudocyst to colon.**
(a) Pancreatic abscess with extraluminal gas loculation displaces splenic flexure of colon. A small amount of contrast material has extravasated into the abscess (arrow).
(b) Fistulogram performed after drainage of abscess demonstrates the irregular cavity (C) with the tract (arrows) extending to the colon.
(Courtesy of J.L. Clements, Jr., M.D., Emory University School of Medicine, Atlanta, GA).

**Fig. 7–21. Acute pancreatitis extending to descending colon.**
Beginning at the level of the anatomic splenic flexure and extending downward, the descending colon shows spasm, limited distensibility, and edematous changes which are more marked on the medial wall. These changes reflect the inferior extension of the pancreatic inflammatory process through the anterior pararenal space. Extraluminal gas stippling is due to early abscess formation.

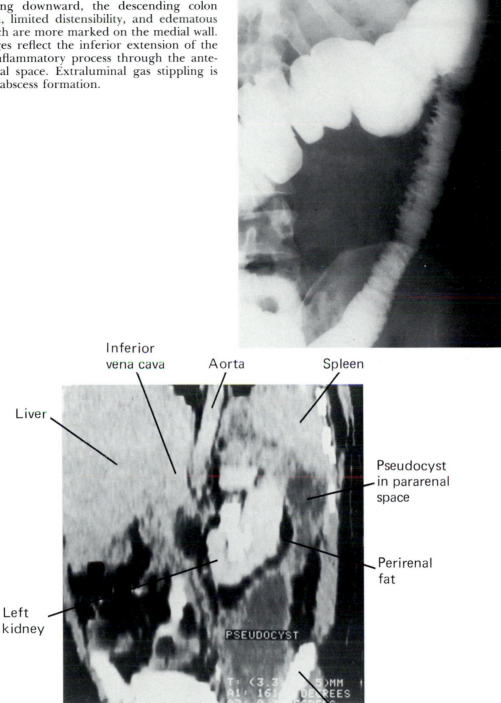

**Fig. 7–22. Extension of pancreatitis into the pelvis.**
Reformatted coronal computed tomography in a patient with a large pancreatic pseudocyst demonstrates inferior extension via the anterior pararenal space into the pelvis. (From Lawson TL, Berland LL, Foley WE: Coronal upper abdominal anatomy: Technique and gastrointestinal applications. Gastrointest Radiol 6: 115–128, 1981)

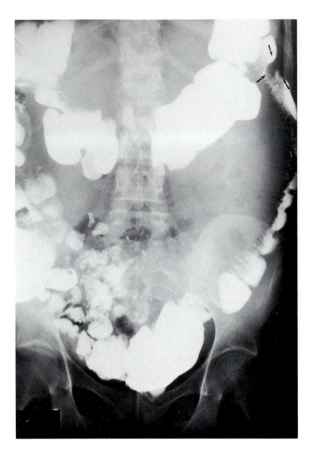

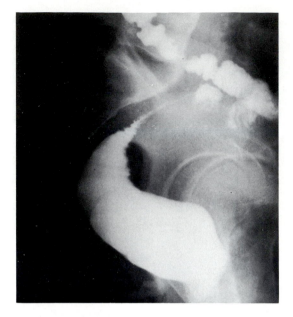

**Fig. 7–25. Extension of pancreatitis into the pelvis.** A pseudocyst of the pancreas extends retroperitoneally to the pelvis with extrinsic compression and partial obstruction of the distal sigmoid colon.

**Fig. 7–23. Extension of pancreatitis into the pelvis.** Effects on the anatomic splenic flexure (arrows) from extravasated enzymes are shown. A large pseudocystic soft-tissue mass extends inferiorly through the left anterior pararenal space to the pelvis, resulting in displacement and mucosal inflammatory changes of the descending colon.

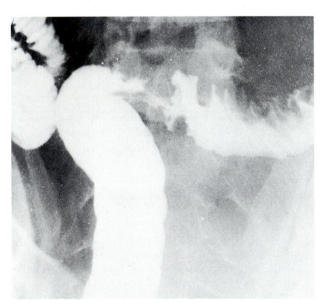

**Fig. 7–24. Extension of pancreatitis into the pelvis.** Massive pancreatitic exudate dissecting along the left retroperitoneum into the pelvis results in extensive edema of the sigmoid colon with mass effect and displacement of the rectum to the right. (From Farman J, Kutcher R, Dallemand S, et al: Unusual pelvic complications of a pancreatic pseudocyst. Gastrointest Radiol 3: 43–45, 1978)

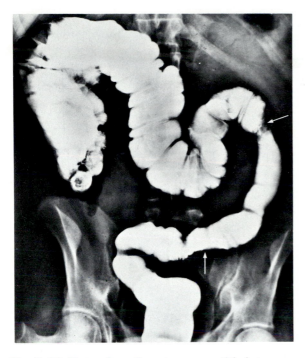

**Fig. 7–26. Extension of acute pancreatitis into scrotum.**
Pseudocyst formation in the tail of the pancreas depresses the distal transverse colon. In addition, extravasated enzymes within the phrenicocolic ligament result in localized narrowing of the anatomic splenic flexure (top arrow). Inferior extension extraperitoneally on the left is revealed by compression of the sigmoid colon (bottom arrow). (Courtesy of Jack Farman, MD, Columbia-Presbyterian Medical Center, New York, N.Y.)

## Effects of Pancreatitis on the Duodenum, Small Bowel, and Cecum: Spread Along Small Bowel Mesentery

The inflammatory process associated with extravasated pancreatic enzymes may disseminate along the root of the small bowel mesentery, either for a portion or for its entire length. Figure 7–27 demonstrates these anatomic relationships near the beginning of the mesentery. Spread through the leaves brings the process to intestinal vessels and to an individual or multiple loops (Fig. 7–28). Figure 7–29 documents communication of the pancreas with the length of the mesenteric root. This pathway provides a plane of spread to the right lower quadrant (Fig. 7–30).

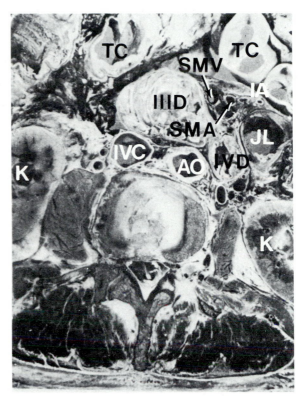

**Fig. 7–27. Anatomic cross-section immediately below the pancreas** shows the relationships of the superior mesenteric artery (SMA) and vein (SMV), in the root of the mesentery, to the third portion of the duodenum (III D) as it continues into the fourth duodenum (IV D). Intestinal arteries (IA) course in the mesentery to loops of jejunum (JL). AO = aorta, K = kidney, IVC = inferior vena cava, TC = transverse colon.

### Duodenum

Compression of the third portion of the duodenum may result from an indurated mesenteric root.[28] This typically occurs in its midportion which may appear sharply cut off (Fig. 7–31), with dilatation and stasis proximally. Such a mechanical process undoubtedly accounts for many instances of the duodenal "ileus" seen in acute pancreatitis.

### Small Bowel and Cecum

As the enzymes progress further down the root of the mesentery, jejunitis may be evident (Fig. 7–32). It has long been recognized that "sentinel loops" from localized paralytic ileus of small bowel may accompany pancreatitis. Jejunal and

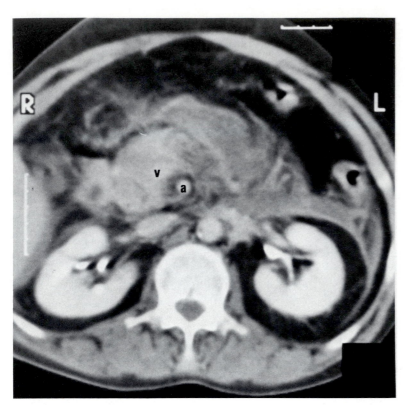

**Fig. 7–28. Spread of pancreatitis through the small bowel mesentery.**
In a case of acute pancreatitis, CT shows the inflammatory reaction extending through the small bowel mesentery, displacing the superior mesenteric artery (a) and vein (v) and intestinal branches. The process also extends within the extraperitoneal anterior pararenal space on the left. (From Meyers et al[5])

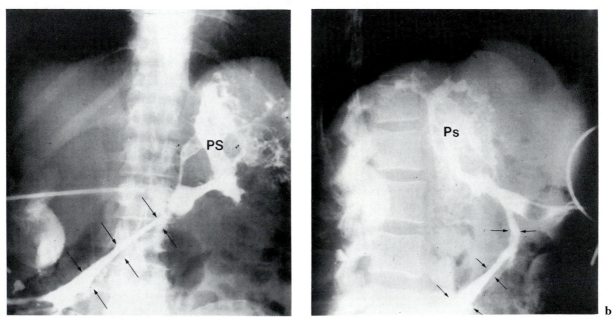

**Fig. 7–29. Opacification of mesenteric root *in vivo*.**
(**a** and **b**) Injection of contrast material through tube draining a loculated pseudocyst (Ps) of the tail of the pancreas demonstrates communication dissecting along the root of the small bowel mesentery (arrows). Note its typically oblique course toward the right lower quadrant in relation to duodenum, jejunum, ileum, and cecum.
(Courtesy of Jack Farman, MD, Columbia-Presbyterian Medical Center, New York, N.Y.)

**Fig. 7–30. Spread of pancreatic pseudocyst down the mesenteric root.**
**(a)** While a large pancreatic pseudocyst (PS$_1$) occupies the lesser sac, a smaller one (PS$_2$) has developed in the region of the uncinate process (U).
**(b)** The smaller pseudocyst has dissected down the root of the small bowel mesentery to reside in the right lower quadrant in relation to a distal ileal loop.
(From Meyers et al[5])

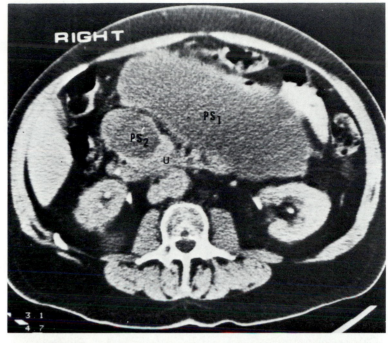

a

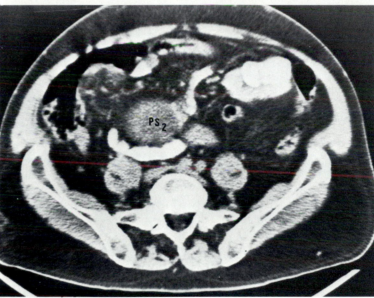

b

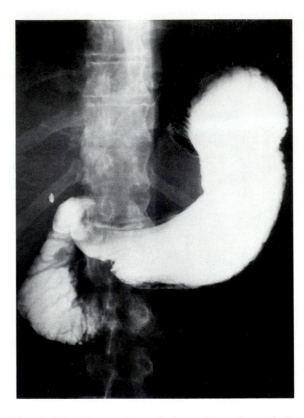

**Fig. 7–31. Obstruction of the midportion of the transverse duodenum by pancreatitis** extending down the mesenteric root. An associated finding is enlargement of the ampulla of Vater. (From Meyers and Evans[2])

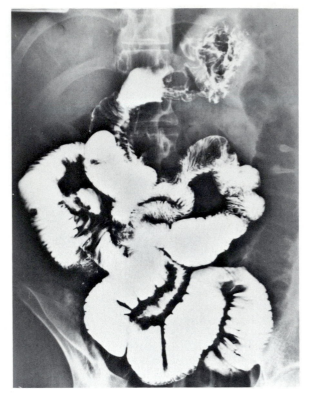

**Fig. 7–33. Acute pancreatitis.**
Jejunitis and ileitis are a consequence of extensive spread of pancreatic enzymes throughout the small bowel mesentery. This is shown by mucosal edema and sites of spastic narrowing with intervening dilatation.

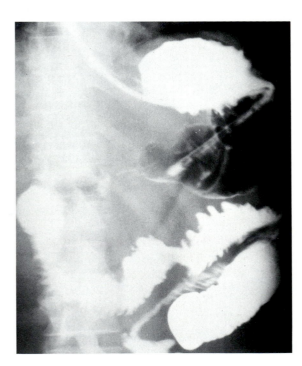

occasionally ileal changes characterized by marked persistent spasm of some segments and dilatation of others, with coarsening of the mucosal folds, may be seen (Figs. 7–33 and 7–34).

Ischemic changes in the intestine as well may be produced by the digestive effects of the liberated enzymes or by thrombosis from areas of fat necrosis. Microaneurysms, pseudoaneurysms, stenoses, and occlusions are being increasingly recognized in mesenteric vessels following pancreatitis.[29,30] The vascular consequences may range from fibrotic strictures[19,31] (Fig. 7–35) to gangrene of the bowel[3,32–35] (Fig. 7–36).

◁ ————————————————

**Fig. 7–32. Acute pancreatitis with jejunitis.**
Besides displacement and mucosal changes in the duodenal loop, evidence of extension of pancreatic enzymes into the small bowel mesentery is shown by their effects on proximal jejunal loops. These demonstrate mucosal edema and sites of spastic narrowing with proximal dilatation.

**Fig. 7–34. Acute pancreatitis.**
CT shows infiltration of the mesentery with severe inflammatory changes of the small bowel and colon.

▷

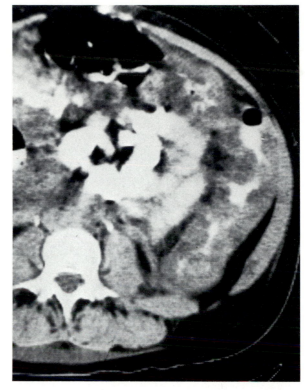

**Fig. 7–35. Pneumatosis intestinalis and ischemic changes secondary to pancreatitis.**
**(a)** Plain film shows three grossly abnormal fixed small bowel loops characterized by (1) bubbly gas collections, (2) thumbprinting and edematous mucosa, and (3) markedly effaced or ulcerated mucosa.
**(b)** Small bowel series. The involved loops show narrowing, ulceration, and pneumatosis.

These features indicate ischemic bowel changes with superimposed pneumatosis. Follow-up 1 month later, following conservative treatment, showed stricture formation in the jejunal segment.
(From Meyers et al[31])

▽

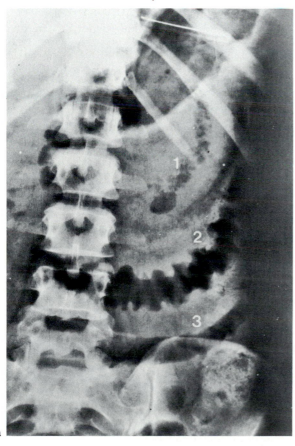

a

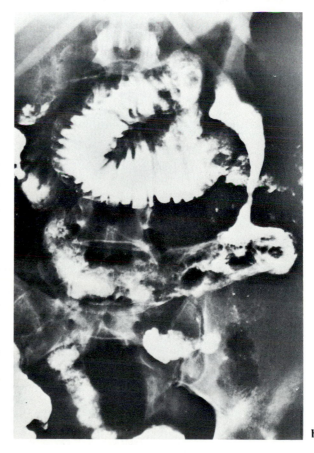

b

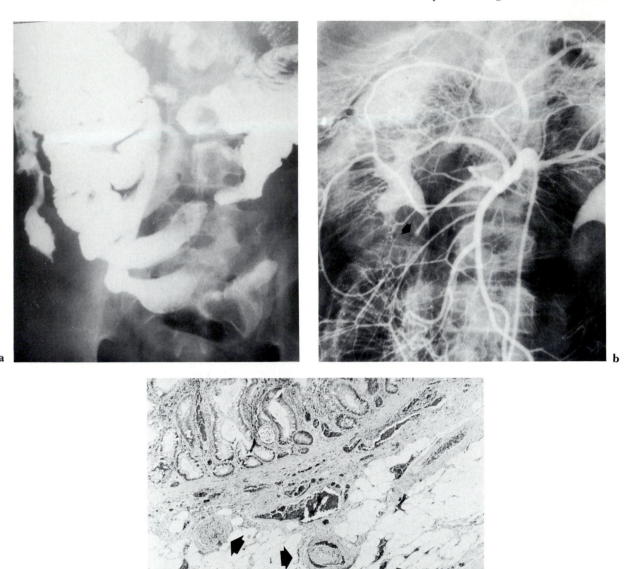

**Fig. 7–36. Colonic necrosis complicating traumatic pancreatitis,** in a 14-year-old male. **(a)** Upper GI and small bowel series reveal ischemic changes in the distal small bowel, cecum, and ascending colon. There is a tubular appearance of distal small bowel with loss of mucosal markings, fixation, and separation of loops. The cecum is conical and there is marked spasm of the ascending colon.

**(b)** Selective superior mesenteric arteriography demonstrates occlusion of ileocolic branches with intraluminal thrombi (arrow).

Laparotomy showed pancreatitis with widespread fat necrosis and necrosis with perforation of the cecum and ascending colon. Thrombi were identified in the ileocolic artery and mesenteric branches to the ascending colon.

**(c)** Histologic examination of the hemicolectomy specimen shows two organizing thrombi (arrows) in the submucosal arterial branches, and severe venous congestion. Mesenteric veins also showed organized and fresh thrombus formation. (Hematoxylin and eosin, ×25)

(Reproduced from Dallemand et al[33])

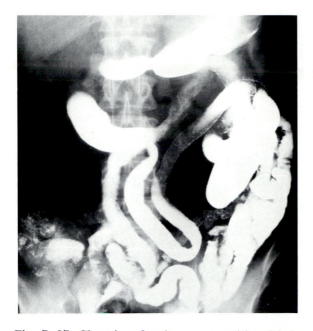

**Fig. 7–37. Chronic relapsing pancreatitis with ischemic atrophy of the intestinal mucosa.**
The most pronounced changes in this case involve the duodenum and proximal jejunum which are strikingly abnormal in appearance. The duodenal loop has a dilated moulagelike appearance. The duodenum and loops of jejunum have a tubular "toothpaste-like" aspect because of the absence of a mucosal relief pattern. Despite the castlike appearance, the involved loops are flaccid, distensible, and lack evidence of fixation, rigidity, or thickening. (From Meyers and Evans[2])

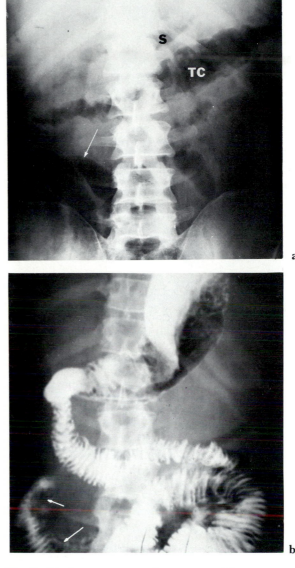

**Fig. 7–39. Acute suppurative pancreatitis.**
**(a)** Admission film shows small bowel ileus predominantly in the right lower quadrant (arrow). Note the normal relationship of the stomach (S) and transverse colon (TC).
**(b)** Barium study 8 days later documents jejunitis and the presence of an exudative abscess displacing distal ileal loops (arrows) at the end of the small bowel mesentery, associated with the development of a large pseudocyst in the tail of the pancreas.
(From Meyers and Evans[2])

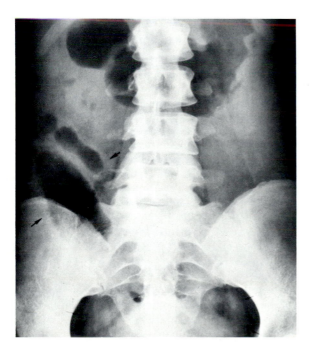

**Fig. 7–38. Acute hemorrhagic pancreatitis.**
Extravasated enzymes passing down the length of the root of the small bowel mesentery produce localized distention of distal ileal loops (arrows). (From Meyers and Evans[2])

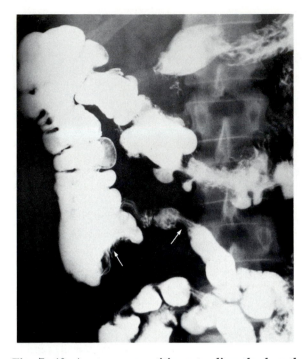

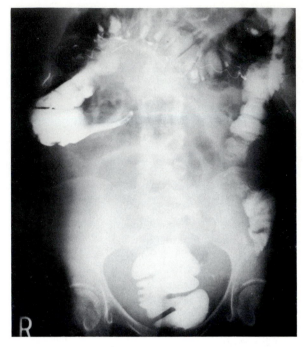

**Fig. 7–40. Acute pancreatitis extending the length of the small bowel mesentery** has resulted in a right lower quadrant pseudocystic collection displacing the terminal ileum and cecum (arrows). Changes are also seen in the midtransverse colon near the confluence of the roots of the transverse mesocolon and small bowel mesentery.
(From Meyers and Evans[2])

**Fig. 7–41. Massive right lower quadrant pancreatic pseudocyst** causes elevation of cecum and appendix.

Figure 7–37 illustrates the findings in a case of malabsorption and jejunal mucosal atrophy secondary to chronic relapsing pancreatitis. Protracted ischemia of the intestine from the vascular effects of pancreatic enzymes in the mesentery underlay the chronic malabsorption in this case. It thus appears that some of the features of pancreatic malabsorption may be on a vascular basis. Localized anatomic changes of mesenteric vessels from the digestive effects of pancreatic enzymes may result in vascular shunts and ischemic malabsorption.

Acute pancreatitis may clinically mimic an acute appendicitis with peritoneal signs localized predominantly in the right lower quadrant. This is a reflection of the process spreading along the length of the root of the small bowel mesentery to result in inflammatory changes of distal ileal loops or the cecum.[2] Plain film findings may then include localized ileus of small bowel loops in the right lower quadrant (Fig. 7–

38). This may be a transient, irritative phenomenon. At times, it may portend the development of a pseudocystic collection that can be demonstrated by its displacement of or mass effects upon ileal loops and the cecum (Figs. 7–39 through 7–41). Since this occurs only with severe pancreatitis, concomitant effects upon other portions of the bowel are usually present.

## References

1. Rich AR, Duff GI: Experimental and pathologic studies on pathogenesis of acute hemorrhagic pancreatitis. Bull Johns Hopkins Hosp 58: 212–259, 1936
2. Meyers MA, Evans JA: Effects of pancreatitis on the small bowel and colon: Spread along mesenteric planes. AJR 119: 151–165, 1973
3. Mendez G, Isikoff MB, Hill MC: CT of acute pancreatitis: Interim assessment. AJR 135: 463–469, 1980
4. Jeffrey RB, Federle MP, Laing FC: Computed tomography of mesenteric involvement in fulminant pancreatitis. Radiology 147: 185–188, 1983
5. Meyers MA, Oliphant M, Berne AS, et al: The

peritoneal ligaments and mesenteries: Pathways of intra-abdominal spread of disease. Annual Oration. Radiology. 163: 593–604, 1987

6. Waring HJ, Griffiths HE: Acute pancreatitis. Br J Surg 11: 476–490, 1924

7. Meyers MA, Whalen JP: Roentgen significance of duodenocolic relationships: Anatomic approach. AJR Rad Ther Nucl Med 117: 263–274, 1973

8. Meyers MA: Roentgen significance of the phrenicocolic ligament. Radiology 95: 539–545, 1970

9. Aronson AR, Davis DA: Obstruction near hepatic flexure in pancreatitis: Rarely reported sign. JAMA 176: 133–134, 1961

10. Price CWR: "Colon cut-off sign" in acute pancreatitis. Med J Australia 1: 313–314, 1956

11. Stuart C: Acute pancreatitis: Preliminary investigation of new radiodiagnostic sign. J Fac Radiologists 8: 50–58, 1956

12. Brascho DJ, Reynolds TN, Zanca P: Radiographic "colon cut-off sign" in acute pancreatitis. Radiology 79: 763–768, 1962

13. Forlini E: Stenosi del colon da pancreatitis. Gior Clin Med 8: 609–620, 1927

14. L'Hermine C, Pringot J, Monnier JP, et al: Le retentissement colique des pancréatites: A propos de 39 observations. J Radiol 61: 27–34, 1980

15. Mohuiddin S, Sakiyalak P, Gullick HD, et al: Stenosing lesions of the colon secondary to pancreatitis. Arch Surg 102: 229–231, 1971

16. Remington JH, Mayo CW, Dockerty MB: Stenosis of colon secondary to chronic pancreatitis. Proc Staff Meet Mayo Clin 22: 260–264, 1947

17. Thompson WM, Kelvin FM, Rice RP: Inflammation and necrosis of the transverse colon secondary to pancreatitis. AJR 128: 943–948, 1977

18. Schwartz S, Nadelhaft J: Simulation of colonic obstruction at splenic flexure by pancreatitis: Roentgen features. AJR Ther Nucl Med 78: 607–616, 1957

19. Hunt DR, Mildenhall P: Etiology of strictures of the colon associated with pancreatitis. Am J Dig Dis 20: 941–946, 1975

20. Meyers MA, Volberg F, Katzen B, et al: Haustral anatomy and pathology: A new look. II. Roentgen interpretation of pathologic alterations. Radiology 108: 505–512, 1973

21. Berne TV, Edmondson HA: Colonic fistulization due to pancreatitis. Am J Surg 111: 359–363, 1966

22. Bohlman TW, Katon RM, Lee TG, et al: Use of endoscopic retrograde cholangiopancreatography in the diagnosis of pancreatic fistula: A case report and review of the literature. Gastroenterology 70: 582–584, 1976.

23. Clements JL, Jr, Bradley EL III, Eaton SB Jr: Spontaneous internal drainage of pancreatic pseudocysts. AJR 126: 985–991, 1976

24. Alexander ES, Clark RA, Federle MP: Pancreatic gas: Indication of pancreatic fistula. AJR 139: 1089–1093, 1982

25. Salvo AF, Nematolahi H: Distant dissection of a pancreatic pseudocyst into the right groin. Am J Surg 126: 430–432, 1973

26. Strax R, Tooms BD, Rauschkolb EN: Correlation of barium enema and CT in acute pancreatitis. AJR 136: 1219–1220, 1981

27. Warshaw AL: Inflammatory masses following acute pancreatitis. Phlegmon, pseudocyst, and abscess. Surg Clin N Am 54: 621–636, 1974

28. Simon M, Lerner MA: Duodenal compression by mesenteric root in acute pancreatitis and inflammatory conditions of bowel. Radiology 79: 75–80, 1962

29. Boijsen E, Tylen U: Vascular changes in chronic pancreatitis. Acta Radiol Diagn 12: 34–38, 1972

30. Walter JF, Chuang VP, Bookstein JJ, et al: Angiography of massive hemorrhage secondary to pancreatic disease. Radiology 124: 337–342, 1977

31. Meyers MA, Ghahremani GG, Clements JL Jr, et al: Pneumatosis intestinalis. Gastrointest Radiol 2: 91–105, 1977

32. Collins JJ Jr, Peterson LM, Wilson RE: Small intestinal infarction as a complication of pancreatitis. Ann Surg 167: 433–436, 1968

33. Dallemand S, Farman J, Stein D, et al: Colonic necrosis complicating pancreatitis. Gastrointest Radiol 2: 27–30, 1977

34. Griffiths RW, Brown PW Jr: Jejunal infarction as a complication of pancreatitis. Gastroenterology 58: 709–712, 1970

35. Katz P, Dorman MJ, Aufses AH Jr: Colonic necrosis complicating postoperative pancreatitis. Ann Surg 179: 403–405, 1974

# 8 The Small Bowel: Normal and Pathologic Anatomy

## General Introduction

The distinctive course, coiled nature, and position of the small bowel are provided by the mesentery. The most characteristic gross anatomic feature of the jejunum and ileum is their organization into a series of bowel loops, compactly arranged in the midabdomen. In the routine interpretation of small intestinal series, little attention is directed to this unique organization of the bowel. Indeed, the confluence or overlapping of small bowel loops often presents a misleading appearance. Their serpentine, undulating course ordinarily poses a diagnostic challenge in identifying the presence of a localized abnormality.

However, the anatomic relationships inherent in this characteristic arrangement of the small intestine into loops of bowel may provide significant diagnostic information.[1,2] Pathologically, many disease processes selectively involve the mesenteric or antimesenteric borders of the small intestine. An understanding of their anatomic definition and relationships permits radiologic identification of the specific borders.[1]

## Anatomic Considerations

The *mesentery* (Fig. 8–1) suspends the jejunum and ileum from the posterior abdominal wall. It is composed of fatty extraperitoneal connective tissue, blood vessels, nerves, lymphatics, and an investment of peritoneum that reflects from the posterior parietal peritoneum. Features associated with the fan-shaped dimensions of the mesentery make it a unique suspensory ligament and contribute to the characteristic nature of small bowel loops.

The attached border, the *root of the mesentery,* extends obliquely from the point of termination of the duodenum, at the lower border of the pancreas on the left side of the second lumbar vertebra, to the cecum in the right iliac fossa near the right sacroiliac articulation. In that

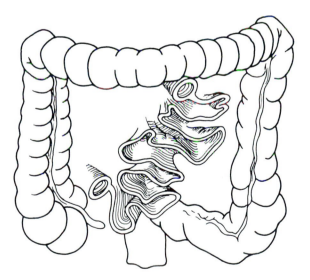

**Fig. 8–1. The small bowel mesentery.** It extends from its line of attachment, or root, in a series of fanlike ruffles to suspend the jejunum and ileum. The undulating course of its intestinal edge constitutes a series of convexities and concavities. Peritoneal recesses extend between the mesenteric reflections.
(From Meyers[1])

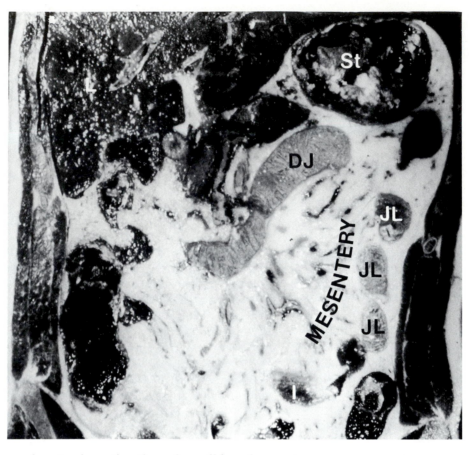

**Fig. 8–2. Coronal anatomic section through small bowel mesentery.**
This section is taken at the level of the third and fourth portions of the duodenum and the duodenojejunal junction (DJ). It demonstrates the fatty elastic nature of the mesentery, which contains the intestinal vessels as it radiates from its root to suspend loops of jejunum (JL) and ileum (I). L = liver, St = stomach. (Courtesy of Manuel Viamonte, MD, Mount Sinai Hospital, Miami Beach, Fla.)
(From Meyers[1])

course the line of attachment passes from the dudodenojejunal flexure down over the front of the third part of the duodenum, then obliquely across the aorta, the inferior vena cava, the right ureter, and the psoas major muscle, to the right iliac region. From the root, the mesentery extends in a series of fanlike ruffles to suspend the jejunum and ileum. There are usually six main folds, from the margins of which secondary folds project in all directions, and from those again even a third series may be formed. A series of peritoneal recesses are formed between the ruffles of the small bowel mesentery. The root of the mesentery is only about 15 cm (6 in.) long and is fixed in position. It is much thicker than the part near the gut, since it contains be-

tween its layers a considerable amount of fatty fibroareolar extraperitoneal tissue and the large vascular trunks that supply the intestine (Fig. 8–2).

The *base*, or unattached border, *of the mesentery* is frilled out to an enormous degree so that, while the root measures only 6–7 in., the free border is extended to 20–22 ft (Fig. 8–3). The great length of the intestinal border is produced by plication of the mesentery along its edge for a depth of from 6 to 8 cm ($2\frac{1}{2}$–$3\frac{1}{2}$ in.).

The *length of the mesentery* (Fig. 8–3), measured from its root to the attached edge of the intestine directly opposite, usually measures 20–22 cm (8–9 in.). It is greater at that part that suspends the coils of the intestine lying between

2 and 3 m (6 and 11 ft) from the duodenum, where it may reach a length of 25 cm (10 in.). It tends to increase in length as age advances.

# Normal Radiologic Observations

From these basic considerations, several principles may be derived[2] that have practical diagnostic application to radiology of the abdomen.

## Axis of the Root of the Small Bowel Mesentery

The plane of attachment of the small bowel mesentery may be drawn by an imaginary line extending from the midtransverse duodenum or duodenojejunal junction to the ileocecal junction. The root of the mesentery most often in-

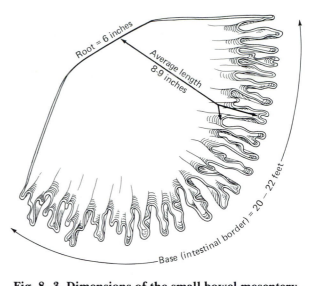

**Fig. 8–3. Dimensions of the small bowel mesentery.** The length of the intestinal border to an extent approximately 40 times that of its root is brought about by its unique frilled nature. This determines the characteristic formation of the small bowel into loops. (From Meyers[1])

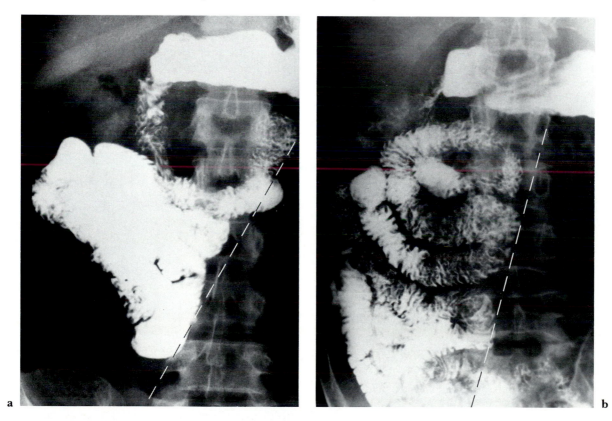

a          b

**Fig. 8–4. Two different cases of nonrotation of the jejunum in the right abdomen.**
The oblique plane which provides the medial demarcation of the loops of bowel identifies the axis of the root of the small bowel mesentery (dashed line). (From Meyers[1])

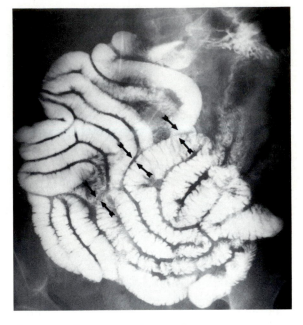

**Fig. 8–5. The root of the small bowel mesentery.**
This is revealed as the oblique plane (arrows) from which the intestinal coils are suspended. In this instance, it provides a line of transition between jejunal loops (shown by their prominent valvulae conniventes), which project to the patient's left, and ileal loops (with less conspicuous valvulae), which extend to the right. (From Meyers[1])

serts at the termination of the ileum with the colon, and only rarely on the ascending colon or the distal ileum. On plain films, the line may be drawn from the left of L2 to the right sacroiliac articulation.

The axis of the root may be defined more clearly by barium contrast studies, which then relates more directly to small bowel loops. Figure 8–4 illustrates two different cases of nonrotation of the jejunum, a common developmental variant. The root of the small bowel mesentery is shown by the oblique plane providing the medial demarcation of these jejunal loops. The root may also be identified in cases of normal development and fixation of the mesentery. In the small bowel series shown in Figure 8–5, the attached border of the mesentery can be appreciated as the oblique plane from which the loops are suspended.

It is these normal relationships of small bowel loops to the supporting mesentery that basically determine the radiologic findings in cases of mechanical obstruction. The dilated loops are then each tensely suspended from the mesenteric root as peristalsis persists; the hydrodynamic consequences lead to the classic "stepladder" configuration (Fig. 8–6).

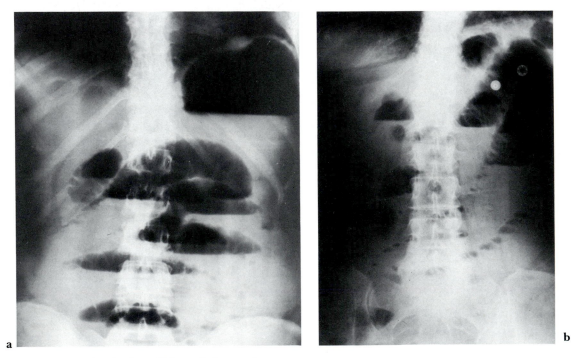

a                                                                                                                                                    b

**Fig. 8–6. Mechanical small bowel obstruction.**
(**a** and **b**) Erect films in two different cases illustrate the "stepladder" arrangement of dilated obstructed loops. This pattern is related to tension anchored on the root of the mesentery.

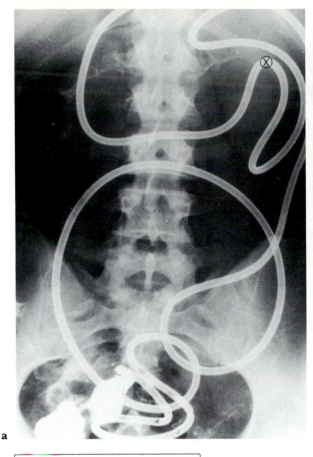

a

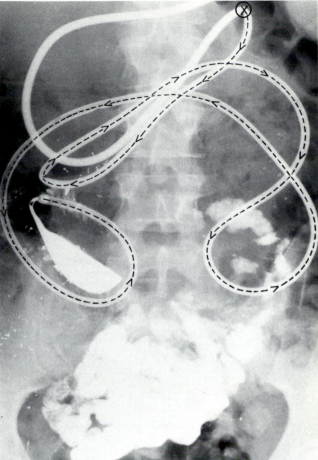

b

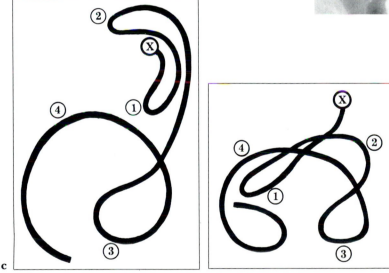

c

d

**Fig. 8–7. Changeable position of small bowel loops.**
(**a** and **b**) Radiographs of the intubated small intestine 1 day apart, demonstrating striking variations in the positions of the bowel loops. (X marks the duodenojejunal junction.)
(**c** and **d**) Tracings illustrate that changes in position and arcing convexities of some bowel segments are more marked than in others.
(From Meyers[1])

## Undulating Changeable Nature of Coils of Bowel Loops

A fan-shaped supporting ligament such as the mesentery, with an attachment of only 6 in. and an average length of 8–9 in., must suspend 20–22 ft of small bowel. This remarkable feat is accomplished by the unique plication or frilling of its intestinal border. The mesentery extends from its root in a series of fanlike ruffles. This geometric arrangement provides an unusually long border to suspend the jejunum and ileum. It is precisely this feature which contributes to the characteristic undulating nature of the coils

369

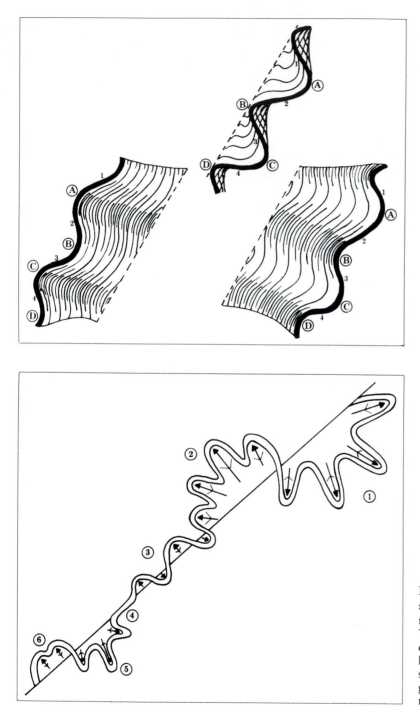

**Fig. 8–8. Diagram of the ruffled edge of the mesentery.**
This immediately suspends the small bowel loops.

(*Top*) Vertical (sagittal). (*Left*) Rotation to the right. (*Right*) Rotation to the left.

(The dashed line indicates the root of the small bowel mesentery.) (From Meyers[1])

**Fig. 8–9. Variable orientations of small bowel loops to mesenteric root.**
The mesenteric border (arrows) constitutes the concave margin of a loop facing the root. The antimesenteric border is the convex margin of a loop facing away from the root. (From Meyers[1])

of small intestine. The mesentery is of such a length that the loops are able to move freely in the abdominal cavity, and consequently the position occupied by any portion of the small bowel, with the usual exception of the beginning of the jejunum and the ending of the ileum, cannot be stated with certainty. Nevertheless, in general, the jejunum occupies the superior and left portions of the peritoneal cavity below the stomach, and the ileum the inferior and right divisions.

The changeable position of jejunal and ileal loops *in vivo* is most easily documented by comparing portions of the intubated small bowel on sequential films as in Figure 8–7. These show the loops are movable on the root of the mesentery, but they maintain the convexities of the ruffles. Specific intestinal segments (Nos. 1 through 4) can be matched and demonstrate varying positions within the peritoneal cavity. The changeable location is difficult to evaluate during routine contrast studies of the small intestine, chiefly because of the common inaccuracy in tracing the continuity of opacified, superimposed bowel loops.

## Identification of Mesenteric and Antimesenteric Borders of Small Bowel Loops

It is necessary to recognize the axis of the root of the mesentery and the undulating, changeable nature of the small bowel loops to understand the basis for the radiologic identification of their mesenteric and antimesenteric borders.[1] Figure 8–8 illustrates certain constant geometric properties of the mesentery. The base of the mesentery, from which the jejunum and ileum are suspended, is essentially a series of alternating convexities and concavities connected by intervening limbs. Any single limb is thus shared by a convexity and a concavity on either side. A limb or straight segment of small bowel, therefore, connects one convex loop with the next concave loop. Any curved line presents basically two surfaces—one convex, the other concave—determined by the point of reference. In the small bowel, the point of reference used is the root of the mesentery. By definition, therefore, the concept of convexity or concavity of bowel loops is determined by the axis of the root of the small bowel mesentery. Figure 8–8 top illustrates that limbs 1 and 2 constitute the convex loop A, limbs 2 and 3 form the concave loop B, and limbs 3 and 4 produce the convex loop C.

Another phenomenon of the ruffled nature of the mesentery and small bowel loops results, depending on positional relationships to the mesenteric root. If rotation occurs toward the left (Fig. 8–8 right), there is no essential change in the convex-concave relationships of bowel loops. However, if rotation on the mesenteric root occurs toward the right (Fig. 8–8 left), there may be a complete reversal of these relationships. Figure 8–8 left shows that now loop A

is concave, B convex, C concave, etc. It must also be recognized that *in vivo* the small bowel loops do not act synchronously in rotating in position on the mesenteric root. One coil may be horizontal (transverse), the next vertical (sagittal), the next in the coronal plane, and the next obliquely oriented between any of these three planes. The variability is further increased by the fact that these mesenteric projections may extend toward the left or toward the right and may alternate. Position of the patient, peristaltic dynamics, and factors of intraabdominal pressure are likely determinants.

Thus, several conclusions can be derived from these observations which can be accurately applied in the radiologic–anatomic identification of small bowel loops.[1] Figure 8–9 illustrates these:

1. *The concave margin of a small bowel loop, facing toward the axis of the root of the mesentery, is the mesenteric border.* This is true whether the loop is positioned to the left or to the right of the mesenteric root. This is shown in segments 1, 2, 5, and 6 in Figure 8–9.

2. *The convex margin of a small bowel loop, facing away from the axis of the root of the mesentery, constitutes the antimesenteric border.* This is also true, of course, whether the loop projects to the left or to the right of the mesenteric root.*

3. Even if loops are suspended in the midline, their mesenteric and antimesenteric borders can be identified similarly if they project in the coronal plane. This is shown in segment 3 in Figure 8–9.

4. When viewed in a frontal x-ray, a loop projecting in the sagittal or horizontal plane does not present its mesenteric and antimesenteric borders for definition. This occurs most often near the midline overlying the mesenteric root, as shown in segment 4 of Figure 8–9. Pressure films or radiographs with the patient positioned obliquely may render such a loop convex and allow delineation of its mesenteric and antime-

---

* It can further be appreciated that consequent to the fixation of the mesenteric ruffles, the convex margin of a bowel loop facing *toward* the axis of the root of the mesentery, may at times also constitute the mesenteric border of that particular loop (Fig. 8–1 and loops A and C in Fig. 8–8b). However, while this may be anatomically true, its radiologic application would be untrustworthy.

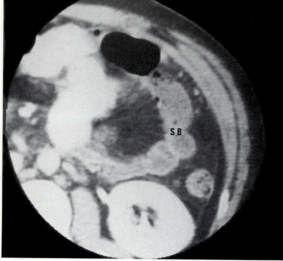

**Fig. 8–10. Intestinal borders.**
Computed tomography identifies fat-containing leaf of mesentery with vascular branches extending to the concave mesenteric border of small bowel loop (SB).

Table 8–1. Pathologic localization.

| Diseases | Mesenteric | Antimesenteric |
|---|:---:|:---:|
| | Sole or predominant border of small bowel involved | |
| Diverticulosis | ■ | |
| Meckel's diverticulum | | ■ |
| Intestinal duplication | ■ | |
| Seeded metastases | ■ | |
| Hematogenous metastases | | ■ |
| Regional enteritis | | |
|   Rigidity, ulcerations, sinus tracts | ■ | |
|   Pseudosacculations | ± | ■ |
| Lymphoma | ■ | |
| Bleeding | | |
|   Intramural thumbprints | ■ | |
|   Postfibrotic pseudodiverticula | | ■ |
|   Intramesenteric | ■ | |

senteric borders. Viewed in the axial plane, these intestinal borders are easily appreciable on computed tomograpy (Fig. 8–10).

# Abnormal Radiologic Features

Many small bowel abnormalities selectively involve either the mesenteric or antimesenteric borders of small intestinal loops solely or predominantly. Precise radiologic distinction between these margins can localize and diagnose a variety of intraabdominal disease states, which otherwise share many common features. Table 8–1 summarizes the characteristic localization of involvement in a variety of conditions. Application of these principles is particularly helpful at any early stage of the lesion or when there may otherwise be an extensive differential diagnosis.

## Diverticulosis of the Small Intestine

Acquired diverticula of the small bowel are usually multiple and are practically limited to the upper part of the jejunum.[3] Examination of a specimen (Fig. 8–11a) documents that the diverticula do not arise randomly from the circumference of the small intestine but are strikingly situated at or immediately alongside the mesenteric border, pushing their way between the leaves of the mesentery. The long axis of their domes, as well as of their elliptical orifices (Fig. 8–11b), tends to parallel the longitudinal axis of the bowel. Such diverticula of the small intestine are of the "pulsion" mucous membrane type. They arise in relation to the sites of penetration of the bowel wall by the vasa recta, which enter on the mesenteric border.[4]

This precise localization of small bowel diverticula to the mesenteric border can be identified radiologically in 75% of the cases.[2] The saccules usually are amorphous, without a mucosal pattern, and characteristically extend from the concave (mesenteric) margins of jejunal loops curved away from the axis of the root of the mesentery (Figs. 8–12 and 8–13). Diverticula of the terminal ileum also follow this pattern (Fig. 8–14).

## Meckel's Diverticulum

A Meckel's diverticulum represents a remnant of the omphalomesenteric (vitelline) duct. This pouchlike persistence had the same anatomic structure as the remainder of the intestine, and thus contains all four histologic layers. It generally follows the "rule of twos": it is present in 2%

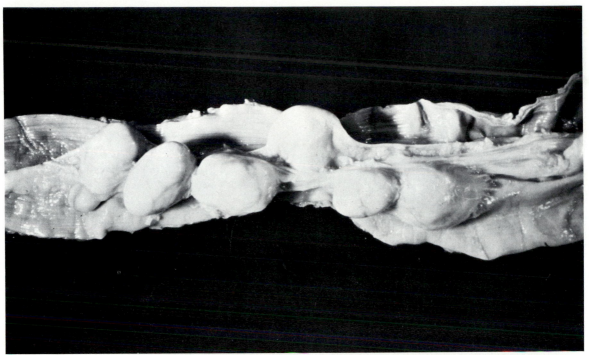

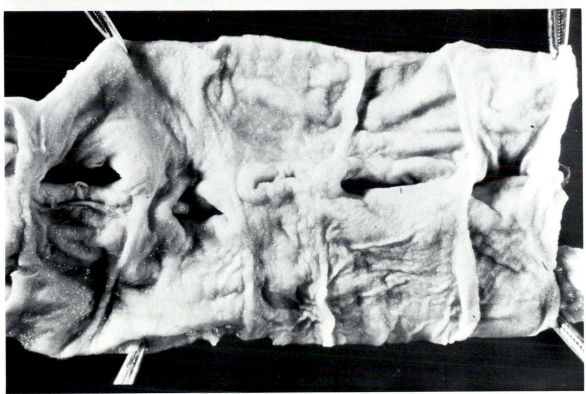

**Fig. 8–11. Gross specimen of diverticulosis of the jejunum.**
(**a**) The loop is opened by cutting along the antimesenteric border. The multiple diverticula arise in a row distinctly from the mesenteric borders, invaginating between the leaves of the mesentery.
(**b**) Viewed from the mucosal aspect, the elliptical orifices extend along the line of attachment of the mesentery.
(From Meyers[2])

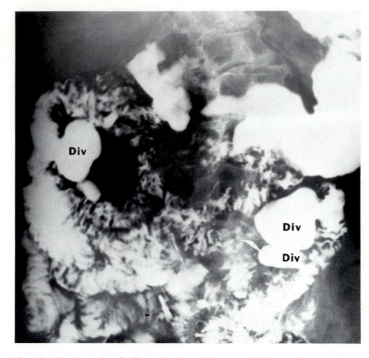

**Fig. 8–12. Acquired diverticula of the small intestine.**
Multiple diverticula (Div) project from the mesenteric borders of jejunal loops. (From Meyers[2])

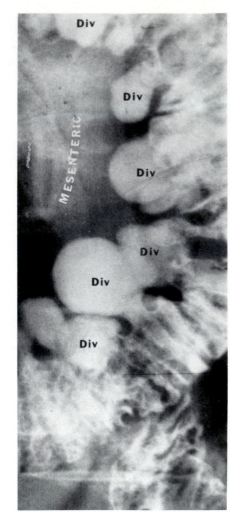

**Fig. 8–13. Diverticulosis of the small bowel.**
Pressure spot film localizes the diverticula (Div) as specifically arising from the concave, mesenteric border of a jejunal loop. (From Meyers[2])

of people, averages 2 in. in length, and is found in the distal ileum about 2 ft proximal to the ileocecal valve.

The radiologic hallmark of a Meckel's diverticulum is thus based on its identification as a saccule extending precisely from the antimesenteric, convex border of a terminal ileal loop (Figs. 8–15 through 8–17), usually in the right lower quadrant. This can be seen in almost two-thirds of instances.[2] Because of the variability in position of small bowel loops, the segment from which a Meckel's diverticulum arises may, at times, project within other areas of the abdomen,[5] but its localization nevertheless to the antimesenteric border can be of great diagnostic value (Fig. 8–18).

## Intestinal Duplication

The cystic structure of an intestinal duplication (also called "enteric cyst" or "enterogenous cyst") may, but usually does not, communicate with the adjacent intestinal lumen. The muscular coats of the duplication are intimately adherent to and, at times, are microscopically an integral part of the muscularis of the alimentary tract. Ladd and Gross[6] noted that it arises most often in relationship to the ileum and typically from its mesenteric border. Symptomatology in children includes obstruction, pain, and hemorrhage because of interference with the intestinal blood supply leading to sloughing of the ileal mucosa. Complete extirpation of the mass along

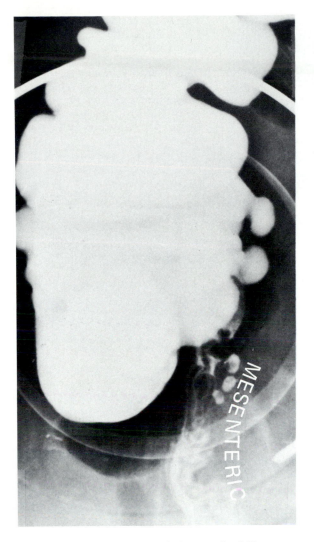

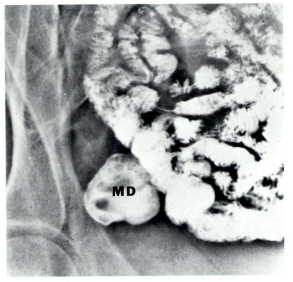

**Fig. 8–15. Meckel's diverticulum.**
The saccule (MD) extends from the antimesenteric convex border of a terminal ileal loop. (The filling defects within it in this instance are secondary to calculus formation.) (From Meyers[2])

**Fig. 8–14. Diverticulosis of the terminal ileum.**
Pressure spot film shows the diverticula arising from the mesenteric border. A few cecal diverticula are also present.

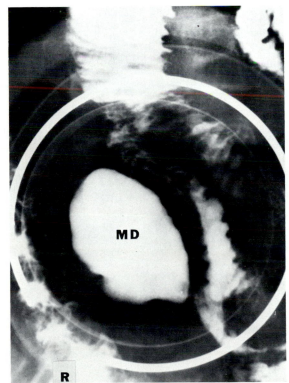

**Fig. 8–16. Meckel's diverticulum.**
The large saccule (MD) extends from the antimesenteric border of a terminal ileal loop, which it indents in the right lower quadrant of the abdomen. (From Meyers[2])

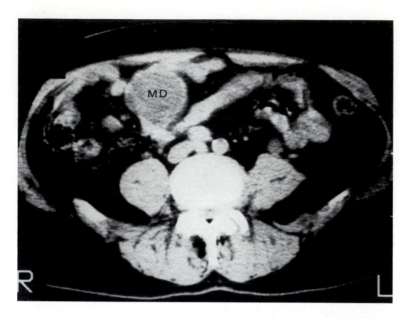

**Fig. 8–17. Meckel's diverticulum.** CT demonstrates a 5-cm Meckel's diverticulum (MD) attached to the antimesenteric side of the ileum. The fibrous remnant of the vitelline duct extends between the diverticulum and the umbilical region. (Courtesy of Gary Ghahremani, MD, Evanston, Ill.)

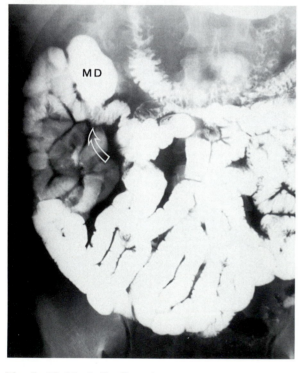

**Fig. 8–18. Meckel's diverticulum.**
The opacified saccule (MD) attached to the antimesenteric border of a midileal loop (curved arrow) occupies the subhepatic region in the right upper quadrant. (Courtesy of Gary Ghahremani, MD, Evanston, Ill.)

with resection of the adjacent portion of the intestine is thus necessary.

With an understanding of the radiologic identification of the mesenteric and antimesenteric borders of small bowel loops, barium contrast studies may be of considerable help in the diagnosis. A noncommunicating intestinal duplication may be revealed as an extrinsic soft-tissue mass displacing an ileal loop upon its mesenteric margin. This precise localization may be seen in 60% of cases.[2] The lumen of a communicating duplication may be opacified to clearly demonstrate it as a tubular or spherical structure, specifically arising in relationship to the mesenteric border (Fig. 8–19).

## Seeded Metastases

The distribution of seeded metastases within the abdomen, as discussed in Chapter 3, has been shown to follow the dynamic pathways of the circulation of ascitic fluid.[7–9] The malignant cells are shed by the primary neoplasm and then transported by the ascites. They are then deposited and subsequently grow as seeded metastases at the sites of stasis or pooling of the ascitic fluid. In the midabdomen, pooling occurs within the peritoneal recesses of the mesenteric ruffles.[10] Flow occurs in a series of rivulets or cascades from one mesenteric recess to the next lower, with the largest and most consistent pool

**Fig. 8–19. Duplication of terminal ileum.**
The intestinal duplication (ID) is identified as a tubular structure without a recognizable mucosal pattern, lying along the mesenteric border of the terminal ileum (TI) with which it communicates. (From Meyers[2])

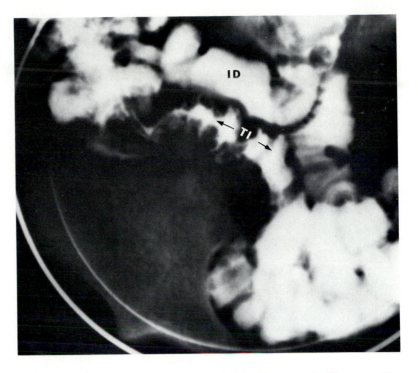

formed at the termination of the small bowel mesentery at the ileocolic junction. The seeded metastases lodge and grow, therefore, on the mesenteric borders and involve distal ileal loops in over 40% of all cases.[8]

The distinctive radiologic feature lies in the localization of changes to the mesenteric border of distal ileal loops, evident in over 75% of seeded metastases in the right lower quadrant of the abdomen.[2] Mass changes and associated desmoplastic tethering of mucosal folds constitute the basic characteristics. Figure 8–20 illustrates multiple masses indenting the mesenteric borders of individual distal ileal loops in a case of seeded metastases from carcinoma of the ovary. They are strikingly oriented in relation to the axis of the small bowel mesentery. The associated desmoplastic response, another sign highly distinctive of seeded lesions,[10] results in angulated tethering of the mucosal folds on the mesenteric borders only. Angulation of the loops themselves at the sites of the serosal masses on the mesenteric borders (Fig. 8–21) further indicates the desmoplastic process.

## Hematogenous Metastases

The vasa recta of the bowel penetrate the wall on the mesenteric border. They then extend intramurally for variable distances before ramifying toward the antimesenteric border to arborize into the rich submucosal plexus.

The most common hematogenous metastasis to the small bowel clinically encountered is metastatic melanoma.[9] Its dissemination can be observed radiologically to follow, at times, the field of a specific arterial distribution.[9] The embolic metastases typically present as submucosal filling defects, often with central ulceration ("bull's-eye" lesions), within a single or multiple intestinal loops. However, when visualized on one wall of a bowel loop, they are localized precisely to its antimesenteric border (Fig. 8–22) in 80% of cases.[2] This correlates with experimental studies indicating that strictly mechanical and circulatory factors can account for the distribution of some secondary tumors.[11] The radiologic–anatomic observation presumably reflects lodgement and subsequent growth of embolic malignant cells within the smaller arterial arborizations on the antimesenteric border.

## Regional Enteritis

The general radiologic findings of regional enteritis correlate closely with the gross pathologic features. The involved bowel, often affected by "skip lesions," is sharply delimited from contig-

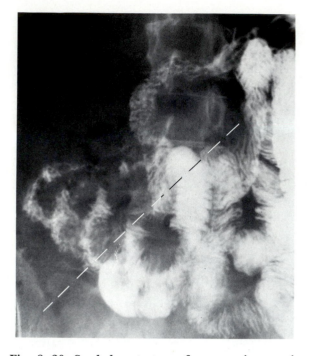

**Fig. 8–20. Seeded metastases from ovarian carcinoma.**
Multiple masses cause scalloped displacement on the mesenteric borders of ileal loops in the right lower quadrant. Mucosal tethering is also localized to the mesenteric margins.

Note the relationship of these changes to the axis of the small bowel mesentery, indicated by the line of dashes. (From Meyers[2])

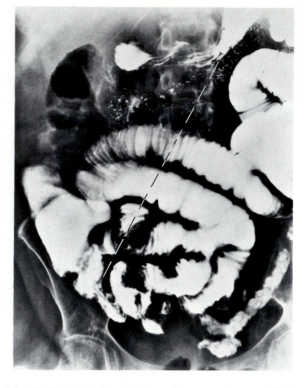

**Fig. 8–21. Seeded metastases from carcinoma of the ovary.**
Multiple serosal masses indent the mesenteric margins of angulated ileal loops in the right lower quadrant. Luminal narrowing and some desmoplastic angulation result in proximal obstruction. (From Meyers[2])

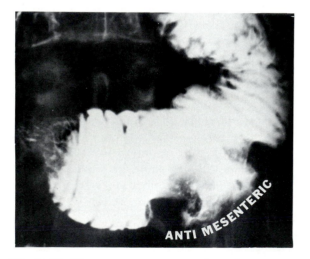

**Fig. 8–22. Hematogenous metastatic melanoma.**
A large submucosal mass with a prominent central ulceration is localized to the convex, antimesenteric margin of a distal jejunal loop. (From Meyers[2])

uous gut and has a narrowed lumen, which is sometimes strictured. The bowel wall is rigid and thick, the mesentery is often markedly thickened and edematous, and the mesenteric lymph nodes are enlarged. The swollen, inflamed mucosa develops a cobblestone appearance as longitudinal and transverse ulcers intersect. As these extend deeply through the wall, sinus tracts and fistulas may be present.

Other specific, more localized changes of regional enteritis have been observed surgically and pathologically. In their pioneering report in 1932, Crohn, Ginzburg, and Oppenheimer noted on opening the intestine that a series of small linear ulcerations lying in a groove on the mesenteric side of the intestine is almost always present.[12] It has also been observed that there is a close relationship between the destructive changes in the mucosa and the extent of in-

**Fig. 8–23. Regional enteritis.**
Diffuse involvement of ileum. One loop demonstrates ulcerations and small sinus tracts along the concave, mesenteric border at the site of mesenteric tumefaction.

Pseudosacculations on the convex margin of the loop indicate that the antimesenteric border retains some pliability.

The dashed line indicates the axis of the root of the mesentery. (From Meyers[2])

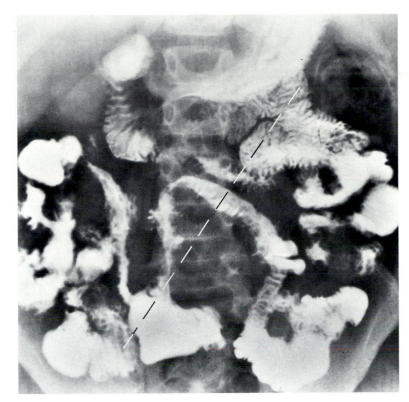

creased mesenteric fat.[13] The development of pseudodiverticula, furthermore, is probably related to eccentric skip areas.[13]

These discrete pathologic observations in regional enteritis may be directly applied to the radiologic alterations for a more definite diagnosis. The process may be identified, particularly in its early stages, as localized predominantly to the mesenteric borders of involved loops. The findings of mucosal irregularities, ulcerations, fixation and rigidity, sinus tracts, and extrinsic mass tumefaction may be confined or most evident on the concave margins (Figs. 8–23 through 8–25). The fact that the antimesenteric wall may not be symmetrically involved at the same time but, rather, retains some degree of pliability may be revealed by the development of pseudosacculations from the convex border.

In severely involved loops, the segmental, skip nature of the lesions may result in pseudosaccular outpouchings from both the mesenteric and antimesenteric borders (Fig. 8–26).

It follows that pseudosacculations or the appearance of diverticula limited solely to the mesenteric borders are not a feature of regional enteritis.

## Lymphoma

Within the small bowel, malignant lymphoma involves the terminal ileum most often (Fig. 8–27). Growth may be predominantly away from the intestinal lumen, in an exoenteric fashion. Mass extension into the mesentery may produce extrinsic compression of the bowel lumen. This form of the disease and primary mesenteric lymphoma are characterized radiologically by the presence of mesenteric masses extrinsically compressing and distorting the concave borders of small bowel loops (Figs. 8–28 and 8–29).

## Intramural and Mesenteric Bleeding

Bleeding into the wall of the small intestine and into the mesentery may be a consequence of many different disorders. It is seen in mesenteric thromboses and emboli, segmental ischemic disease, abdominal trauma, anticoagulation medication, underlying diseases associated

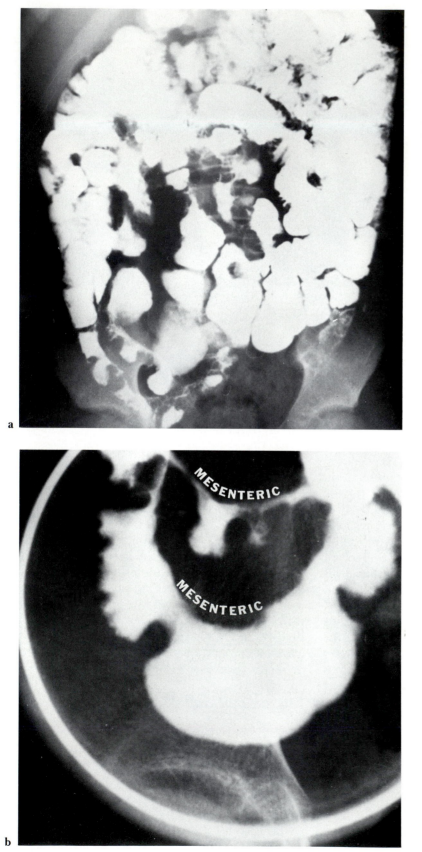

a

b

**Fig. 8–24. Regional enteritis in an 11-year-old male.**
Small bowel series (**a**) with pressure spot film of distal ileum (**b**) show rigidity from the ulcerative process clearly limited to the mesenteric borders, and pseudosaccular out-pouchings from the more pliable antimesenteric margins.
(From Meyers[2])

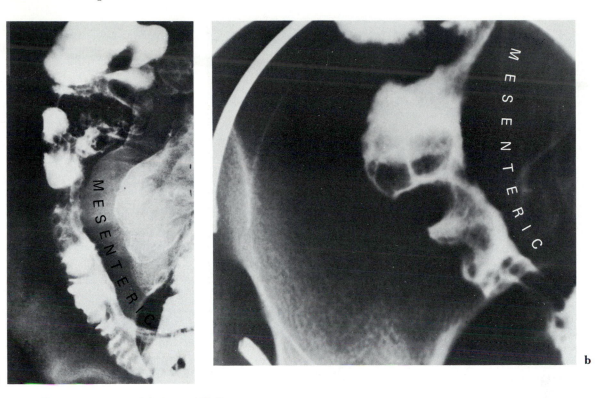

**Fig. 8–25. Regional enteritis in two different cases.**
(**a** and **b**) Flattening and rigidity are conspicuously localized to the mesenteric border of the terminal ileum. The antimesenteric border retains some pliability as shown by pseudosaccular outpouchings.

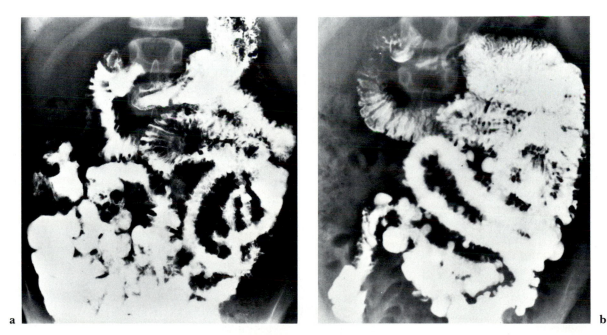

**Fig. 8–26. Regional enteritis.**
(**a**) Extensive involvement of small bowel in a 10-year-old male.
(**b**) Six months later, the skip nature of the severe lesions involving various segments of the circumference of the bowel has resulted in striking pseudosacculations extending from both the mesenteric and antimesenteric borders.
(From Meyers[2])

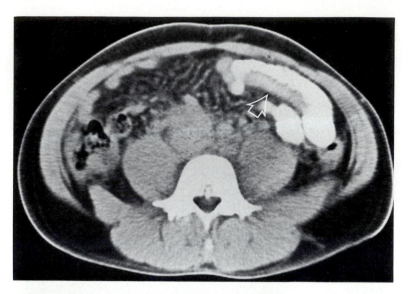

**Fig. 8–27. Hodgkin's lymphoma.** CT demonstrates mural thickening of an opacified ileal loop in the left lower quadrant strikingly limited to its mesenteric border (arrow). This is accompanied by retroperitoneal adenopathy and stellate infiltration of the mesentery.

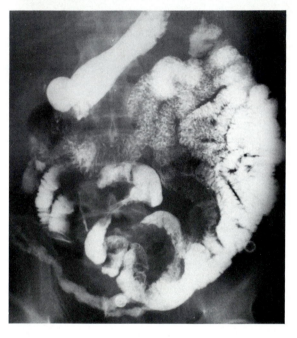

**Fig. 8–28. Lymphosarcoma.** The process is revealed as masses discretely separating and pressing on the concave mesenteric borders of distal ileal loops in the right lower quadrant. (From Meyers[2])

with coagulation defects (hemophilia, leukemia, multiple myeloma, lymphoma, and metastatic carcinoma), and the vasculitis of collagen diseases (polyarteritis nodosa, systemic lupus erythematosus), thromboangiitis obliterans (Buerger's disease), and the Henoch–Schönlein syndrome.

While diffuse intramural fluid results in a compact appearance of prominent mucosal folds, sometimes described as the "stacked-coin" or "picket-fence" arrangement, coalescence of the submucosal edema and hemorrhage produces the characteristic scalloped or nodular filling defects along the contours of the bowel referred to as "thumbprinting."

These distinctive "thumbprint" defects in intramural intestinal bleeding are by far most consistently localized to the mesenteric borders of the loops (Figs. 8–30 through 8–32). In advanced cases, the defects may randomly involve both margins of the involved loops, but in early or limited stages, the nodular masses are clearly localized to the concave borders in 75% of patients.[2] These defects are typically superimposed on a pattern indicating diffuse intramural fluid. If fibrosis progresses, the antimesenteric border then forms multiple sacculations or pseudodiverticula. Severe involvement may result in a concentric stricture.

Mesenteric bleeding exaggerates and tends to fix the coiled nature of the small intestine. It is further revealed by mass separation and extrinsic compression on the mesenteric borders of the loops (Fig. 8–33).

**Fig. 8–29. Mesenteric lymphoma.**
Computed tomography shows huge lymphomatous mass which is contiguous with the root of the mesentery (arrows) grossly displacing contrast-filled small bowel loops.

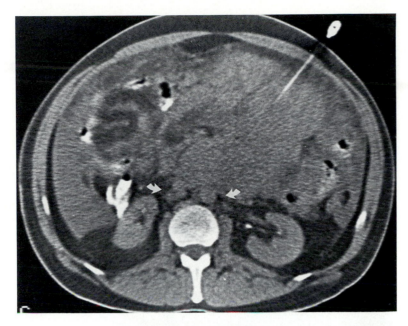

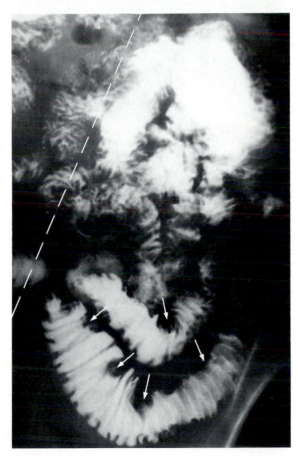

**Fig. 8–30. Intramural bleeding, secondary to over-anticoagulation.**
Rectal bleeding in a 56-year-old male on anticoagulants while recovering from a myocardial infarction prompted this small intestinal series. Note that the thumbprint defects (arrows) of coalescent intramural blood are localized specifically to the concave, mesenteric borders. (The dashed line indicates the mesenteric root.) Diffuse submucosal fluid is also present. (From Meyers[2])

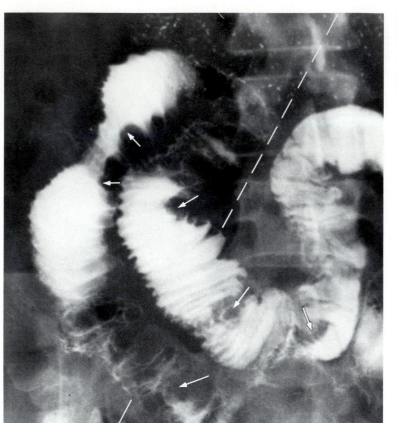

**Fig. 8–31. Intramural bleeding in a heroin addict.**
The thumbprint filling defects (arrows) of intramural bleeding are confined to the concave mesenteric borders. (From Meyers[2])

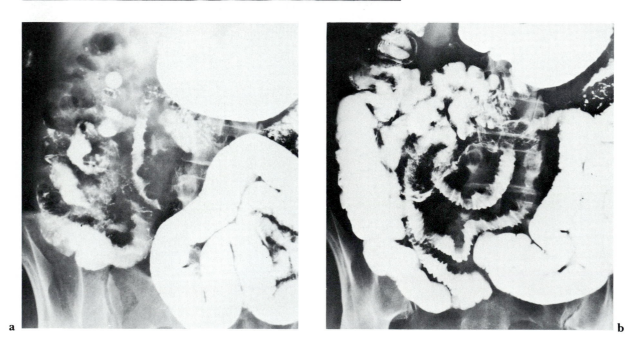

a                                                                                                          b

**Fig. 8–32. Ischemic enteritis.**
(**a** and **b**)  Small bowel series (45 minutes and 2 hours, respectively) in a female taking oral contraceptive pills show the features of ischemic enteritis involving several ileal loops, with the changes most prominent on their mesenteric borders.

**Fig. 8–33. (a** and **b) Two different cases of mesenteric bleeding secondary to Henoch–Schönlein purpura.**
Bleeding into the mesentery has resulted in mass separation and displacement upon the concave, mesenteric borders of small bowel loops. Accompanying intramural fluid is also evident. (From Meyers[2])

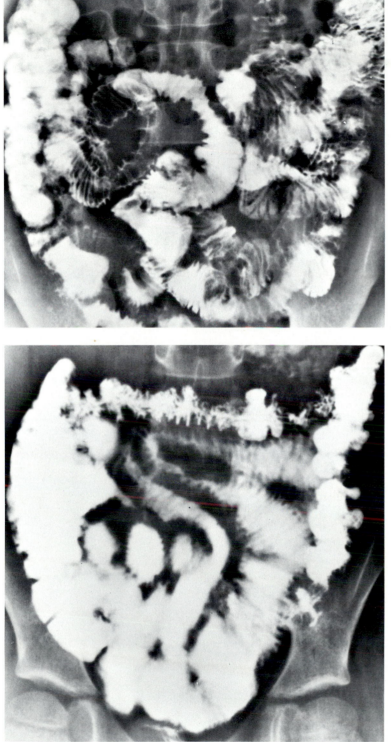

a

b

# References

1. Meyers MA: Clinical involvement of mesenteric and antimesenteric borders of small bowel loops. I. Normal pattern and relationships. Gastrointest Radiol 1: 41–48, 1976
2. Meyers MA: Clinical involvement of mesenteric and antimesenteric borders of small bowel loops. II. Roentgen interpretation of pathological alterations. Gastrointest Radiol 1: 49–58, 1976
3. Maglinte DDT, Chernish SM, DeWeese R, et al: Acquired jejunoileal diverticular disease: Subject review. Radiology 158: 577–580, 1986
4. Edwards HC: Diverticulosis of the small intestine. Ann Surg 103: 230–254, 1936
5. Ghahremani GG: Radiology of Meckel's diverticulum. Crit Rev Diagn Imag 26(1): 1–43, 1986
6. Ladd WE, Gross RE: Surgical treatment of duplications of the alimentary tract: Enterogenous cysts, enteric cysts, or ileum duplex. Surg Gynecol Obstet 70: 295–307, 1940
7. Meyers MA: The spread and localization of acute intraperitoneal effusions. Radiology 95: 547–554, 1970
8. Meyers MA: Distribution of intra-abdominal malignant seeding: Dependency on dynamics of flow of ascitic fluid. AJR Rad Ther Nucl Med 119: 198–206, 1973
9. Meyers MA, McSweeney J: Secondary neoplasms of the bowel. Radiology 105: 1–11, 1972
10. Meyers MA: Malignant seeding along small bowel mesentery: Roentgen features. AJR Rad Ther Nucl Med 123: 67–73, 1975
11. Coman DR, deLong RP, McCutcheon M: Studies on the mechanisms of metastasis. The distribution of tumors in various organs in relation to the distribution of arterial emboli. Cancer Res 11: 648–651, 1951
12. Crohn BB, Ginzburg L, Oppenheimer GD: Regional ileitis. JAMA 99: 1323–1329, 1932
13. Marshak RH, Wolf BS: Chronic ulcerative granulomatous jejunitis and ileojejunitis. AJR 70: 93–112, 1953

# 9 The Colon: Normal and Pathologic Anatomy

## General Introduction

The distinctive haustral contour of the large intestine is provided by three bands of longitudinal muscle—the taeniae coli. Since the taeniae are shorter than the length of the colon itself, their tethering action in relation to the circular muscle results in the characteristic haustral sacculations. The colonic haustra are thus organized into three distinct rows, each of which has characteristic anatomic relationships.[5]

The development and action of the taeniae have been carefully studied by Lineback.[2] In the embryo, the outer layer of muscle originates in the caudal end of the bowel and extends upward until it eventually encases the colon. The three taenial bands are well marked by the 100-mm stage. Haustra are not often seen in infancy, however. It is not until the third year of life that the disproportionate increase in length between the colon and its longitudinal muscle bands results in the colon being consistently bunched up, forming its characteristic saccular haustrations.

Internally, the colon presents a relatively smooth surface, except for the semicircular folds of the haustral pouches. Section of a longitudinal muscle band at the level of a haustration obliterates the haustration and causes the bowel segment to lengthen. The taniae function not only as shortening bands for the colon but as strong, fixed longitudinal cables on which the circular fibers are fixed (Fig. 9–1). The waves of contraction in the circular muscle occur independently and asynchronously in each of the three intertaenial regions[2,3] and it is this contraction that further produces the haustral clefts. The contribution of both the longitudinal muscle bands and the contraction of the circular muscle to the formation of the haustral folds accounts to some degree for their variable appearance on barium enema examination.[4,5]

In the routine interpretation of barium enema studies, little attention is ordinarily directed to the organization of the large intestine into three constituent rows of haustra. Indeed, the overlapping of the contours of the sacculations is generally considered a bothersome feature in contrast to the more readily apparent outlines of the stomach or small bowel loops. Careful evaluation of the anatomic profiles of the haustra, however, provides a precise basis for the radiologic analysis of a variety of abdominal diseases. In cases of extrinsic mass impressions on the colon or extension of an adjacent process to the large intestine, detailed analysis of the specific group of haustral sacculations first or principally involved leads to more precise localization and thereby identification of the primary process.[6] Basic to an appreciation of pathologic alterations, however, is an understanding of the normal haustral anatomy and relationships.

## Anatomic Considerations

The colon has a complete outer longitudinal muscle coat, less than half the thickness of the inner circular muscle.[2,7] The outer longitudinal layer is thickened by three bands of muscle, the taeniae coli, each 0.5–1.0 cm in width. They are most distinct in the ascending and transverse

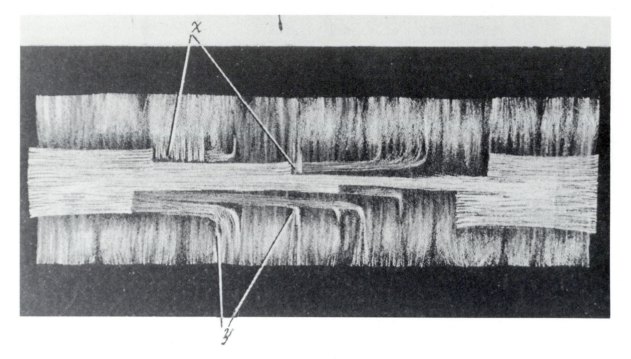

**Fig. 9–1. Interconnections of colonic muscle between the layers.**
Longitudinal muscle fibers (y) of the taenia turn at right angles and fuse with the circular muscle layer (x). This linkage provides a point for contraction, limiting the formation of interhaustral clefts to the zones between adjacent taeniae. (From Lineback[2])

colon. In the lower descending and sigmoid colon, they increase at the expense of the rest of the outer longitudinal muscle coat and at the level of the rectum become merged into broad diffuse bands.

Figure 9–2a shows that each of the taeniae is named according to its topographic situation relative to the transverse colon:

1. The *taenia mesocolica* (TM) is situated on the posterosuperior surface of the transverse colon at the line of attachment of the transverse mesocolon.
2. The *taenia omentalis* (TO) runs along the anterosuperior surface of the transverse colon and is in relation to the line of attachment of the greater omentum extending inferiorly and of the gastrocolic ligament above.
3. The *taenia libera* (TL), so-called because it is free and not related to any mesenteric or omental attachment, is found on the postero-inferior aspect of the transverse colon.

These relationships of the taeniae are not maintained on the ascending and descending portions of the colon (Fig. 9–2b). Here the TM

lies posteromedial, the TO posterolateral, and the TL anterior. The changing relationships of the taeniae are most simply understood if it is recalled that there is some anterior rotation of the transverse colon on its mesocolon relative to the flexures (Figs. 9–3 and 9–4). Nevertheless, continuity of the taeniae and thereby of the haustral rows can be easily traced.

## Classification of Organization of Haustral Rows

Three distinct rows of haustral sacculations are thus produced (Fig. 9–2), which can be referred to by the taeniae which give their form:

1. TM-TO. In the transverse colon this row provides the superior (mesenteric) contour. Here the haustra bear two important relationships: (a) they face the inferior recess of the lesser sac, providing its lower boundary and (b) they are in most direct continuity with the gastrocolic ligament extending downward from the stomach.

In the ascending and descending colon, these sacculations occupy the posterior third. This

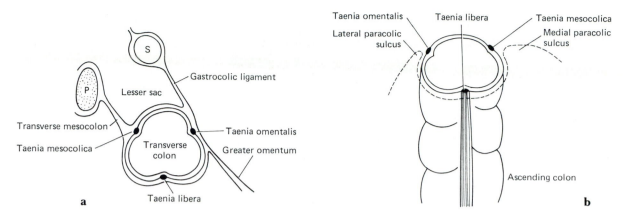

**Fig. 9–2. Position and relationships of the taeniae and haustra of the colon.**
(a) Sagittal diagram of transverse colon. P = pancreas, S = stomach.
(b) Horizontal diagram of ascending colon. The peritoneal reflections (dashed line) are shown in relation to the haustra. In the descending colon, the relationships are mirrorlike.
(From Meyers et al[5])

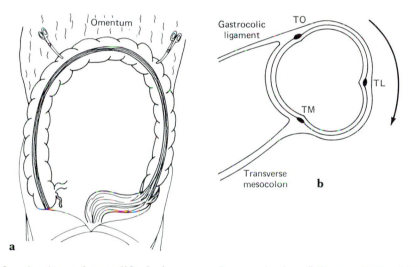

**Fig. 9–3. (a) Colon *in situ*, colon uplifted,** demonstrating continuity of the taenia libera from the ventral surface of the ascending and descending colon to the undersurface of the transverse colon.
**(b) Position of the three taeniae** in the uplifted transverse colon and the anterior rotation (indicated by arrow) which occurs when it assumes its normal position in the body. The taeniae and haustral rows then have the relationships shown in Fig. 9–2a.
(From Meyers et al[5])

row of haustra is unique in that their contour completely faces extraperitoneal structures only.

2. TM-TL. In the transverse colon this haustral row faces posteriorly and is in most direct continuity with the transverse mesocolon.

In the ascending and descending colon, these haustra constitute the medial third of the colonic contour (mesenteric border) and are in re-lation to the shallow intraperitoneal recess of the medial paracolic gutter.

3. TO-TL. In the transverse colon this group of sacculations provides the inferior (antimesenteric) contour and is the most anterior row. It is thus in relation to the greater omentum and anterior abdominal wall.

In the ascending and descending colon, these haustra constitute the lateral (antimesenteric)

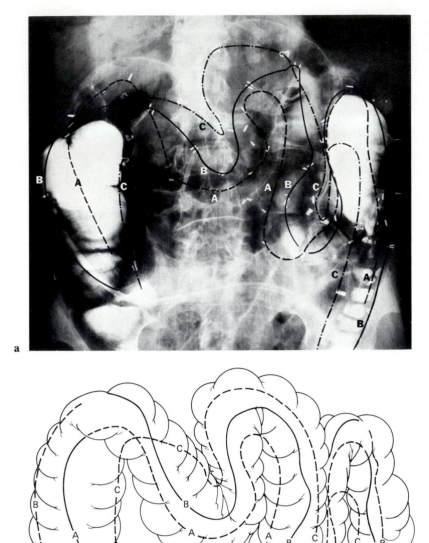

a

b

**Fig. 9–4. Postmortem double contrast radiograph marked *in situ* with metallic clips.**
The change in both course and relative position between the ascending, transverse, and descending colon is shown. A = taenia libera, B = taenia omentalis, C = taenia mesocolica. (From Meyers et al[5])

contour and are in most intimate relationship to the deep intraperitoneal lateral paracolic gutter.

## Normal Radiologic Observations

The haustral recesses, bordered by the course of the taeniae, can be identified easily by routine barium enema examination, particularly with air-contrast studies.[5] Their distinctive organization into rows and the position and anatomic limits as well as the relationships of each row are clearly delineated.

In the supine position, barium gravitates to the dependent posterior row of sacculations in the middle third. This outlines the TM-TO row in the ascending colon (Fig. 9–5) and the TM-TL row in the transverse colon (Figs. 9–5 and 9–6). At the same time, air tends to outline the border-forming haustral rows.

**Fig. 9–5. Barium enema examination with air contrast.**
Supine projection. The three taeniae and the organization of the haustra into three identifiable rows are clearly shown. TL = taenia libera, TO = taenia omentalis, TM = taenia mesocolica. (From Meyers et al[5])

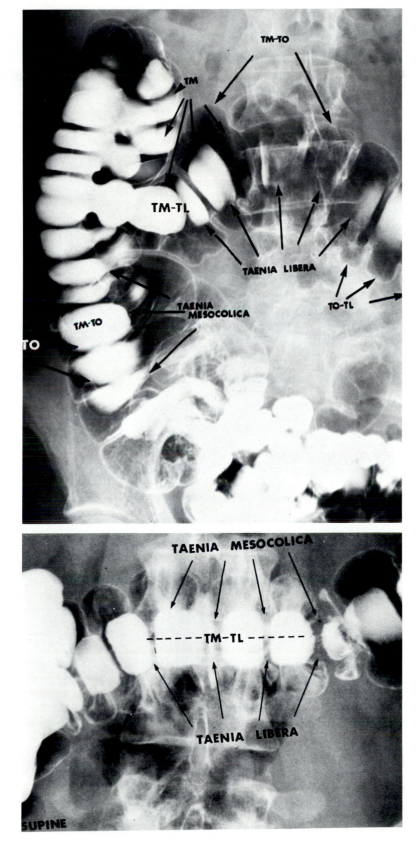

**Fig. 9–6. Barium enema with air contrast.**
In the supine position, barium fills the posterior TM-TL row of haustra in the internal third of the transverse colon, while air outlines the border-forming TM-TO row superiorly and the TO-TL row inferiorly. (From Meyers et al[5])

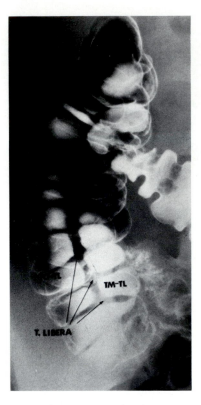

**Fig. 9–7. Prone projection.**
The TO-TL and TM-TL rows in the ascending colon are delineated by the indentation of the taenia libera. (From Meyers et al[5])

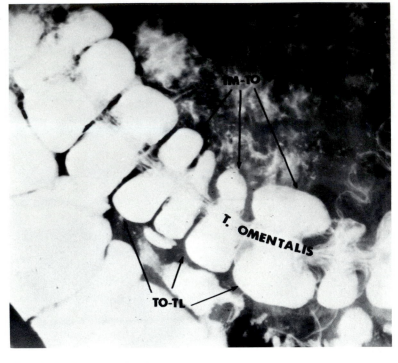

**Fig. 9–8. Prone projection.**
The TM-TO and TO-TL rows in the transverse colon are delineated by the taenia omentalis. (From Meyers et al[5])

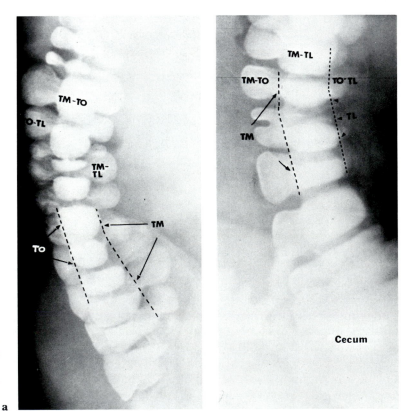

**Fig. 9–9. Ascending colon.**
(a) Supine.
(b) Left lateral. Note that the three rows of haustra can be identified clearly in the lateral view. Multiple projections afford clearer visualization of their complete contour. (From Meyers et al[5])

a

b

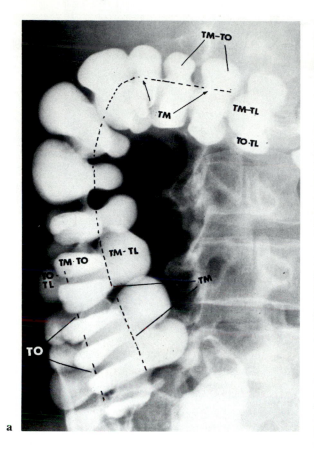

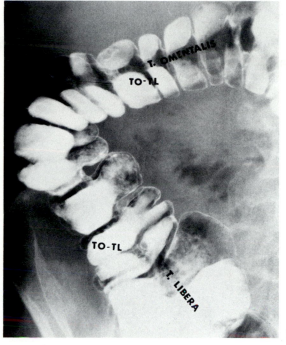

**Fig. 9–10. The altered relationships of the taeniae and the haustral rows** around the hepatic flexure are demonstrated.
**(a)** Prone.
**(b)** Left posterior oblique projection.
(From Meyers et al[5])

In the prone position, the more ventral haustral groups are visualized more clearly. These include the TO-TL and TM-TL haustra of the ascending colon (Fig. 9–7) and the TO-TL and TM-TO haustra of the transverse colon (Fig. 9–8). Demarcation is provided by their shared taenia.

Precise correlation of the relative position of the haustral rows is further provided in lateral projections (Fig. 9–9).

The haustra are almost invariably demarcated clearly in the ascending and transverse colon, and less often in the descending colon. The size of the haustra in each row is roughly equal, except in the lower descending colon. Here the TO and TL broaden and quickly approximate each other, reducing their intervening lateral haustral row. Sigmoid loops only rarely demonstrate haustral delineation. Because of their shape and the effects of gravity, the entire contour of a haustrum is not visualized in a single view. Yet, with the multiple views conventionally employed in a barium-contrast study, the complete contours of all of the haustral rows are usually seen. Decubitus and optimally obliqued or lateral projections adequately complement frontal views.

The appearance of the altered relations of the rows of haustra as they continue around the hepatic flexure from the ascending colon to the transverse colon is best appreciated on oblique projections (Fig. 9–10). It can then be noted that the TM, for example, curves around the flexure from a posteromedial position on the ascending colon to assume a posterosuperior course on the transverse colon. Similarly, because of the rotation at the flexure, the other taeniae alter their course. In this way, continuity of the rows of haustra themselves can be traced.

Even with contractions of portions of the colon, the haustral rows may still be identified (Fig. 9–11). In a mass peristaltic movement, the wave of contraction may involve only one haustral row (Fig. 9–12). This may simulate a filling defect unless the haustral relationships are recognized.

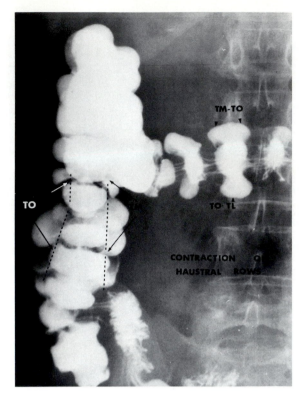

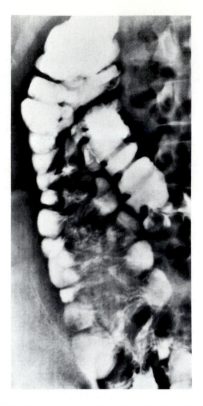

**Fig. 9–11. Contraction of haustra.**
Each row remains identifiable. Note that in the transverse colon the rows are aligned transiently. (From Meyers et al[5])

**Fig. 9–12. Mass contraction limited to the TM-TO haustral row** of the ascending colon mimics a filling defect due to a lesion.

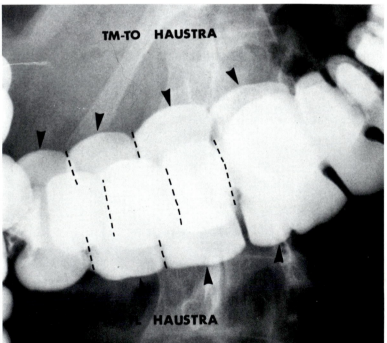

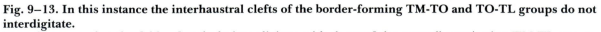

**Fig. 9–13. In this instance the interhaustral clefts of the border-forming TM-TO and TO-TL groups do not interdigitate.**
Note, however, that the folds of each do interdigitate with those of the centrally projecting TM-TL group. (From Meyers et al[5])

Classically, interdigitation of haustral folds has been considered a plain-film landmark for the identification of the large intestine and particularly in the differentiation from gas-distended small bowel loops. However, reliance on this feature, without an understanding of the haustral anatomy, may be misleading. While it is true that the folds between two adjacent rows of haustra often interdigitate, it must be recognized that each row of sacculations may contract independently of the other two. In this way, the third row of haustra may not be appreciated on a single projection, either because it is in a state of contraction or obscured by superimposed shadows or densities (Figs. 9–13 and 9–14). The haustral folds visualized at the contours of the colon may then project in the same plane, rather than in an interdigitating manner, and be mistaken for the semicircular folds of a distended small bowel loop.

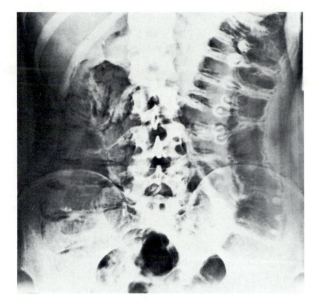

**Fig. 9–14. This example of pneumatosis coli with gas within the interhaustral septae illustrates clearly that the clefts on the two opposing walls do not interdigitate.**

## Abnormal Radiologic Features

Specific haustral rows of the colon may be involved by a variety of intraabdominal lesions. Characteristic groups of sacculations are affected by mesenteric pathways of extension of disease to the colon, extrinsic compression by organomegaly and masses, a spectrum of intra- and extraperitoneal processes, and intrinsic colonic diseases. Radiologic identification of pathologic alterations involving predominantly one haustral row allows precise localization and diagnosis.[6]

### *Lesions Within the Gastrocolic Ligament*

Figure 9–15 shows that processes extending along or arising within the gastrocolic ligament may be clearly identified by their specific effect on the transverse colon. Anatomic dissections have shown that the point of attachment of the gastrocolic ligament is actually within a couple of centimeters cephalad to the taenia omentalis. Injection experiments consistently demonstrate that the mesenteric plane of extension is preferentially upward along the TM-TO haustral row.[6] This constitutes the superior border of the transverse colon.

Selective involvement of this row of sacculations may thus reveal extension of a carcinoma of the stomach along the gastrocolic ligament (Figs. 9–16 and 9–17). With even greater mural invasion and consequent fixation, the haustral pattern of the uninvolved TO-TL row on the inferior contour of the transverse colon is often thrown into a pseudosaccular appearance (Fig. 9–16).

The pseudosacculations of the haustral row opposite to that primarily involved by fixation are basically a functional phenomenon. They are largely a consequence of disordered peristaltic contractions and thus change in size, shape, and axis. In contrast, the pseudosacculations of scleroderma of the colon are constant structures brought about by atrophy of the muscle and collagenous replacement. Characteristically, they have wide mouths, contain fecaliths, and fail to contract on postevacuation studies. They are most consistently seen arising from the TO-TL haustra of the transverse colon (Fig. 9–18).

Lesions originating within the gastrocolic ligament may produce similar changes of the TM-TO haustra, but characteristically, they are either more localized or lack the tethering of

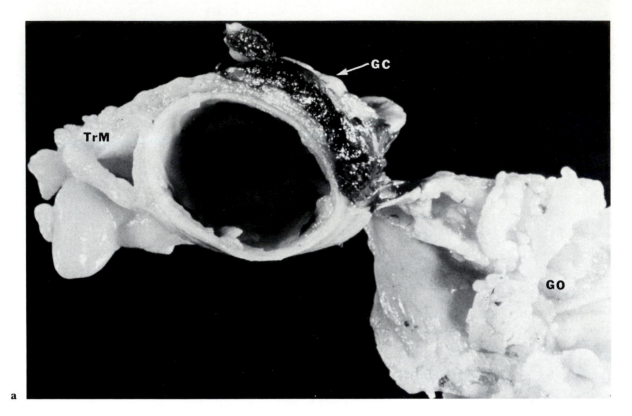

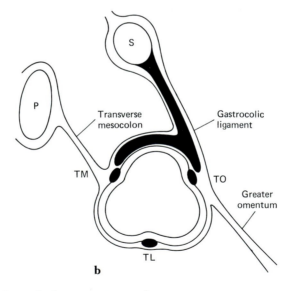

**Fig. 9–15. Sagittal section through the transverse colon.**
Specimen shows that injection of contrast material into the gastrocolic ligament spreads preferentially to the superior TM-TO haustral row. GC = gastrocolic ligament, GO = greater omentum, TrM = transverse mesocolon, S = stomach, P = pancreas. (From Meyers et al[6])

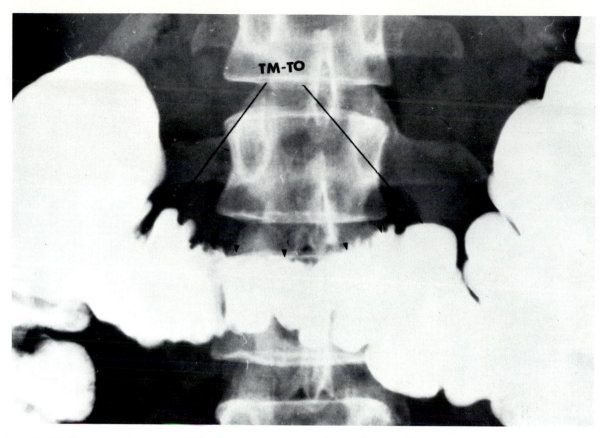

**Fig. 9–16. Extensive invasion of the TM-TO row** (arrowheads) **by gastric carcinoma spreading down the gastrocolic ligament.**
The fixation results in pseudosaccular haustral outpouchings from the uninvolved TO-TL row on the inferior border. (From Meyers et al[6])

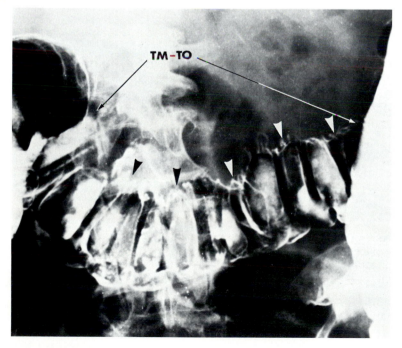

**Fig. 9–17. Carcinoma of the stomach extending down the gastrocolic ligament** involves the TM-TO haustral row on the superior contour of the transverse colon (arrowheads). The TM-TL and TO-TL rows are not affected. (From Meyers et al[6])

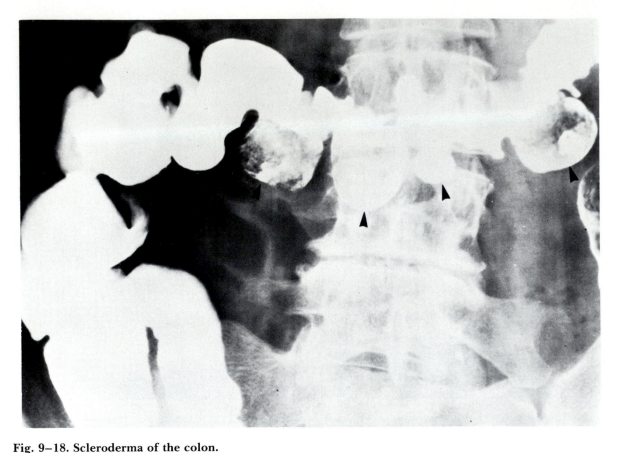

**Fig. 9–18. Scleroderma of the colon.**
Fecalith-containing pseudosacculations (arrowheads) arise characteristically from the TO-TL haustral row.
(From Meyers et al[6])

mucosal folds. Figure 9–19 illustrates localized changes involving only three haustra of the TM-TO row secondary to an actinomycotic abscess within the gastrocolic ligament. If a mass within the ligament bulges anteriorly, it may characteristically extend to depress the TO-TL haustral row as well (Fig. 9–20).

Not all instances of extrinsic involvement of the TM-TO row reflect a lesion within the gastrocolic ligament. The normal gallbladder may locally indent the superior border of this row in the hepatic flexure. Conspicuous depression, however, indicates enlargement of the gallbladder as may be seen in hydrops, empyema, or a Courvoisier condition (Fig. 9–21). Figure 9–22 illustrates the value of haustral analysis in the diagnosis of choledochal cyst.

## Lesions Within the Transverse Mesocolon

Anatomic dissections and injection experiments have documented that the mesenteric plane of the transverse mesocolon extends preferentially downward along the TM-TL haustra toward the TO-TL row[6] (Fig. 9–23). This constitutes the inferior border of the transverse colon.

Pancreatic lesions, by extending along the leaves of the transverse mesocolon, may then be revealed by their characteristic effects on the inferior haustral row. In severe pancreatitis, extravasated enzymes typically flatten the lower contours of the TO-TL row (Fig. 9–24). The enzymes may spread along the limits of the transverse mesocolon toward the left, so that the effects on the colon may end specifically at the level of the phrenicocolic ligament. The haustral pattern of the uninvolved TM-TO row on

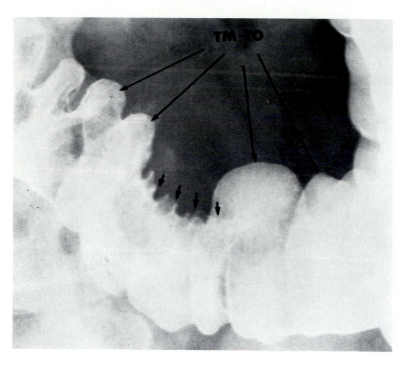

**Fig. 9–19. Localized abscess in the gastrocolic ligament** results in effacement, depression, and mucosal irregularities of TM-TO haustra (arrows) in the transverse colon. (From Meyers et al[6])

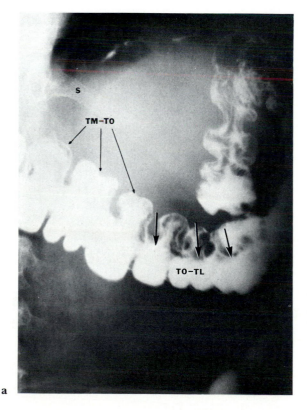

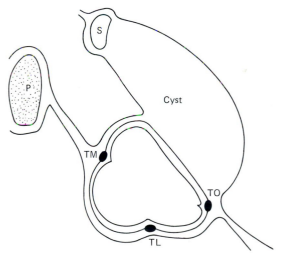

**Fig. 9–20. Hemorrhagic cyst of the gastrocolic ligament.**
(a) Mass in the region of the gastrocolic ligament bulges anteriorly into the greater peritoneal cavity. It elevates the stomach (S), compresses the TM-TO row from in front, and depresses the superior contour of the TO-TL row (arrows).
(b) Haustral changes. S = stomach, P = pancreas.

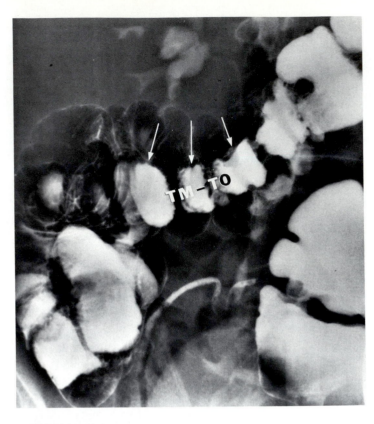

Double contrast barium enema. Prone film demonstrates extrinsic mass compression on the superior borders of the TM-TO haustral row of the hepatic flexure.

**Fig. 9–22. Choledochal cyst.**
**(a)** Supine radiograph, oral cholecystogram. There is nonopacification of the gallbladder. Residual Telepaque outlines unaffected TM-TL haustra (arrows). However, the TM-TO row shows a double convex depression (arrowheads). (From Meyers et al[6])
**(b)** At surgery, an enlarged gallbladder containing stones accounted for the lateral depression. The T-tube study shows that a choledochal cyst accounts for the medial depression of the TM-TO row.

▽

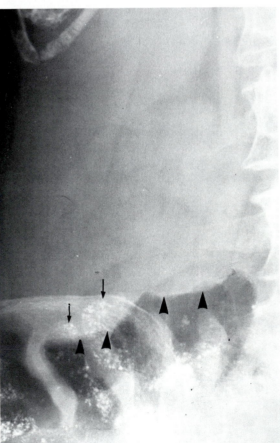

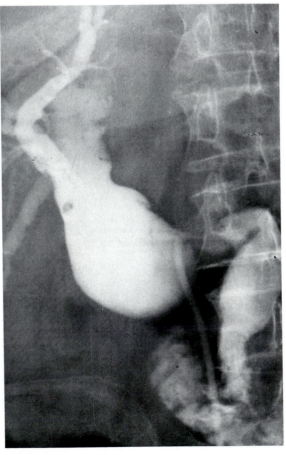

a

b

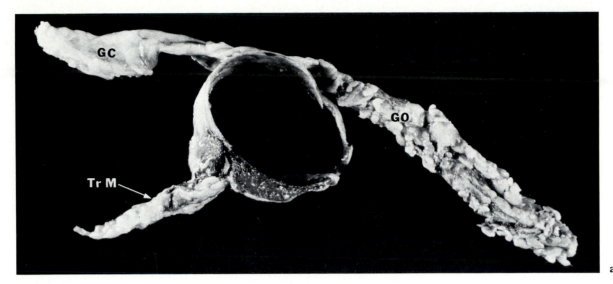

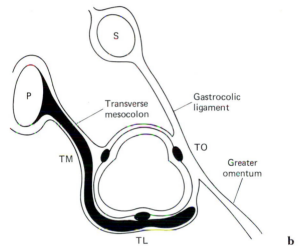

**Fig. 9–23. Sagittal section through transverse colon.**
Specimen shows that contrast material injected into the transverse mesocolon spreads preferentially down-ward along the TM-TL haustra toward the TO-TL row. TrM = transverse mesocolon, GC = gastrocolic ligament, GO = greater omentum, S = stomach, P = pancreas. (From Meyers et al[6])

the superior contour of the transverse colon is often thrown into a pseudosaccular appearance.

In a similar manner, direct extension of carcinoma of the pancreas to the transverse colon along the mesocolon characteristically involves the TO-TL row first or predominantly (Fig. 9–25).

## Distinction Between Intra- and Extraperitoneal Processes

Figure 9–26 illustrates that in the ascending or descending colon, two of the haustral rows face intraperitoneal structures. The TO-TL sacculations are in relation to the lateral paracolic gutter and the TM-TL row to the medial paracolic sulcus and the small bowel loops. Intraperitoneal processes in these areas, then, produce predominant changes on these haustra. In contrast, the posterior TM-TO row is unique in bearing relationship only to extraperitoneal processes, which are often clinically occult and radiologically confusing. Changes limited to this haustral row thus clearly indicate the site of the abnormality as extraperitoneal in nature.

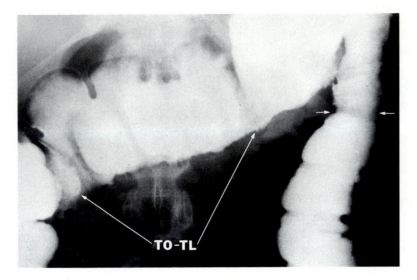

**Fig. 9–24. Traumatic pancreatitis.**
The extravasated enzymes have spread along the transverse mesocolon to involve the TO-TL row on the inferior contour with irregular flattening and rigidity. The process ends laterally at the level of the phrenicocolic ligament (arrows). The fixation results in pseudosaccular haustral outpouchings from the uninvolved TM-TO row on the superior border. (From Meyers et al[6])

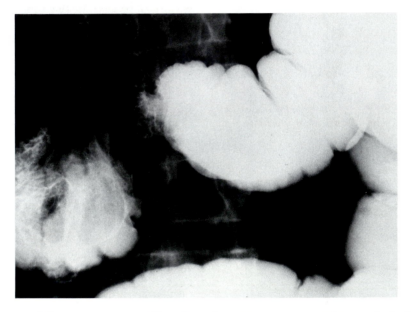

**Fig. 9–25. Carcinoma of the pancreas extending along the transverse mesocolon** results in fixation and mass along the inferior border of the transverse colon.

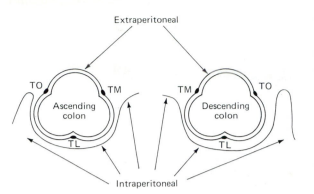

**Fig. 9–26. Intraperitoneal and extraperitoneal relationships.**
In the ascending and descending colon, the TO-TL and TM-TL rows bear intraperitoneal relationships and the TM-TO haustra face extraperitoneal structures. (From Meyers et al[6])

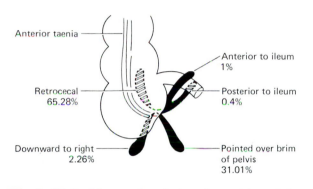

**Fig. 9–27. Incidence of variations in position of the appendix,** as determined by Wakely.[10]

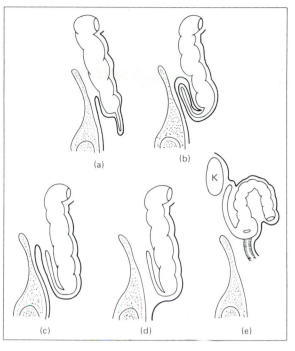

**Fig. 9–28. Normal variations in the position and peritoneal fixation of the appendix.**
**(a)** Intraperitoneal, pointing over the brim of the pelvis.
**(b)** Intraperitoneal, ascending retrocecal.
**(c)** Extraperitoneal, ascending retrocecal. A paracecal fossa is present.
**(d)** Extraperitoneal, ascending retrocecal.
**(e)** Extraperitoneal, ascending retrocecal, lying anterior to the right kidney (K) deep to the liver, associated with an undescended subhepatic cecum. The terminal ileum, also extraperitoneal, enters the cecum from behind.
(From Meyers and Oliphant[8])

## Ascending Retrocecal Appendicitis

These observations have been most useful in the diagnosis of ascending retrocecal appendicitis.[8] An ascending retrocecal position of the appendix is surprisingly common; its incidence ranges from 26% in surgical cases[9] to 65% in an autopsy series[10] (Fig. 9–27). In this position the appendix may be intraperitoneal or extraperitoneal (Fig. 9–28).

Many complications of appendicitis are related to anatomic variations in the position of the appendix, reflected clinically in the problem of differential diagnosis of acute appendiceal disease and lesions of the gallbladder, liver, right kidney, and base of the right lung or pleura. The radiologic features, however, constitute a characteristic pattern that permits precise localization and diagnosis. Inflammation as-

sociated with an intraperitoneal ascending retrocecal appendix occurs in the right paracolic gutter and involves the lateral (TO-TL) haustral row of the ascending colon (Fig. 9–29). In contrast, inflammation associated with an extraperitoneal ascending retrocecal appendix affects primarily the posterior (TM-TO) haustral row (Figs. 9–30 through 9–33). Computed tomography may readily demonstrate the extraperitoneal inflammatory collection and its effect upon the colon[1,11] (Fig. 9–34). The appendix itself may show definite abnormalities, including mass displacement (Fig. 9–29), sinus tracts (Fig. 9–32), and opacification of the abscess cavity.

If the appendix is not visible, its location can still be confidently inferred by the position of the ileocecal valve, due to the embryologic de-

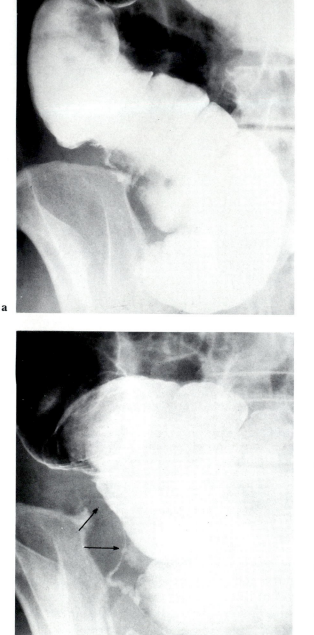

a

b

**Fig. 9–29. Intraperitoneal ascending retrocecal appendicitis.**
(a) Frontal view shows mass displacement and nodular deformity of the lateral contour of the proximal ascending colon.
(b) Oblique view reveals gentle arcuate mass displacement of an ascending retrocecal appendix (arrows). The posterior wall of the proximal ascending colon is grossly intact.
(From Meyers and Oliphant[8])

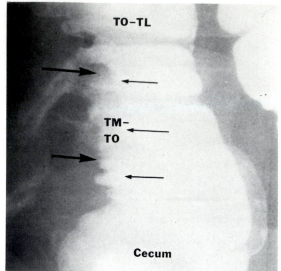

**Fig. 9–30. Extraperitoneal appendicitis.**
Lateral view. The extraperitoneal nature of the inflammatory process associated with an ascending retrocecal appendix is revealed by the predominant involvement of the TM-TO row (large arrows). The posterior border of the TO-TL row is relatively unaffected (small arrows).
(From Meyers et al[6])

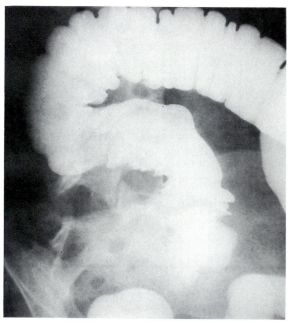

**Fig. 9–31. Extraperitoneal appendicitis.**
Oblique view of barium enema study demonstrates anterior and medial displacement of the cecum and proximal ascending colon by a large abscess secondary to a perforated retrocecal appendix. The appendix is not opacified but note the position of the ileocecal valve.

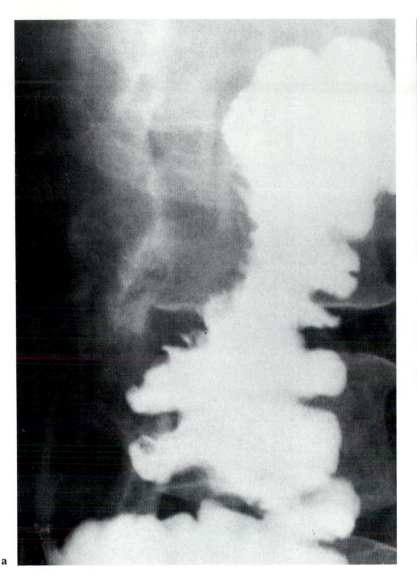

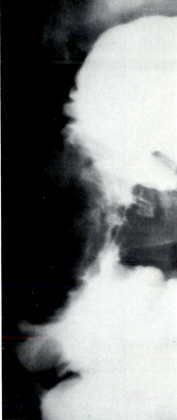

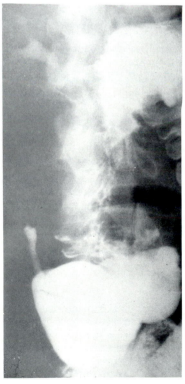

**Fig. 9–32. Extraperitoneal appendicitis.**
(a) A prominent fixed irregular mass involves the posterolateral contour of the ascending colon, accompanied by some deformity of the opposing haustra.
(b and c) Associated inflammatory findings are suggested by the frequent spastic changes, producing further narrowing of the lumen over varying lengths. Minute sinus tracts extend from the tip of an ascending retrocecal appendix.
(From Meyers and Oliphant[8])

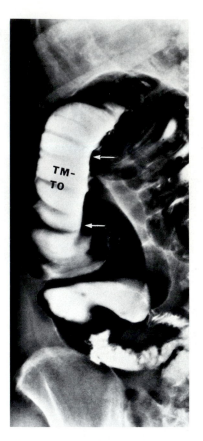

**Fig. 9–33. Extraperitoneal appendicitis.**
Supine study demonstrates extrinsic flattening of the medial border of the TM-TO haustral row of the ascending colon (arrows). This change localizes the primary process to the extraperitoneal space. There is reflux into the terminal ileum but no opacification of the appendix.

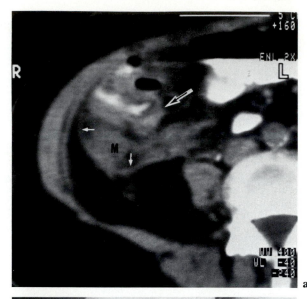

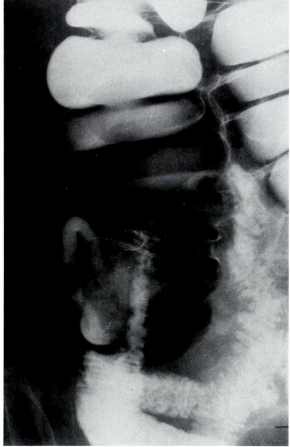

▷

**Figure 9–34. Extraperitoneal appendicitis.**
(a) CT demonstrates an inflammatory mass (M) in the right anterior pararenal space below the level of the kidney. The ascending colon, filled with oral contrast medium, shows irregular bowel-wall thickening posteriorly due to inflammatory edema (large arrow).

There is associated thickening of the lateroconal and anterior renal fasciae (small arrows).
(b) A barium enema study performed two years earlier demonstrates a retrocecal position of the appendix. (Courtesy of Michiel Feldberg, M.D., Utrecht, The Netherlands.)

**Fig. 9–35. Extraperitoneal hematoma.**
**(a)** The descending colon is medially displaced, but significantly, there is no pressure effect on its lateral TO-TL row.
**(b)** Oblique view shows some anterior displacement but with definite straightening of the contours of the posterior TM-TO row (arrows) by the mass. This finding localizes the mass to the extraperitoneal space and distinguishes it from an intraperitoneal fluid mass occupying the lateral paracolic gutter.
(From Meyers et al[6])

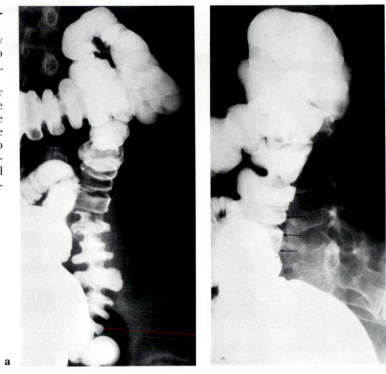

a                                            b

velopment of rotation and fixation.[8] If the appendix is intraperitoneal and points inferiorly toward the pelvis, the ileum enters the cecum from the medial aspect so that the customary position of the ileocecal valve is on the medial wall. However, with an ascending retrocecal appendix, the ileum enters from behind so that the ileocecal valve may be seen on the posterior wall.

## Abdominal Trauma

In cases of abdominal trauma with medial displacement of the ascending or descending colon, identification of the haustral row primarily affected may be the key in the differential diagnosis between intra- and extraperitoneal bleeding. Intraperitoneal fluid in the lateral paracolic gutter tends to compress the TO-TL row. In contrast, extraperitoneal blood in relationship to the colon flattens particularly the TM-TO haustral row (Fig. 9–35).

## Malignant Seeding

Malignant intraperitoneal seeding, following the pathways of flow of ascitic fluid as described in Chapter 3, tends to localize to the TO-TL row

of the ascending colon. Embolic metastases, in accord with the intramural arterial distribution, also tend to develop in the antimesenteric row of haustra.

## Duplication of the Colon

Duplications of the colon have a well-developed smooth muscle layer, are lined by colonic mucosa, and are adherent to and often communicate with the large intestine.[12] They typically displace the colon along the mesenteric border and thus lie in relationship to the TM-TL haustral row of the ascending or descending colon and the TM-TO row of the transverse colon (Figs. 9–36 and 9–37). Because the two colons share a common blood supply and in most cases there is only a single mesentery, resection of the supernumerary colon or microcolon is usually impossible.[13,14]

## *Diverticulosis and Diverticulitis*

Colonic diverticula do not arise randomly from the circumference of the large intestine but tend to originate in four distinct rows (Fig. 9–38): (a) on either side of the TM and (b) near the mes-

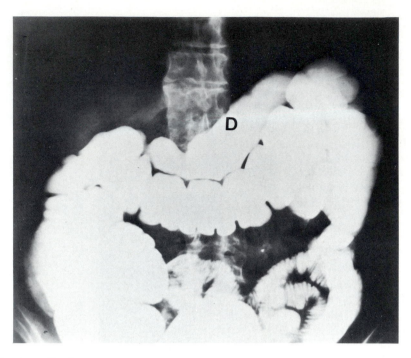

**Fig. 9–36. Duplication of colon.**
Barium enema study demonstrates a tubular communicating duplication (D) within the mesentery of the transverse colon. Its lower border conforms to the superior haustral row of the transverse colon.

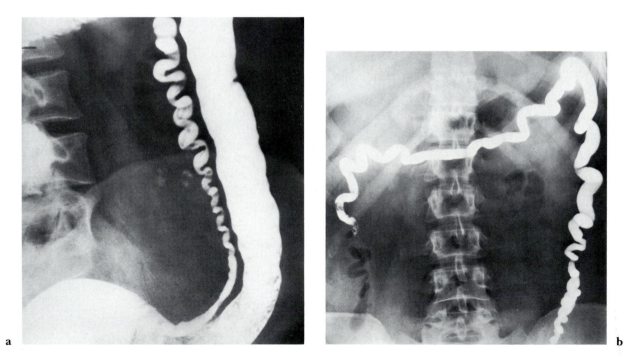

a

b

**Fig. 9–37. Duplication of colon.**
(a) Barium enema study demonstrates a narrow tortuous duplication in the mesentery of the descending colon.
(b) Following selective opacification of the duplication, the "microcolon" is outlined throughout the mesenteric border of the large intestine, ending blindly at the level of the cecum. (From Beyer et al[13])

**Fig. 9–38. Sites of origin of colonic diverticula.**
Note that the antimesenteric TO-TL haustral row does not give rise to diverticula. (From Meyers et al[6])

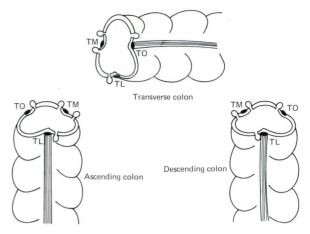

enteric borders of the TO and TL.[6,15] These are related to the points of intramural penetration through connective tissue septa of the colonic wall.[15] Their sites of origin from the TM-TL and TM-TO haustra can be identified clearly on routine radiographic studies (Fig. 9–39).

Bona fide diverticula do not arise from the TO-TL antimesenteric row of sacculations. At surgery or autopsy, only pinhead protrusions may be noted occasionally in association with this row, but they are not identifiable on contrast studies, and no clinical significance has been attributed to them. On frontal and even oblique views, diverticula may project laterally from the lower descending and sigmoid colon. This appearance is related to the fact that the TO and TL anatomically approach each other in this region, reducing the dimensions of their intervening haustra. Lateral views, however, consistently show that these diverticula actually arise from the posterior wall (TM-TO).

## Colonic Diverticular Angioarchitecture and Hemorrhage

Colonic diverticulosis increases in incidence with each decade of adult life and occurs in as high as 35–50% of individuals over 60 years of age.[16] Diverticula of the large intestine constitute a common source of lower gastrointestinal bleeding, both occult and massive, and are a particularly common cause of right-sided colonic hemorrhage.[15,17,18] Colonic diverticulosis is the most frequent cause of severe rectal bleeding.[19] The hemorrhage is typically acute, massive, and life threatening, in contrast to the mild and often intermittent bleeding secondary to diverticulitis, which apparently originates from highly vascularized granulation tissue lining inflamed diverticula.[20]

*Angioarchitecture and Pathogenesis of Bleeding.* Meyers et al have defined the characteristic an-

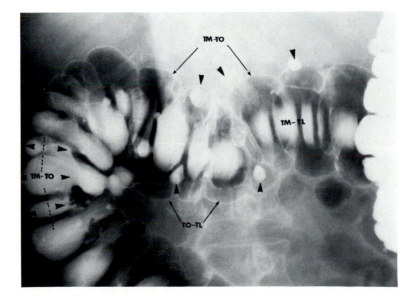

**Fig. 9–39. Diverticula** (arrowheads) arise from the TM-TO and TM-TL rows but none originates from the antimesenteric TO-TL haustra. (From Meyers et al[6])

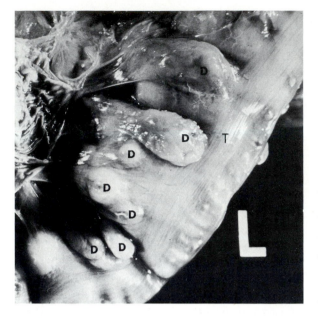

**Fig. 9–40. Photograph of descending colon showing multiple diverticula** (D) **arising in a row adjacent to a taenia** (T). (From Meyers et al[15])

gioarchitecture of colonic diverticula[15] and shown their structural predisposition to massive bleeding.[21,22] The four distinct longitudinal rows from which diverticula arise (Fig. 9–40) correspond closely with the four sites of penetration of the major branches of the vasa recta, the colonic branches of the marginal artery (Fig. 9–41).

Injection studies have shown that a prominent long vasa recta courses in an intimate subserosal position over the dome of every colonic diverticulum (Figs. 9–42 and 9–43a) to reappear as either a single or multiple submucosal branches along the antimesenteric side of its orifice (Fig. 9–43b). Rather than the point of vascular penetration directly leading to a weakness (locus minoris resistentiae) in the bowel wall predisposing to the formation of diverticula,[23] we have shown that it is the obliquely oriented connective-tissue septa separating the circular smooth muscle bundles of the colonic walls that constitute the common plane of least resistance.

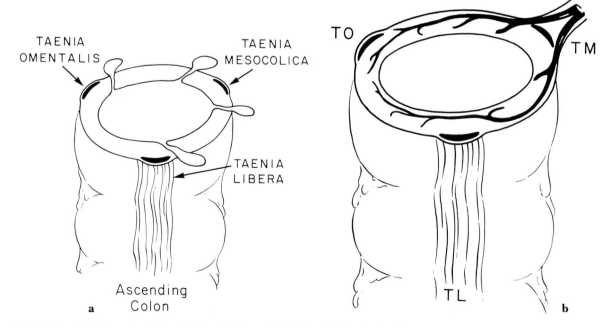

**Fig. 9–41. (a) Sites of origin of colonic diverticula in relation to taenia.**
Diverticula point toward mesenteric border.
**(b) Intramural blood supply of colon.**
Vasa recta reach bowel wall and divide into long subserosal branches which then penetrate obliquely through bowel wall. Short branches penetrate near the taenia mesocolica (TM). They continue in submucosa, finally ramifying into rich plexus.
(From Meyers et al[21])

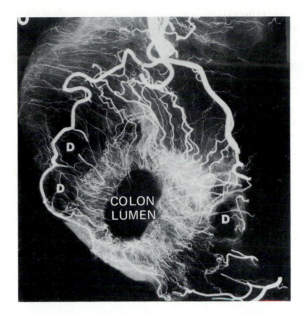

**Fig. 9–42. Radiograph of sigmoid colon with injected arterial supply.**
The circumferential branches of the vasa recta are deflected immediately over the domes of diverticula (D), and short branches of these are displaced around their necks. (From Meyers et al[15])

It is clearly through these septa that both the vasa recta consistently penetrate the colonic wall from the serosa to the submucosa (Fig. 9–44) and the diverticula form from mucosal protrusions.[15] Segmentation of the colon produced by muscular contraction leads to localized increased intraluminal pressure which results in herniation of mucosa and submucosa through these natural weaknesses in the colonic wall.[24,25]

These anatomic relationships result in a remarkably constant angioarchitecture of colonic diverticula (Figs. 9–45 and 9–46). An artery of considerable relative size, the vas rectum, intimately courses in the serosa over the dome of the diverticulum; at this point, it is separated from the lumen of the diverticulum by only mucosa and a few strands of attenuated muscle fibers. The vas rectum then penetrates the colonic wall along the antimesenteric margin of the diverticulum, lying close to its neck and orifice.

The pathogenesis of massively bleeding diverticulosis is primarily determined by their distinctive angioarchitecture.[21,22] Histologic changes at the precise site of bleeding show asymmetric rupture of the vas rectum toward the lumen of the diverticulum precisely at its dome or antimesenteric margin. The changes are associated with conspicuous eccentric intimal thickening of the vas rectum, often with medial thinning and duplication of the internal elastic lamina (Figs. 9–47 through 9–49). The mechanism involves injurious factors arising within the diverticular or colonic lumen which induce eccentric intimal proliferation and weakening of the associated vasa recta, predisposing to rupture and massive bleeding (Fig. 9–50). It is important to recognize that smooth muscle cells of the media develop the intimal layer, so that intimal proliferation results in attenuation and weakening of the muscular component of the vas rectum. This explains why rectal hemorrhage, rather than intra- or extraperitoneal bleeding, is a consequence of this condition.

The predominance of hemorrhage from right-sided diverticula is noteworthy since the majority of diverticula are located in the descending and sigmoid colon, and only about one-third of patients with diverticulosis have diffuse involvement of the large intestine. One anatomic feature distinguishes right-sided from left-sided diverticula, which may explain their increased frequency of bleeding. Because the diverticula arising in the right colon have wider necks and domes, their vasa recta are exposed over a greater length to injurious factors arising from the colon.[21,22]

*Arteriographic Diagnosis and Management.* In the diagnosis and management of massive diverticular hemorrhage, the primary problem is accurate localization of the bleeding point. Selective arteriography may readily accomplish this, allowing a trial of nonoperative control of hemorrhage by infusion of vasopressin, permitting more specific and limited colonic resection when bleeding is uncontrolled or recurrent.[18,26,27] Extravasation is shown in virtually all cases of acutely bleeding diverticula[17,18] as a circular accumulation of the contrast medium within the confines of the diverticulum (Fig. 9–51) which, in the presence of extremely brisk bleeding, may overflow to opacify the lumen of one or several haustral sacculations. The feeding vas rectum itself can be identified and, at times, its precise point of rupture[15] (Fig. 9–51).

Vasoconstrictive therapy immediately following arteriographic diagnosis and localization

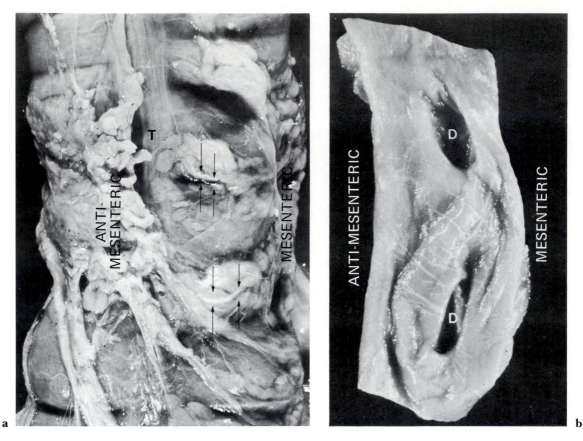

**Fig. 9–43. Gross vascular relationships of colonic diverticula.**
**(a)** Photograph of serosal surface of ascending colon. Prominent injected vasa recta (arrows) course from the mesenteric side on the right over the domes of two diverticula. In penetrating the colonic wall, they disappear from view on the antimesenteric borders of the diverticula, near a taenia (T).
**(b)** Enlarged photograph of the mucosal surface of two diverticula. The branches of the injected vasa recta reappear in the submucosa on the antimesenteric side of the orifices of the diverticula (D).
(From Meyers et al[15])

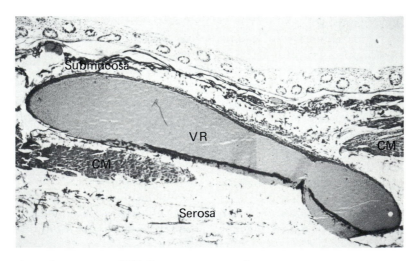

**Fig. 9–44. Penetration of vasa recta** (VR) **from serosa to submucosa.**
Transverse histologic section shows that it occurs through a widened, obliquely oriented connective-tissue cleft between fascicles of circular muscle (CM). (From Meyers et al[15])

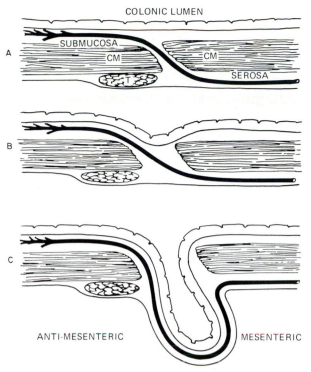

COLONIC LUMEN

SUBMUCOSA

A   CM                    CM

SEROSA

T

B

C

ANTI-MESENTERIC                    MESENTERIC

**Fig. 9–45. Structural dynamics of diverticular formation and vascular relationships.**
**(a)** The vas rectum normally penetrates the colonic wall from the serosa to the submucosa through an obliquely oriented connective-tissue septum in the circular muscle (CM). This occurs near the mesenteric side of a taenia (T).
**(b)** The mucosal protrusion marking the development of a diverticulum occurs through, and consequently widens, the connective-tissue cleft. In doing this, it begins to lift up the artery.
**(c)** With transmural extension of the diverticulum, the vas rectum is displaced over its dome, and therefore penetrates to the submucosa on the antimesenteric border of its neck and orifice.
(Modified from Meyers et al[15])

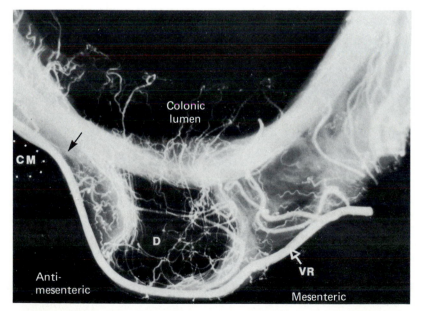

**Fig. 9–46. Characteristic angioarchitecture of colonic diverticula.**
Radiograph of colonic diverticulum with injected vas rectum. The vas rectum (VR) approaches the diverticulum (D) from its mesenteric border, arches in the serosa immediately over its dome, and penetrates the colonic wall on its antimesenteric margin (arrow). CM designates the approximate location of circular muscle. (×8)
(Modified from Meyers et al[15])

413

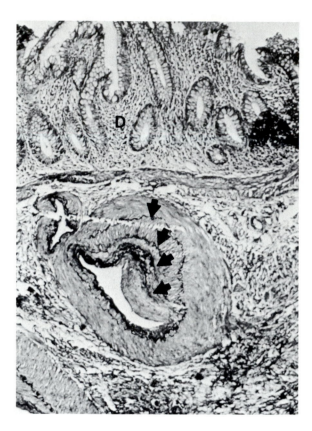

**Fig. 9–47. Eccentric mural changes in vas rectum in case of bleeding diverticulum.**
Vas rectum in area of hemorrhage demonstrates duplication of internal elastic lamina (arrows) with lamellar arrangement and marked eccentric thickening of intima. D = mucosa of diverticulum. (Elastic Van Giesson ×65). (From Meyers et al[22])

provides an effective method which may make operation avoidable.[17,26,27]

Bleeding may recur within hours or days of the initial control,[17,27] but the temporary cessation of bleeding provides time for stabilization of the patient's clinical condition before segmental colectomy. Occasionally, rebleeding has been encountered within several months[17] which may be a consequence of dislodgment of the thrombus which characteristically extends into the lumen of the diverticulum.[15,21,22] Recurrent bleeding from a second distant diverticulum has been documented only rarely.[28]

If vasopressin fails to control diverticular bleeding in a patient who is a poor surgical risk, embolization of the bleeding artery may be carried out,[28] but this incurs the risk of potential

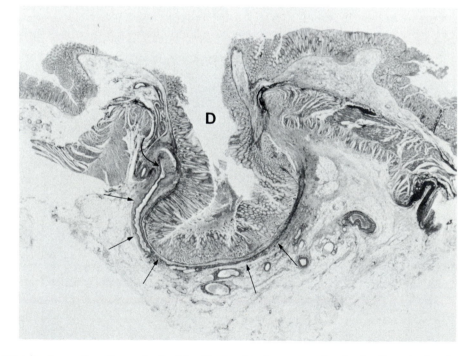

**Fig. 9–48. Histologic section through the bleeding point in a case of colonic diverticular hemorrhage.**
The vas rectum (arrows) courses over the dome of the diverticulum from the right, extends along its antimesenteric margin, and has ruptured (curved arrow) near the neck of the diverticulum. (Elastic Van Giesson ×65). (From Meyers et al[22])

**Fig. 9–49. Histologic section through the bleeding point in a case of colonic diverticular hemorrhage.** A thrombus (T) projects from the lumen of the ruptured vas rectum (VR) through a small mucosal erosion into the lumen of the diverticulum (D). The vas rectum shows marked intimal thickening (arrows) which is visible deep to the darkly stained internal elastic lamina. The thickening is strikingly eccentric toward the lumen of the diverticulum, and the media of the artery is absent in this area. (Elastic Van Giesson ×65). (From Meyers et al[22])

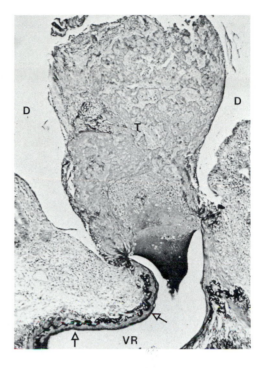

ischemic injury to the colon[29,30] because of the relative lack of collateral blood supply.

## Diverticulitis

The majority of diverticula are related to extraperitoneal tissues (Fig. 9–38). Diverticulitis may thus result in a localized inflammatory process involving only the TM-TL or TM-TO haustra (Fig. 9–52). Mesenteric abscesses and extraperitoneal gas or abscesses are well-recognized complications of diverticulitis.[31] Many cases of intestinovesical fistulas are secondary to extraperitoneal extension of an inflammatory or suppurative process from the diverticulum and then perforation through the base of the urinary bladder. Furthermore, the absence of diverticular origin from the lateral haustral rows facing the intraperitoneal lateral paracolic gutters provides an explanation for the low incidence of subhepatic and subphrenic abscesses secondary to diverticulitis. Thus, localized involvement of the TO-TL haustra alone can not be secondary to diverticulitis. Inflammatory re-

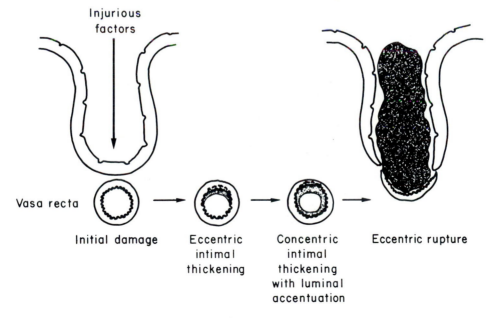

**Fig. 9–50. Pathogenesis of colonic diverticular hemorrhage.**
Progressive eccentric changes weaken the wall of the vas rectum, which finally ruptures into the lumen of the diverticulum. (From Meyers et al[22])

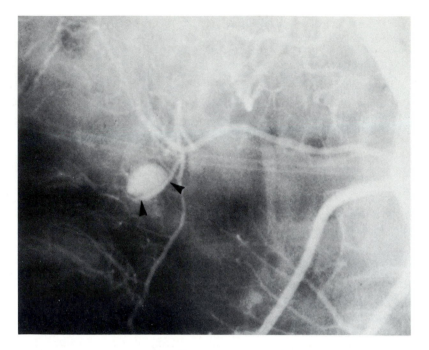

**Fig. 9–51. Extravasation into an acutely bleeding right colon diverticulum shown by selective superior mesenteric arteriography.**
A vas rectum (arrowheads) courses typically over the dome of the diverticulum and appears intact in this segment, indicating its point of arterial rupture to be on the antimesenteric margin of the diverticulum. (From Meyers et al[15])

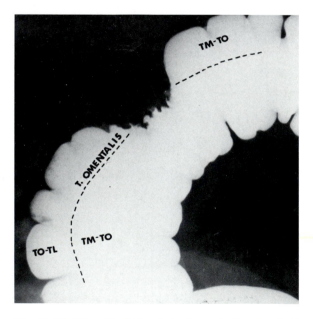

**Fig. 9–52. Diverticulitis** of the hepatic flexure. Left posterior oblique projection. Localized inflammatory changes involve the TM-TO haustra. (From Meyers[6])

action of these haustra consequent to diverticulitis affecting one or both of the mesenteric rows indicates an extensive paracolic abscess.

## Diverticulitis Complicating Granulomatous Colitis

Granulomatous colitis (Crohn's disease of the colon) is not unusual in patients over the age of 50 years and may affect any segment of the colon. The sigmoid colon is involved in 72% of primary Crohn's colitis and in 35% of granulomatous ileocolitis.[32] Diverticulosis is also common in this age group, particularly involving the sigmoid colon. The clinical and radiologic difficulty in distinguishing between segmental granulomatous colitis and diverticulitis has been described.[33,34] Clinically, either may present with pain, partial obstruction, a lower abdominal mass, rectal bleeding, fever, and leukocytosis. Often, however, "the diagnostic problem is not primarily the distinguishing of Crohn's colitis from diverticular disease, but recognizing when the diseases coexist."[35] I have shown, however, that the relationship is not one of chance coex-

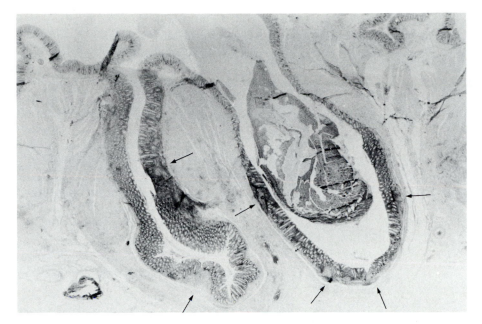

**Fig. 9–53. Diverticular involvement by Crohn's disease.**
Noncaseating granulomas (arrows) involve the mucosa of two sigmoid diverticula. (×8). (From Meyers et al[36])

istence, but rather that the involvement of diverticula by granulomatous colitis causes a 2- to 10-fold increased incidence of diverticulitis.[36]

Granulomatous colitis is characterized by transmural inflammation, mucosal ulceration, and fissuring of the bowel wall, typically accompanied by the presence of a granulomatous tissue response.[37] In contrast, diverticulitis results from a micro- or macroperforation of a diverticulum with sequelae such as deep sigmoiditis, perisigmoiditis (peridiverticulitis), or frank peritonitis.[38]

Because diverticula represent protrusions of mucosa and submucosa into and through the bowel wall, their involvement by Crohn's disease facilitates the transmural extension and paracolic complications of this disease process. The mucosal lining of diverticula may be the site of giant cell granulomas (Fig. 9–53) and aphthous ulcerations overlying lymphoid follicles, which may extend as dissecting intramural tracts (Fig. 9–54) and lead to the formation of pericolic abscesses.

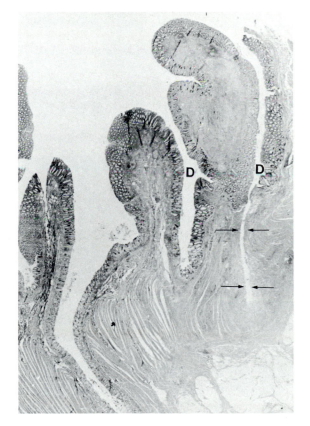

**Fig. 9–54. Diverticular involvement by Crohn's disease.**
Dissecting intramural tract (arrows) extends from ulcerated diverticulum (D). (×18). (From Meyers et al[36])

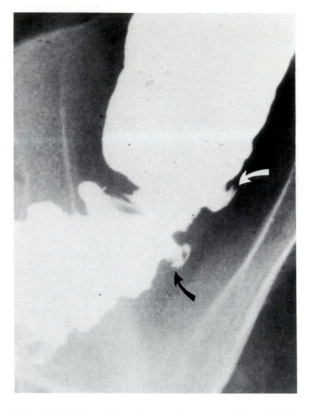

The radiologic signs of peridiverticulitis complicating granulomatous colitis usually show clear evidence of the underlying pathologic changes. These include (1) the presence of aphthous ulcers, superficial ulcerations overlying areas of lymphoid hyperplasia, within diverticula which may indicate a predisposition to their rupture (Fig. 9–55); (2) localized diverticular perforation, perhaps with multiple communications (Figs. 9–56 and 9–57); and (3) mass pressure on the sigmoid colon from the paracolic abscess. Any extraluminal longitudinal sinus tract is thus almost invariably on the mesenteric border of the colon (Fig. 9–58).

Based on these histologic and radiologic observations, the pathogenic mechanisms of diverticulitis complicating granulomatous colitis are established (Fig. 9–59):

1. The earliest lesion of Crohn's disease is lymphoid hyperplasia followed by superficial ulceration.[39,40] When this type of aphthous ulcer involves the mucosa of a diverticulum, it may undergo infection to result in peridiverticulitis.
2. The deep fissuring characteristic of Crohn's disease may establish communication with one or several diverticula which may then be followed by peridiverticulitis and/or abscess formation.
3. A paracolic abscess secondary to transmural fissuring ulcerations of severe Crohn's disease

**Fig. 9–55. Granulomatous colitis with ulcerated diverticulosis.**
Aphthous ulcerations are present within two diverticula (arrows) adjacent to a localized area of colonic mural induration containing minute mucosal ulcerations. (From Meyers et al[36])

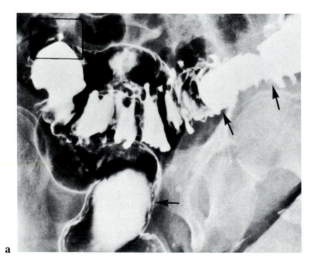
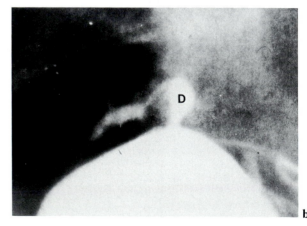

**Fig. 9–56. Diverticulitis complicating granulomatous colitis.**
(a) Crohn's disease is evident by the indentation and ulceration on the left side of the rectum and the gross changes in the proximal sigmoid colon (arrows). Multiple diverticula are present.
(b) Enlargement of boxed area shows 8 × 1-mm sinus tract penetrating from a sigmoid diverticulum (D). (From Meyers et al[36])

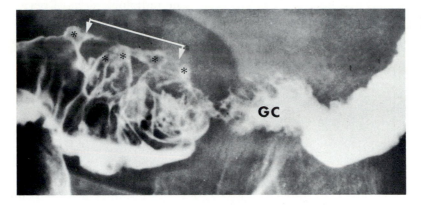

**Fig. 9–57. Diverticulitis complicating granulomatous colitis.**
A 4.5-cm sinus tract (bracket) in the paracolic tissues communicates with five sigmoid diverticula (*). The surrounding abscess produces a mild mass impression on the colon. Proximally, granulomatous colitis is shown by a narrowed lumen and a grossly distorted mucosa with multiple ulcerations (GC). (From Meyers et al[36])

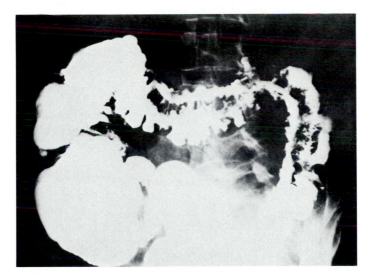

**Fig. 9–58. Granulomatous colitis with extraluminal longitudinal sinus tract.** An extremely long continuous tract follows the mesenteric border of the sigmoid, descending, and transverse colon. It can be presumed that this striking paracolic localization is due to the communicating form of peridiverticulitis as a consequence of involvement by Crohn's disease.
(From Marshak et al[33])

may penetrate through the domes of adjacent diverticula with further dissecting peridiverticulitis.

# Summary

Table 9–1 summarizes the basic features that enable identification of the specific haustral rows and the most common conditions resulting in localized involvement. Application of these principles is particularly helpful in the diagnosis of a variety of disease processes at a stage before gross displacement and distortion of the colon result. These concepts allow the precise localization and often the specific diagnosis of an extracolonic lesion at its earliest stage of extension to the large intestine and permit the radiologist to

**Table 9–1.** Haustral anatomy and pathology.

| | Ascending and descending colon | | | Transverse colon | | |
|---|---|---|---|---|---|---|
| | TM-TO | TO-TL | TM-TL | TM-TO | TO-TL | TM-TL |
| Position | Posterior | Lateral | Medial | Superior | Inferior | Posterior |
| Major relationship | Extraperitoneal structures | Lateral paracolic sulcus | Medial paracolic sulcus | Gastrocolic ligament (stomach, lesser sac) | Greater omentum, anterior abdominal wall | Transverse mesocolon (pancreas) |
| Outlining on double-contrast studies | | | | | | |
| Supine | Barium | Air | Air | Air | Air | Barium |
| Prone | Air | Barium | Barium | Barium | Barium | Air |
| Gross designation | | Antimesenteric border | Mesenteric border | Mesenteric border | Antimesenteric border | |
| Localized or predominant involvement | Primary extraperitoneal lesions | Exudate, malignant seeding in lateral intraperitoneal gutter | Extension from primary small bowel process | Extension of gastric carcinoma | Extension of pancreatic carcinoma and pancreatitis | Extension of pancreatic carcinoma and pancreatitis |
| | Diverticulitis | Embolic metastases | Diverticulitis | Primary masses of gastrocolic ligament | Primary masses of transverse mesocolon | Primary masses of transverse mesocolon |
| | | Never localized diverticulitis; in association with involvement of other haustral rows, indicates an extensive paracolic abscess | | Enlarged gallbladder | Scleroderma | Diverticulitis |
| | | | | Choledochal cyst | Never localized diverticulitis; in association with involvement of other haustral rows, indicates an extensive paracolic abscess | |
| | | | | Diverticulitis | | |

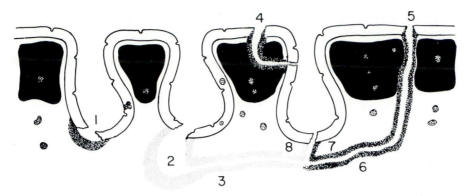

**Fig. 9–59. Pathogenesis of diverticulitis complicating granulomatous colitis.**
An aphthous ulcer involving the mucosal lining of a diverticulum (1) may lead to perforation, with the formation of a peridiverticular abscess (2). This may then extend as a longitudinal paracolic sinus tract (3). A fissuring ulcer of granulomatous colitis may directly perforate into a diverticulum (4). Complete transmural fissuring (5) may result in an abscess, deep to the muscularis propria, which may take the form of a longitudinal sinus tract (6). Perforation of the domes of diverticula with peridiverticulitis may occur secondary to extension from either granulomatous colitis (7) or dissecting diverticulitis (8). (From Meyers et al[36])

further refine the diagnosis of intraabdominal disease.

# References

1. Feldberg MAM, Hendriks MJ, van Waes P: Computed tomography in complicated acute appendicitis. Gastrointest Radiol 10: 289–295, 1985
2. Lineback PE: Studies on the musculature of the human colon with special reference to the taeniae. Am J Anat 36–37: 357–383, 1925–1926
3. Ritchie JA: Movement of segmental constrictions in the human colon. Gut 12: 35–355, 1971
4. Hawkins CF, Hardy TL: On the nature of haustration of the colon. J Fac Radiol 2: 95–98, 1950
5. Meyers MA, Volberg F, Katzen B, et al: Haustral anatomy and pathology: A new look. I. Roentgen identification of normal patterns and relationships. Radiology 108: 497–504, 1973
6. Meyers MA, Volberg F, Katzen B, et al: Haustral anatomy and pathology: A new look. II. Roentgen interpretation of pathologic alterations. Radiology 108: 505–512, 1973
7. Pace JL, Williams I: Organization of the muscular wall of the human colon. Gut 10: 352–359, 1969
8. Meyers MA, Oliphant M: Ascending retrocecal appendicitis. Radiology 110: 295–299, 1974
9. Collins DC: 71,000 human appendix specimens. A final report summarizing forty years' study. Am J Proctol 14: 365–381, 1963
10. Wakely CPG: The position of the vermiform appendix as ascertained by an analysis of 10,000 cases. J Anat 67: 277–283, 1933
11. Balthazar EG, Megibow AJ, Hulnick D, et al: CT of appendicitis. AJR 147: 705–710, 1986
12. Kottra JJ, Dodds WJ: Duplication of the large bowel. AJR 113: 310–315, 1971
13. Beyer D, Friedmann G, Müller J: Duplication of the colon: Report of two cases and review of the literature. Gastrointest Radiol 6: 151–156, 1981
14. Ravitch MM: Hind gut duplication: Doubling of colon and genital urinary tracts. Ann Surg 137: 588–601, 1953
15. Meyers MA, Volberg F, Katzen B, et al: Angioarchitecture of colonic diverticula: Significance in bleeding diverticulosis. Radiology 108: 249–261, 1973
16. Hughes LE: Postmortem survey of diverticular disease of the colon. I. Diverticulosis and diverticulitis. Gut 10: 336–344, 1969
17. Athanasoulis CA, Baum S. Rosch J, et al: Mesenteric arterial infusions of vasopressin for hemorrhage from colonic diverticulosis. Am J Surg 129: 212–216, 1975
18. Casarella WJ, Kanter IE, Seaman WB: Right-sided colonic diverticula as a cause of acute rectal hemorrhage. N Engl J Med 286: 450–453, 1972
19. Noer RJ, Hamilton JE, Williams DJ, et al: Rectal hemorrhage: Moderate and severe. Ann Surg 155: 794–805, 1962
20. Mobley JE, Dockerty MB, Waugh JM: Bleeding in colonic diverticulitis. Am J Surg 94: 44–51, 1957
21. Meyers MA, Alonso DR, Baer JW: Pathogenesis of massively bleeding colonic diverticulosis: New observations. AJR 127: 901–908, 1976
22. Meyers MA, Alonso DR, Gray GF, et al: Pathogenesis of bleeding colonic diverticulosis. Gastroenterology 71: 577–583, 1976

23. Drummond H: Sacculi of the large intestine, with special reference to their relations to the blood vessels of the bowel wall. Br J Surg 4: 407–413, 1916

24. Arfwidsson S, Dock NG: Pathogenesis of multiple diverticula of the sigmoid colon in diverticular disease. Acta Chir Scand (Suppl) 342: 5–68, 1964

25. Painter NS, Truelove SC, Ardran GM, et al: Segmentation and the localization of intraluminal pressures in the human colon, with special reference to the pathogenesis of colonic diverticula. Gastroenterology 49: 169–177, 1965

26. Baum S, Rosch J, Dotter CT, et al: Selective mesenteric arterial infusions in the management of massive diverticular hemorrhage. N Engl J Med 288: 1269–1272, 1973

27. Eisenberg H, Laufer I, Skillman JJ: Arteriographic diagnosis and management of suspected colonic diverticular hemorrhage. Gastroenterology 64: 1091–1100, 1973

28. Goldberger LE, Bookstein JJ: Transcatheter embolization for treatment of diverticular hemorrhage. Radiology 122: 613–617, 1977

29. Mitty HA, Efremidis S, Keller RJ: Colonic stricture after transcatheter embolization for diverticular bleeding. AJR 133: 519–521, 1979

30. Rosenkrantz H, Bookstein JJ, Rosen RJ, et al: Postembolic colonic infarction. Radiology 142: 47–51, 1982

31. Feldberg MAM, Hendricks MJ, van Waes PFGM: Role of CT in diagnosis and management of complications of diverticular disease. Gastrointest Radiol 10: 370–377, 1985

32. Sleisenger MH, Fordtran JS: Gastrointestinal Disease. WB Saunders, Philadelphia, 1973, pp 1353–1354

33. Marshak RH, Lindner AE, Pochaczevsky R, et al: Longitudinal sinus tracts in granulomatous colitis and diverticulitis. Semin Roentgenol 11: 101–110, 1976

34. Schmidt GT, Lennard-Jones JE, Morson BC, et al: Crohn's disease of the colon and its distinction from diverticulitis. Gut 9: 7–16, 1968

35. Johnson WD, Roth JLA: Diagnosis and differential diagnosis of chronic ulcerative colitis and Crohn's colitis. In Inflammatory Bowel Disease. Edited by JB Kirsner, RG Shorter. Lea & Febiger, Philadelphia, 1975

36. Meyers MA, Alonso DR, Morson BC, et al: Pathogenesis of diverticulitis complicating granulomatous colitis. Gastroenterology 74: 24–31, 1978

37. Lockhart-Mummery HE, Morson BC: Crohn's disease of the large intestine. Gut 5: 493–509, 1964

38. Fleischner FG: Diverticular disease of the colon. New observations and revised concepts. Gastroenterology 60: 316–324, 1971

39. McGovern VJ, Goulston SJM: Crohn's disease of the colon. Gut 9: 164–176, 1968

40. Morson BC: The muscle abnormality in diverticular disease of the sigmoid colon. Br J Radiol 36: 385–392, 1963

# 10 Internal Abdominal Hernias

## General Introduction

An internal abdominal hernia is defined as the protrusion of a viscus through a normal or abnormal aperture within the confines of the peritoneal cavity. The hernial orifice may be a preexisting anatomic structure, such as the foramen of Winslow, or a pathologic defect of congenital or acquired origin.

The literature on the subject has been composed principally of case reports, often based on observations made at surgery or autopsy. The role of preoperative radiologic diagnosis of internal hernias has generally not been appreciated. Indeed, in the differential diagnosis of radiographic findings of intestinal obstruction or unusual-appearing grouping of bowel loops,[1-5] "some type of internal hernia" is often loosely entertained without a precise appreciation of types and distinctive findings. However, with an awareness of the underlying anatomic features and of the dynamics of intestinal entrapment, the correct diagnosis of an internal hernia can be made in most instances.

The nomenclature of a specific hernia is determined by the location of the hernial ring and not by the eventual position of the sac or the involved intestinal loops. Internal hernias within the lesser sac, for example, may occur from various directions, namely, through the foramen of Winslow or through defects in the transverse mesocolon or lesser omentum. Based on their anatomic location of origin, internal hernias may be conveniently classified into the following groups:

1. Paraduodenal
2. Foramen of Winslow
3. Pericecal
4. Intersigmoid
5. Transmesenteric and transmesocolic
6. Retroanastomotic

The majority of internal hernias result from congenital anomalies of intestinal rotation and peritoneal attachment.[6-9] Acquired defects of the mesentery or peritoneum secondary to abdominal surgery or trauma may also serve as the hernial ring.[10-13] The retroperitoneal group of internal hernias is more frequently encountered in adults, whereas the transmesenteric types are more commonly present in the pediatric age group.[6,8,14]

The autopsy incidence of internal hernia has been reported to be between 0.2 and 0.9%.[6,15] Many are small and easily reducible, so that they may remain relatively asymptomatic during life.[16,17] In other cases, the patients present with a history of intermittent attacks of vague epigastric discomfort, colicky periumbilical pain, nausea, vomiting—especially after intake of a large meal—and recurrent intestinal obstruction. The discomfort may be altered or relieved by change in position. Internal hernias account for 0.5–3% of all cases of intestinal obstruction,[6,18] with a very high rate of mortality, exceeding 50% in most series.[6,12,19] Delayed diagnosis leads to extensive and often irreparable intestinal damage. Adhesions between the intestinal loops or between the bowel and hernial sac develop, further resulting in obstruction or circulatory compromise.[20]

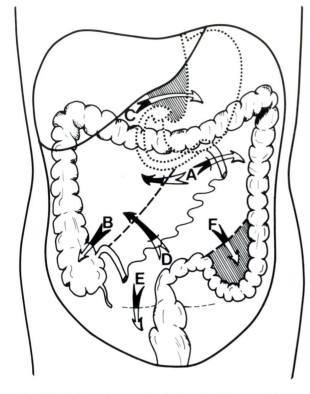

**Fig. 10–1. Location and relative incidence of internal hernias** according to the collective review by Hansmann and Morton[21]: (a) paraduodenal hernias, 53%; (b) pericecal hernias, 13%; (c) foramen of Winslow hernias, 8%; (d) transmesenteric hernias, 8%; (e) hernias into pelvic structures, 7%; (f) transmesosigmoid hernias, 6%. (From Ghahremani and Meyers[16])

Figure 10–1 summarizes the relative incidence of internal hernias at the various susceptible sites. In general, the small bowel examination provides the most useful diagnostic hallmarks, which include (1) abnormal location and disturbed arrangement of the small intestine; (2) sacculation and crowding of several small bowel loops due to encapsulation within the hernial sac (serial radiographs and fluoroscopy with palpation and change in the patient's position may disclose that the loops cannot be separated but rather move *in toto*); and (3) segmental dilatation and prolonged stasis within the herniated loops.

Without a specific radiologic diagnosis a small internal hernia may not be evident at laparotomy for a variety of reasons: the hernia may reduce spontaneously or following inadvertent traction on small bowel loops at the time of surgery; the usual exploratory laparotomy is often inadequate for evaluation of all significant peritoneal fossae and possible mesenteric defects which represent the potential sites of herniation; and the potential space of a peritoneal fossa is generally not evident from the relatively small size of its orifice.[17,20,22]

# Paraduodenal Hernias

Paraduodenal hernias are the most common type of internal abdominal hernias, accounting for over half of reported cases. They are basically congenital in origin, representing entrapment of the small intestine beneath the mesentery of the colon related to embryologic rotation of the midgut and variations in peritoneal fixation and vascular folds.[9,24,25] Nevertheless, repeated encapsulations of intestinal loops can increase the size of the peritoneal defect and result in total or subtotal herniation of the small bowel.[20,22] Seventy-five percent occur on the left side and 25% on the right.[6,17]

## *Anatomic Considerations*

### Left Paraduodenal Hernias

Although nine normal and aberrant paraduodenal folds and fossae have been classically described,[26] there is only one fossa to the left of the duodenum capable of developing into the sac of a hernia, termed the paraduodenal fossa (fossa of Landzert)[27] (Fig. 10–2). This fossa, present in about 2% of autopsy cases,[20] is situated at some distance to the left of the ascending or fourth portion of the duodenum and is caused by the raising up of a peritoneal fold by the inferior mesenteric vein as it runs along the lateral side of the fossa and then above it. Small intestine may herniate through the orifice posteriorly and downward toward the left, lateral to the ascending limb of the duodenum, extending into the descending mesocolon and left portion of the transverse mesocolon. The free edge of the hernia thus contains the inferior mesenteric vein and the ascending left colic artery. Confusion can be minimized if it is understood that

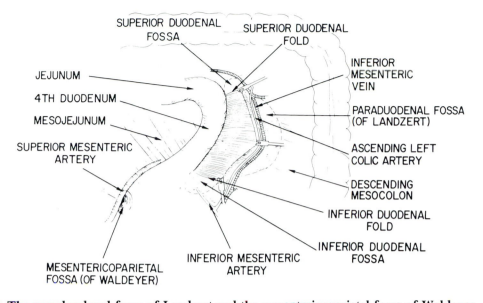

**Fig. 10–2. The paraduodenal fossa of Landzert and the mesentericoparietal fossa of Waldeyer.**
The transverse colon and mesocolon have been elevated and the proximal jejunal loop deflected medially in order to identify the fossae clearly. Behind the fossae lie the parietal peritoneum and retroperitoneal organs. (From Meyers[23])

the hernial orifice is in a paraduodenal location but the herniated loops present at a distance—more clearly, as a hernia into the descending mesocolon[24] (Fig. 10–3).

The hernia may contain only a few loops and be spontaneously reducible. Evaluation during symptom-free intervals is likely to be misleadingly negative. Since the afferent loop enters the sac from behind where the duodenum emerges from its fixed retroperitoneal position, only the efferent loop of the intestine truly passes through the hernial orifice.

## Right Paraduodenal Hernias

The mesentericoparietal fossa (fossa of Waldeyer)[28] is in the first part of the mesentery of the jejunum, immediately behind the superior mesenteric artery and inferior to the transverse duodenum (Figs. 10–2 and 10–4). The fossa's orifice looks to the left, its blind extremity to the right and downward, directly in front of the posterior parietal peritoneum. This fossa is present in 1% of cases.[20] Right paraduodenal hernias most commonly involve the mesentericoparietal fossa (Fig. 10–5), representing an entrapment of the small bowel behind the ascending mesocolon and the right half of the transverse mesocolon, more accurately conceived therefore as hernias into the ascending mesocolon. The superior mesenteric and ileocolic arteries are then in the free edge of the sac.[9,24] Because both afferent and efferent loops pass through the hernial orifice, right paraduodenal hernias are usually more massive and fixed than those occurring on the left side.[16,17]

## Clinical Features

The clinical manifestations of paraduodenal hernias may range from chronic or intermittent mild digestive complaints to acute intestinal obstruction with perhaps gangrene and peritonitis.[17,29,30] A history of indigestion or periodic cramps, vomiting, and distention frequently dating back to childhood may be elicited. Postprandial pain is a characteristic symptom and may be relieved by postural changes. Distention is typically of a mild degree because the obstruction is usually high in the intestinal tract. Compression of the inferior mesenteric vein in the neck of the left hernial sac may result in vascular obstruction with the development of hemorrhoids, dilated anterior abdominal veins, and venous congestion and infarction of the bowel.[31]

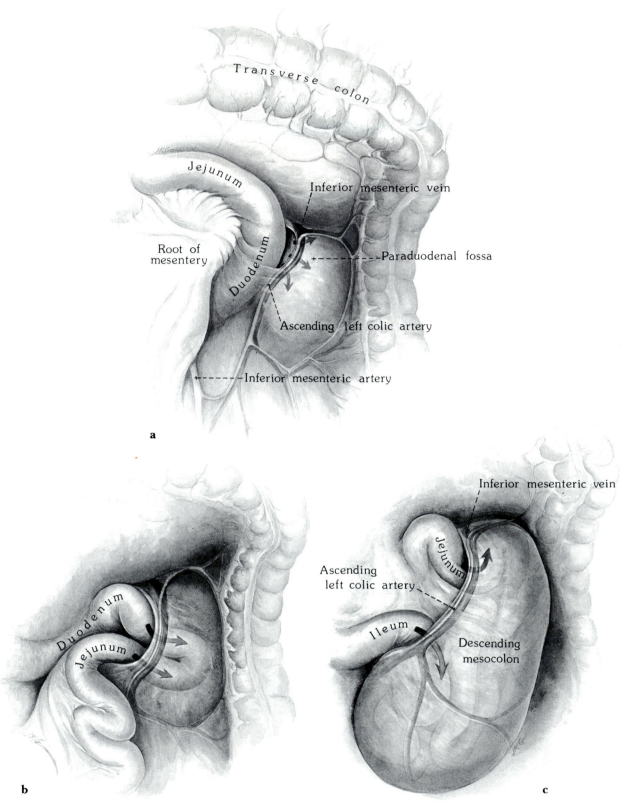

**Fig. 10–3. Development of a left paraduodenal hernia.**
The small bowel loops herniate via the fossa of Landzert into the descending mesocolon. Note the position of the inferior mesenteric vein and ascending left colic artery in the anterior margin of the neck of the sac.

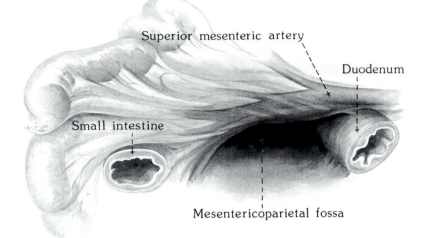

**Fig. 10–4. Lateral drawing of the mesentericoparietal fossa of Waldeyer** showing its position behind the superior mesenteric artery and small bowel mesentery. Note also its infraduodenal position.

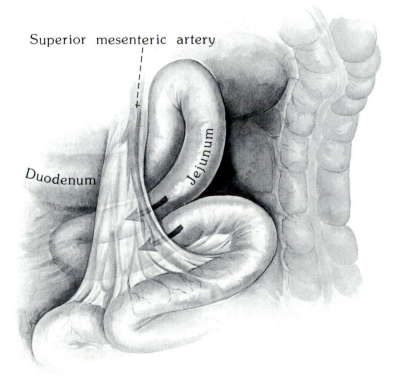

**Fig. 10–5. Development of a right paraduodenal hernia** via the fossa of Waldeyer toward the ascending mesocolon. Note the position of the superior mesenteric artery anterior to the hernia and in the leading edge of the sac.

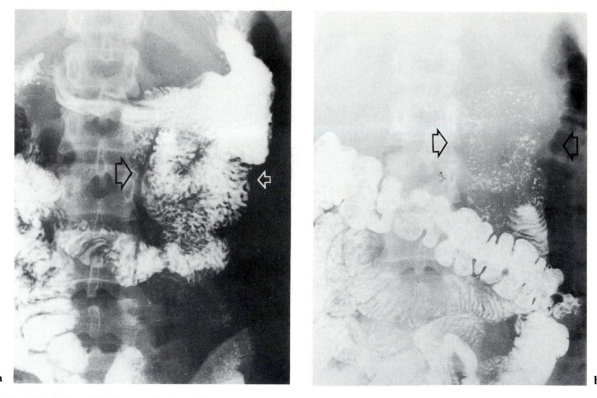

**Fig. 10–6. Small left paraduodenal hernia.**
**(a)** Small bowel series shows a circumscribed ovoid mass of herniated jejunal loops immediately lateral to the ascending duodenum (arrows).
**(b)** Two-hour film demonstrates stasis of barium within these loops (arrows) and depression of the distal transverse colon. At surgery the hernial sac contained only a couple feet of jejunum. This was readily reduced, and the peritoneal defect was repaired.
(From Meyers[17])

## *Radiologic and Arteriographic Features*

The preoperative diagnosis of paraduodenal hernia can be established only by radiologic evaluation. Studies are best performed during a symptomatic period. Examination in intervals between recurrent internal herniation may be negative or may demonstrate mild degrees of dilatation, stasis, and perhaps edematous mucosal folds which may be falsely attributed solely to adhesions. Diligent serial filming is essential to diagnosis.

In patients with a small left paraduodenal hernia (Figs. 10–6 through 10–9) a circumscribed mass of a few loops—most typically, jejunal—may be seen in the left upper quadrant immediately lateral to the ascending duodenum. The herniated loops may depress the dis-

tal transverse colon and indent the posterior wall of the stomach. Stasis of barium within the hernial contents and mild dilatation of the duodenum may be associated findings. Small right paraduodenal hernias present a similar ovoid grouping of small bowel loops lateral and inferior to the descending duodenum (Figs. 10–10 and 10–11).

Large paraduodenal hernias can contain several or most of the small bowel loops. These form a circumscribed ovoid mass having its main axis lateral to the midline and its inferior border convex downward (Figs. 10–12 through 10–14). The encapsulation within the hernial sac prevents separation or displacement of the individual loops from the rest of the hernial contents during fluoroscopic manipulation. Stasis of the contrast material and dilatation of the herniated loops may also be evident. At the her-

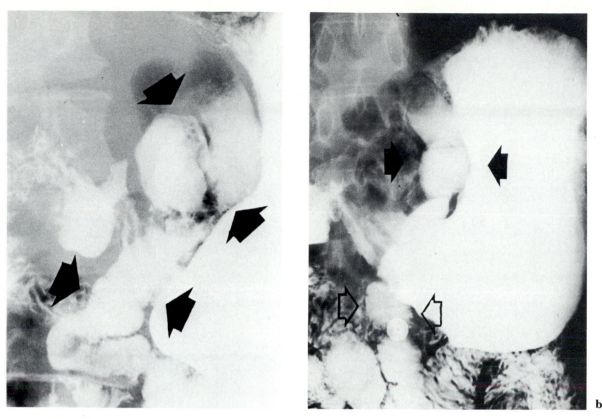

a

b

**Fig. 10–7. Small left paraduodenal hernia.**
**(a** and **b)** Prone oblique and frontal projections demonstrate a proximal jejunal loop within the hernial sac (arrows) behind the stomach, rising above the duodenojejunal junction into the descending mesocolon and especially into the left half of the transverse mesocolon. Note the pressure of the loop on the posterior wall of the stomach. A chronically deformed duodenal bulb is also present.
(From Meyers[17])

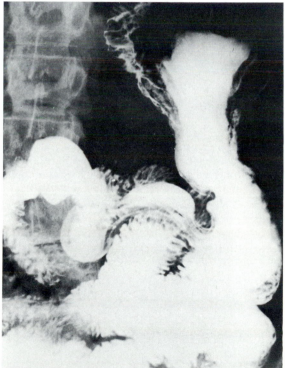

**Fig. 10–8. Small left paraduodenal hernia.**
A dilated jejunal loop resides abnormally high lateral to the fourth portion of the duodenum and mildly displaces the duodenojejunal junction medially. Its degree of dilatation and encapsulation is sufficient to produce pressure deformity on the posterior wall of the adjacent stomach.

Although no hernia was present at the time of autopsy, a paraduodenal fossa admitting three to four fingers was found. This would readily allow intermittent herniation of jejunum as illustrated. (From Meyers[17])

429

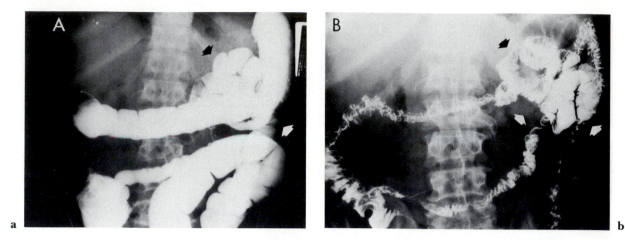

**Fig. 10–9. Left paraduodenal hernia.**
(**a** and **b**) Filled and postevacuation barium enema study demonstrates refluxed proximal ileal loops forming a circumscribed ovoid mass (arrows) with stasis within the left paraduodenal fossa.

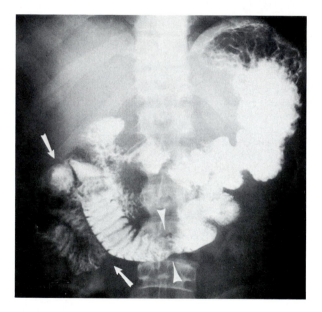

**Fig. 10–10. Small right paraduodenal hernia.**
A circumscribed grouping of jejunal loops (arrows) has herniated into the ascending mesocolon and the right portion of the transverse mesocolon. The dilated afferent jejunal limb shows a localized constriction (arrowheads) at the hernial orifice behind the superior mesenteric artery. (Reproduced from Ghahremani GG, Meyers MA[32])

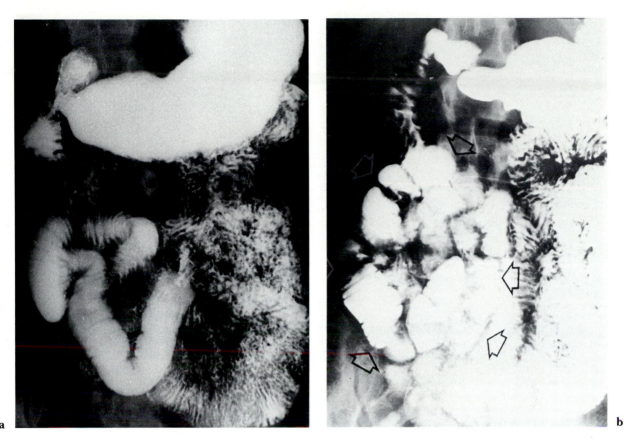

**Fig. 10–11. Right paraduodenal hernia.**
**(a)** The afferent and efferent limbs which lie close together both appear obstructed.
**(b)** Later the small intestinal loops within the circumscribed ovoid hernial sac (arrows) into the ascending mesocolon are still dilated but with a smaller degree of obstruction. The alternating sites of narrowing represent adhesions between loops.
(From Meyers[17])

nial orifice the efferent loop of the left para-duodenal hernia shows an abrupt change of caliber. In a right paraduodenal hernia, however, both the afferent and the efferent loops appear closely apposed and narrowed. Lateral films are particularly useful for detection of retroperito-neal displacement of the hernial content, showing the loops projecting well over the spine.[17,20] On barium enema examination, the descending colon may be seen to be anterior, to the left, or posterior to a left paraduodenal hernia. The ascending colon always lies lateral to a right para-duodenal hernia, however, and the cecum is found in its normal position.[17]

The position of the major mesenteric vessels in the anterior margin of the neck of the para-duodenal hernial sac is important embryologi-cally, surgically, and radiologically. Not only the intestinal loops, but their mesentery and vessels are incorporated into the hernia. Arterio-graphic visualization of these vessels, particu-larly of the position of their branches supplying the small bowel loops, can assist in the radiologic diagnosis of paraduodenal hernias.[17,23] In a right paraduodenal hernia, the jejunal arteries that normally arise from the left side of the superior mesenteric artery reverse their direction and course behind the parent vessel to supply the herniated jejunal loops within the fossa of Waldeyer (Figs. 10–13b and c and 10–14b). In a left paraduodenal hernia, the proximal jejunal arteries show an abrupt change of course along the medial border of the hernial orifice, where they are redirected posteriorly behind the infe-

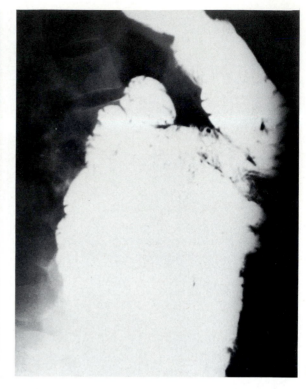

a

b

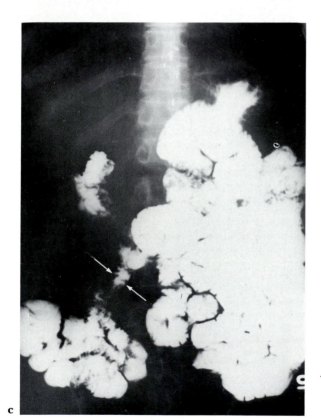

c

**Fig. 10–12. Large left paraduodenal hernia** in a 42-year-old female with persistent postprandial pains despite multiple abdominal operations.

**(a)** Most of the small bowel loops are gathered in the left side of the abdomen, forming a circumscribed mass with a convex inferior margin. Internal adhesions within the sac narrow bowel loops at multiple sites.

**(b)** Lateral projection shows retroperitoneal displacement of the herniated intestine.

**(c)** A serial film demonstrates that the efferent loop (arrows) leads from the hernial sac to the normally situated distal ileum. Despite multiple postural changes, the grouped position of the small bowel loops remained unchanged.

**(d** and **e)** Aortogram shows that the upper jejunal arteries are redirected medially and posteriorly just beyond their origins from the superior mesenteric artery (arrows). This characteristic reversal of their course indicates the posteromedial border of the hernial orifice, beyond which the intestinal loops herniate.

**(f)** Horizontal diagram of anatomic relationships of jejunal arteries redirected medially and posteriorly to left paraduodenal hernia into the descending mesocolon.

(From Meyers[23])

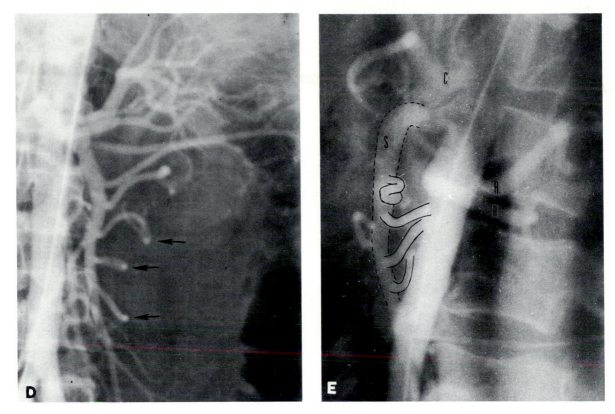

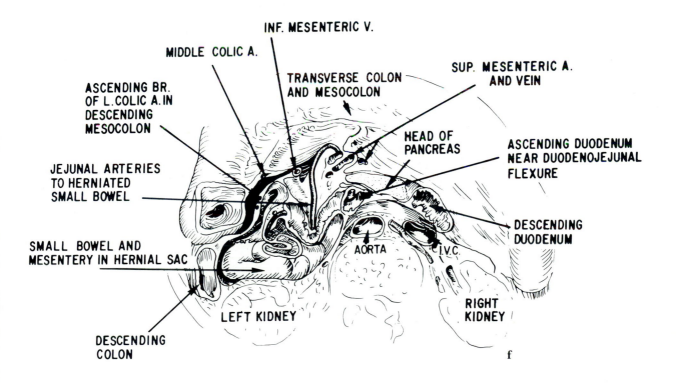

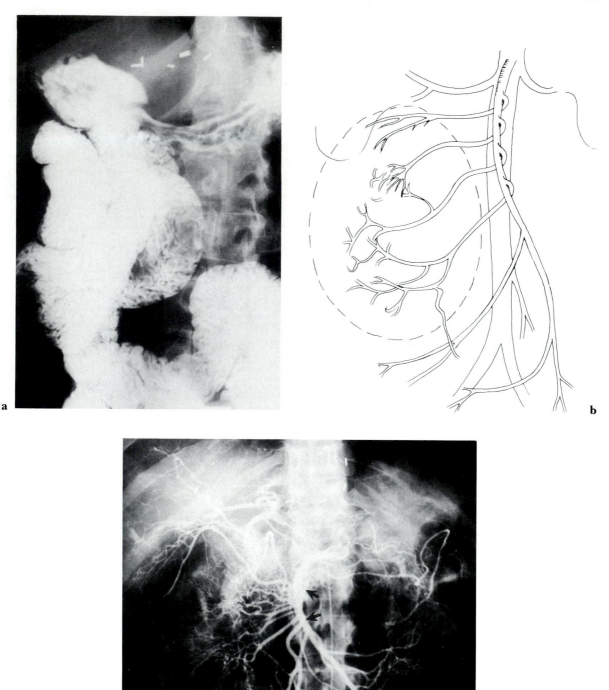

**Fig. 10–13. Large right paraduodenal hernia.**
(a) An ovoid grouping of jejunal loops in the right midabdomen resides within a hernial sac.
(b) Diagram of course of jejunal arteries accompanying the herniation via the mesentericoparietal fossa.
(c) Selective superior mesenteric arteriogram. The jejunal branches originate normally from the left side but abruptly change their direction (arrows) behind and toward the right of the parent vessel to accompany the herniated jejunal loops.

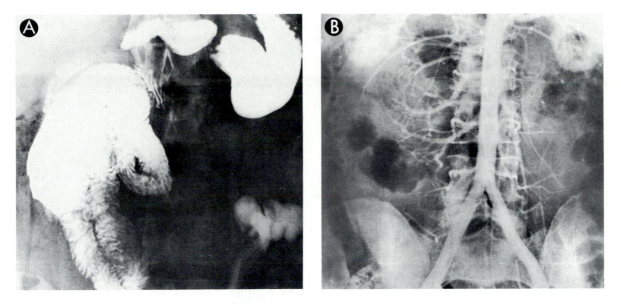

**Fig. 10–14. Large right paraduodenal hernia.**
**(a)** The right midabdomen is occupied by a circumscribed grouping of virtually all of the intestinal loops, representing a total herniation into the ascending mesocolon and right portion of the transverse mesocolon. The cecum was normally positioned.
**(b)** On aortography, the jejunal arteries are demonstrated to course to the right, accompanying the circumscribed herniated loops and their mesentery.
(Reproduced from Lechner and Gebhardt[33])

rior mesenteric vessels to accompany the herniated loops (Fig. 10–12d–f). A line connecting the points at which these arteries suddenly change their course indicates the medial border of the hernial orifice beyond which the small intestinal loops herniate.[17,23]

On computed tomography, the herniated bowel loops are positioned in an unusual relationship to the pancreas[34,35] (Figs. 10–15 and 10–16).

## Internal Hernias Through the Foramen of Winslow

The greater peritoneal cavity communicates with the omental bursa (lesser peritoneal sac) through the epiploic foramen of Winslow. This potential opening is situated beneath the free edge of the lesser omentum, cephalad to the duodenal bulb and deep to the liver, and usually admits one and occasionally two fingers. In life, its anterior and posterior boundaries are usually in contact. The foramen may open to some extent when the trunk is flexed, as in the sitting

position.[36] The omental bursa is limited in front by the stomach, lesser omentum, and the gastrocolic ligament, and behind by the posterior abdominal wall. Herniation of bowel through the foramen of Winslow accounts for 8% of all internal hernias.[6,21] The small intestine alone is involved in the herniation in 60–70% of cases and the terminal small bowel, cecum, and ascending colon in 25–30%. Other viscera such as the transverse colon, omentum, or gallbladder are found occasionally.[6,37,38]

Predisposing causes include a common or abnormally long mesentery or persistence of the ascending mesocolon permitting excessive mobility of the bowel and enlargement of the foramen. Alterations in intraabdominal pressure including parturition, straining, and large meals may tend to provoke the onset of the herniation,[36] which may also be facilitated by an elongated right lobe of the liver directing the mobile intestinal loops toward the foramen of Winslow.[39] The onset is usually acute with severe progressive pain and signs of bowel obstruction. Some relief of pain may be achieved with forward bending or the knee-chest position.[36] The pressure and stretching of the com-

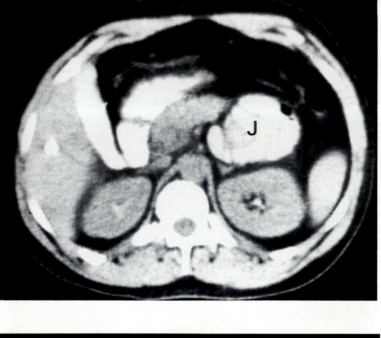

**Fig. 10–15. Left paraduodenal hernia.**
CT gastrografin study shows a cluster of opacified loops of jejunum (J) behind and to the left of the pancreas anterior to the left kidney. (Reproduced from Passas et al[35])

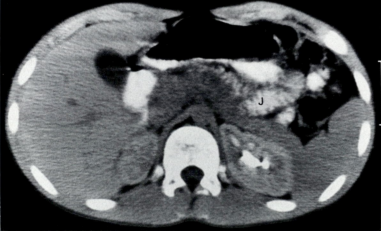

**Fig. 10–16. Left paraduodenal hernia.**
CT scan in a 13-year-old boy identifies a single loop of jejunum (J) between the stomach and the body of the pancreas. (Reproduced from Day et al[34])

mon bile duct by herniated colon may rarely produce an enlarged gallbladder[40] or jaundice.[36]

The characteristic plain-film findings are demonstration of a circumscribed collection of gas-containing intestinal loops high in the abdomen medial and posterior to the stomach, associated with mechanical small bowel obstruction (Figs. 10–17 through 10–19). Distinction from other conditions which can present with gas in the lesser sac (e.g., perforated peptic ulcer or abscess) is possible by identification of the presence of a mucosal pattern and fluid levels within the herniated bowel. The fluid levels do not con-

form precisely to the anatomic recesses of the lesser omental cavity. If the colon is involved in the hernia, there may be a single air–fluid level, but several fluid levels may be present if a segment of small intestine is involved. The stomach is displaced to the left and anteriorly. Dilated small bowel loops generally develop throughout the abdomen. When the cecum and ascending colon are involved in the hernia, the right iliac fossa appears empty[41–43] and interhaustral septa rather than valvulae conniventes may be identified within the herniated loop (Fig. 10–20). When the small intestine is the segment involved in the hernia, it can sometimes be identi-

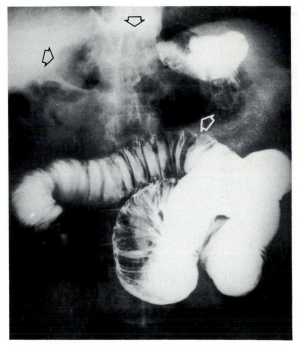

**Fig. 10–17. Foramen of Winslow hernia.**
Small bowel examination demonstrates marked dilatation of jejunum proximal to an obstruction in the right upper abdomen. The gas-containing herniated small bowel loops are visible within the lesser sac (arrows) medial to the stomach. (Reproduced from Ghahremani and Meyers[16])

fied progressing anterior to the hepatic flexure of the colon as it passes up to the foramen (Fig. 10–18b). Compression at this site then leads to distention of the ascending colon and cecum as well.

Barium studies readily confirm the diagnosis.[36,39,42,44] The stomach is characteristically displaced anteriorly and to the left, and the first and second portions of the duodenum may also be displaced to the left[41] (Figs. 10–19b, 10–21, and 10–22). Small bowel series documents the site of obstruction corresponding to the anatomic location of the foramen of Winslow between the duodenal bulb and the hilus of the liver. A barium enema study reveals obstruction with a tapered point near the hepatic flexure if the herniation contains the cecum and ascending colon[36,39,43,46] (Figs. 10–22 and 10–23). If the small bowel alone is herniated, retrograde flow may be arrested in the transverse colon because of traction on the mesentery by the herniating small bowel.[36,44]

The radiographic presentation may be com-

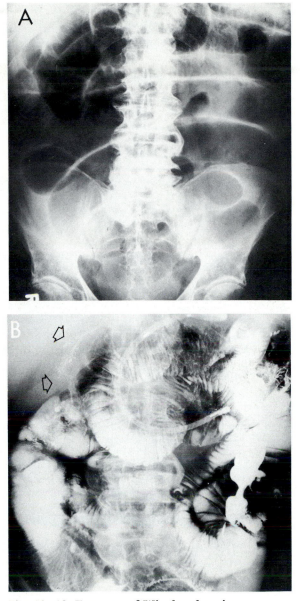

**Fig. 10–18. Foramen of Winslow hernia.**
**(a)** Supine film of the abdomen reveals massive distention of the small bowel and absence of gas in the colon.
**(b)** A subsequent study with contrast material delineates the specific cause of the distal small bowel obstruction. The partially reduced and collapsed ileum and proximal colon (arrows) are seen to pass between the liver and duodenum in the direction of the foramen of Winslow.
(Reproduced from Ghahremani and Meyers[32])

plicated at times if there are associated defects in the gastrocolic or gastrohepatic omentum allowing reentry of the herniated loops into the greater peritoneal cavity.[36]

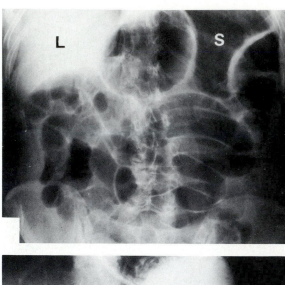

a

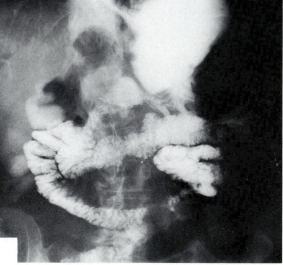

b

**Fig. 10–19. Cecal herniation through the foramen of Winslow.**
**(a)** Supine abdominal film shows marked dilatation of the small bowel. An abnormal collection of gas is seen in the lesser peritoneal sac between the liver (L) and the stomach (S).
**(b)** Upper GI series reveals displacement of the stomach and the first and second parts of the duodenum to the left. There is less gas in the small intestine and within the lesser sac owing to partial spontaneous reduction of the hernia.
(From Henisz et al[41])

**Fig. 10–20. Cecal herniation through the foramen of Winslow.**
Plain film demonstrates gas-containing cecum with identifiable interhaustral septa within the lesser sac, displacing the stomach toward the left.

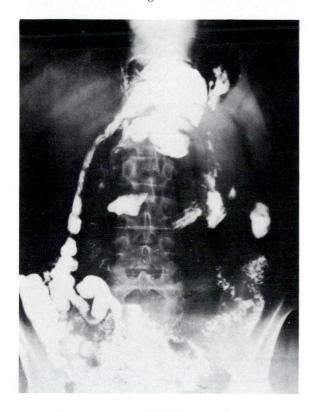

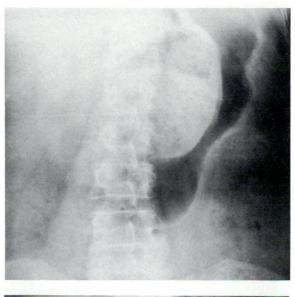

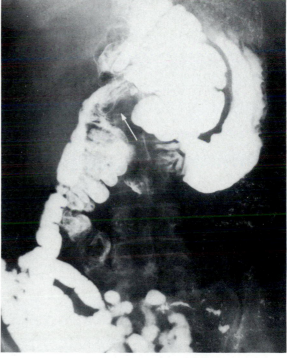

**Fig. 10–21. Foramen of Winslow hernia.**
Delayed film from upper GI series demonstrates
stretched terminal ileum ascending through foramen
of Winslow with the cecum and ascending colon
within the lesser sac medial to the stomach.
(From Schwartz and Feuchtwanger[45])

**Fig. 10–22. Foramen of Winslow hernia.**
(a) Plain film shows mottled gas density consistent
with large bowel impressing upon the lesser curvature of the stomach.
(b) Small bowel follow-through confirms herniation
of the cecum and ascending colon into the lesser sac.
Note the compression of the ascending colon at the
foramen of Winslow (arrow).
(From Goldberger and Berk[46])

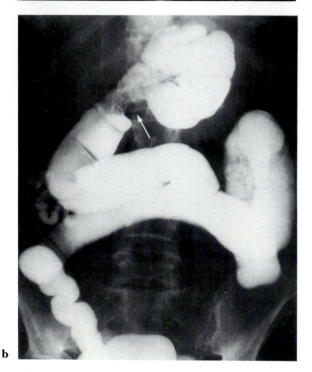

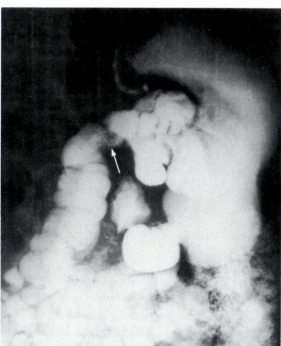

**Fig. 10–23. Foramen of Winslow hernia.**
(a) Barium enema shows failure of fixation of the right colon. The cecum and appendix arise into the right upper quadrant of the abdomen.
(b and c) Barium enema study and small bowel follow-through 4 years later. The cecum and ascending colon have herniated into the lesser sac, indenting the stomach. Compression of the ascending colon as it passes through the foramen of Winslow can be identified (arrows).

A large ovarian cyst which has developed since the preliminary study causes elevation and stretching of the sigmoid colon. This may have contributed to increased intraabdominal pressure and the formation of the internal herniation.
(From Goldberger and Berk[46])

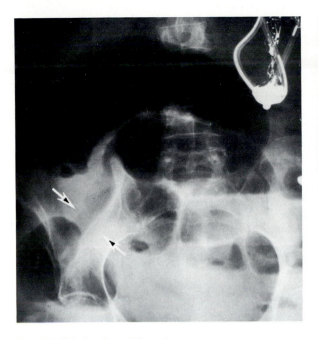

**Fig. 10–24. Pericecal hernia.**
The distal ileum protruding through a defect in the mesentery of the cecum is seen in the right lower abdomen, and there is gaseous distention of the proximal small intestine. The narrowed afferent segment of the herniated ileal loop (arrow) is identified. (From Ghahremani and Meyers[16])

# Pericecal Hernias

Four peritoneal fossae in the ileocecal region, as well as congenital and acquired defects in the mesentery of the cecum or appendix, may lead to development of a pericecal hernia.[7,9,19,47] The variety of other terms (ileocolic, retrocecal, ileocecal, paracecal) used to classify these hernias appear to have limited practical value in the radiologic differential diagnosis and surgical management.[16]

In the collective review of 467 internal hernias by Hansmann and Morton,[21] 13% involved the ileocecal region. The clinical manifestations are usually intermittent episodes of right lower abdominal pain, tenderness, small bowel distention, nausea, and vomiting. Chronic incarceration may produce symptoms compatible with a periappendiceal abscess, Crohn's disease, or intestinal obstruction due to adhesions.[9,19]

In most cases, a portion of ileum passes through defects in the mesentery of the cecum to occupy the right paracolic gutter. The correct

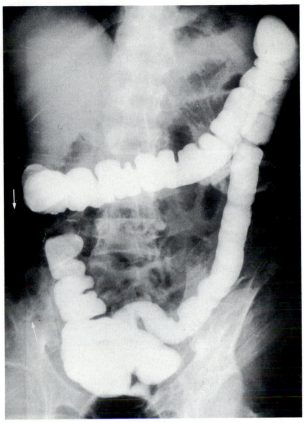

**Fig. 10–25. Herniation of the ileal loops through a defect in a persistent ascending mesocolon.**
There is moderate dilatation of the proximal small bowel, and there are gas-containing loops in the right paracolic gutter (arrows) displacing the ascending colon medially. (From Ghahremani and Meyers[16])

diagnosis may be suggested on plain radiographs of the abdomen (Fig. 10–24). More useful are the delayed films of the small bowel series, or a barium enema examination in which reflux into the terminal ileum has been achieved. Careful fluoroscopic evaluation and radiographs in lateral and oblique projections are particularly valuable for the demonstration of the fixed position of herniated loops posterolateral to the cecum.[16] This is also true for the diagnosis of internal hernias which rarely develop through defects in a persistent ascending mesocolon[18] (Fig. 10–25). In this condition, the radiologic differentiation from a transitory transmigration of the small intestine anteriorly over the ascending colon into the right paracolic gutter has clinical and prognostic significance.

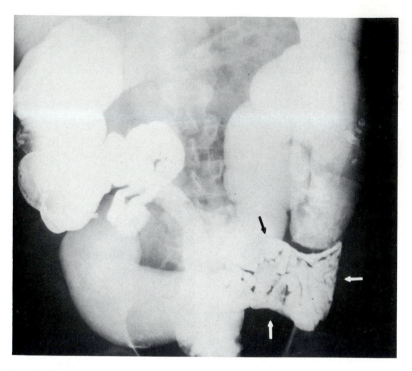

**Fig. 10–26. Intersigmoid hernia.**
Barium enema examination, with retrograde filling of the small bowel, shows encapsulation of several ileal loops (arrows) within the intersigmoid fossa. (From Ghahremani and Meyers[32])

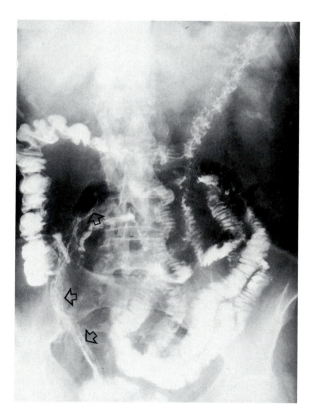

# Intersigmoid Hernias

The intersigmoid fossa is a peritoneal pouch formed between the two loops of the sigmoid colon and its mesentery. This pocket is found in 65% of cadavers and serves as a potential site for an intersigmoid hernia.[9,16,18] This is usually a reducible hernia containing a few small bowel loops. Incarceration is uncommon.

The radiologic diagnosis of intersigmoid hernia is best made by retrograde filling of the small intestine during barium enema examination. Figure 10–26 shows the encapsulated ileal loops in a characteristic relationship to the sigmoid colon.

Two other similar, but rare, entities are (1) the *intramesosigmoid hernia*, which involves a de-

**Fig. 10–27. Transmesosigmoid hernia.**
The postevacuation film of a barium enema study demonstrates herniated small bowel loops occupying the left lower abdomen. The sigmoid colon (arrows) is elevated and displaced to the right. (From Ghahremani and Meyers[16])

fect of only one of the constituent mesenteric leaves, the separation of which forms the hernial sac,[18] and (2) the *transmesosigmoid hernia*, in which a usually large defect in both layers of the sigmoid mesentery allows herniation of the small bowel loops toward the left lower abdomen posterolateral to the sigmoid colon[18,19] (Fig. 10–27).

Radiologic differentiation of the three types of hernia involving the mesosigmoid is often difficult and irrelevant in terms of their ultimate surgical management. Observation of an intimate relationship between the sigmoid colon and intestinal loops clumped or fixed posterior and lateral to it can serve as a useful criterion to indicate the probability of an internal hernia involving the mesosigmoid.[16]

The findings are to be distinguished from a persistent descending mesocolon[7,18,40a] which may occasionally contain defects involving both layers; small bowel loops may then pass behind the descending colon and fill the left paracolic gutter (Fig. 10–28).

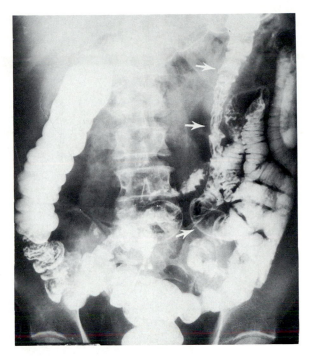

**Fig. 10–28. Persistent descending mesocolon.** The ileal loops opacified by reflux during barium enema examination occupy the left paracolic gutter. The descending colon (arrows) is displaced toward the midline. The presence of a probable defect in the mesocolon is not yet verified surgically in this patient. (From Ghahremani and Meyers[16])

# Transmesenteric and Transmesocolic Hernias

About 5–10% of all internal hernias occur through defects in the mesentery of the small intestine.[12,13,21] An etiologic relationship to prenatal intestinal ischemic accidents seems probable, because in infants with atretic intestinal segments such defects and herniation are frequently associated.[14] In fact, nearly 35% of these hernias occur in the pediatric age group, in which they constitute the most common type of internal hernias.[8,14] In adults, however, most mesenteric defects serving as the hernial ring are probably the result of previous surgery, abdominal trauma, or intraperitoneal inflammation.[12,13]

The mesenteric defects are often located close to the ligament of Treitz or the ileocecal valve. The rather small size of the defect (usually 2–5 cm) and the absence of a limiting hernial sac account for a relatively high incidence of strangulation and intestinal gangrene with a mortality rate of about 50% for surgically

treated patients and 100% for those without surgical treatment.[12]

Radiographs of the abdomen usually demonstrate mechanical small bowel obstruction and, occasionally, a single distended "closed loop" (Fig. 10–29). The small bowel series or barium enema study with reflux may further assist in the diagnosis by showing a constriction around the closely approximated afferent and efferent loops of the herniated intestine[47] (Fig. 10–30). These findings invariably signal a surgical emergency, although clinical and radiologic differentiation of the hernia from small bowel volvulus or entrapment beneath peritoneal adhesions may be impossible.[16] Arteriography may reveal an abrupt change in the course of the superior mesenteric artery and displacement of the visceral branches, indicating an internal hernia with the site of the herniation suggested by the change in the course of the vessels[49,50] (Fig. 10–31).

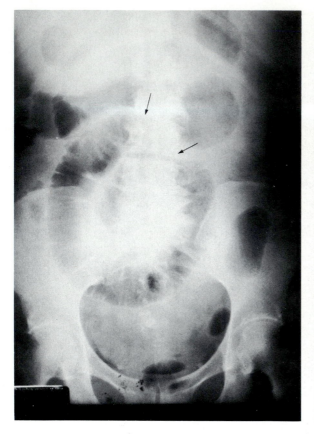

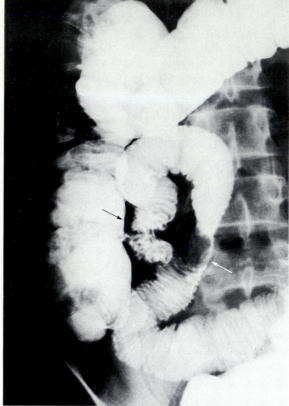

**Fig. 10–29. Transmesenteric hernia.**
Herniation of a jejunal loop through a defect in the
small bowel mesentery. Note the typical presentation
of a distended closed loop with approximation of its
ends at the hernial orifice (arrows). (From Ghahremani and Meyers[16])

**Fig. 10–30. Transmesenteric hernia.**
Herniation of the distal ileum through a congenital
defect in the mesentery of a Meckel's diverticulum.
Barium enema study with reflux shows constriction
around the closely approximated afferent and efferent loops (arrows) of the ileum. (From Dalinka MK et
al[48])

Defects in the transverse mesocolon may
rarely provide access for internal herniation of
small bowel loops posterior to the transverse colon into the lesser sac[7,51,52] (Fig. 10–32). Although these defects may result from trauma,
inflammation, or operative procedures, most
are probably congenital in origin. Since the orifice is usually very large with an avascular space
in the base of the mesocolon, many loops may
herniate without strangulation, gangrene, or
even significant obstruction. Reentry into the
greater peritoneal cavity is frequent, via the
routes of the foramen of Winslow, the gastrohepatic ligament, and the gastrocolic ligament[53]
(Fig. 10–33).

## Retroanastomotic Hernias

Retroanastomotic hernias occur usually in patients who have undergone partial gastrectomy
and gastrojejunostomy, particularly of the antecolic variety.[11,54] The superior border of the
hernial ring is formed by the transverse mesocolon, the inferior border by the ligament of
Treitz, and the anterior aspect by the gastrojejunostomy together with the afferent limb of the
jejunum[11] (Fig. 10–34). The herniated loop is
usually the efferent jejunal segment or, less
commonly, an excessively long afferent limb
that protrudes into the retroanastomotic space.

About half of these hernias manifest themselves within 1 month and another 25% within 1
year after the operation,[55] with symptoms of

**Fig. 10–31. Transmesenteric hernia.**
Arteriogram in a 48-year-old female with acute abdominal symptoms shows an abrupt change in the course of the superior mesenteric artery which is seen to fold back on itself. The terminal ileal and ileocolic branches course in a twisting fashion toward the left upper quadrant and fan toward the right flank instead of distributing in the normal lower abdominal course from the left to the right.

At surgery, herniation of the entire right colon and half of the small bowel with a twist through a 10-cm congenital defect in the small bowel mesentery was found. This was reduced manually and the defect closed. (From Cohen and Patel[49])

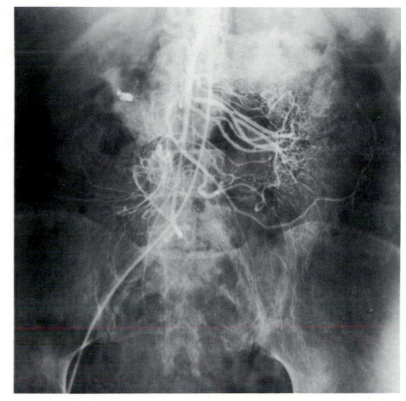

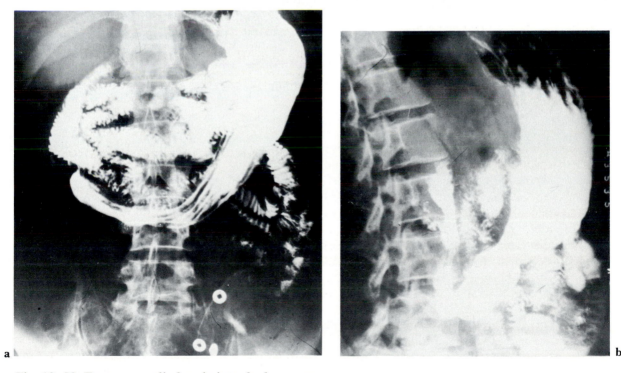

a                                                                                                                                    b

**Fig. 10–32. Transmesocolic hernia into the lesser sac.**
**(a)** Prone and **(b)** oblique radiographs demonstrate multiple small bowel loops above and posterior to the displaced stomach. They have entered the lesser sac through a large defect in the transverse mesocolon. (From Meyers and Whalen[52])

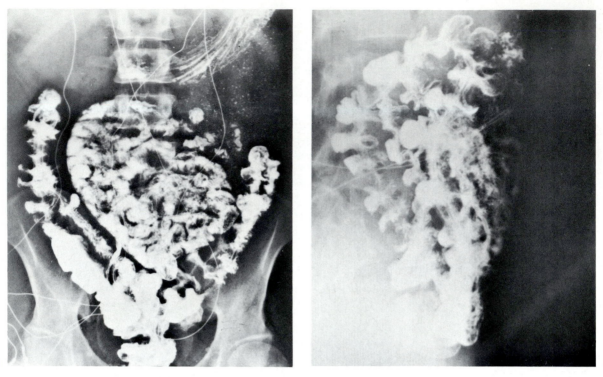

a                                                                                                                   b

**Fig. 10–33. Transmesocolic hernia.**
Supine **(a)** and lateral **(b)** radiographs demonstrate virtually the entire small bowel loops have herniated through a large defect in the transverse mesocolon into the lesser sac. They have then bulged anteriorly into or through the gastrocolic ligament to displace the transverse colon inferiorly and posteriorly.
(Courtesy of Alan Herschman, MD, New Brunswick, N.J.)

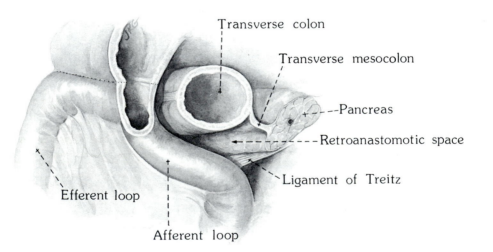

**Fig. 10–34. Lateral drawing of the retroanastomotic hernial ring in the antecolic gastrojejunostomy.**

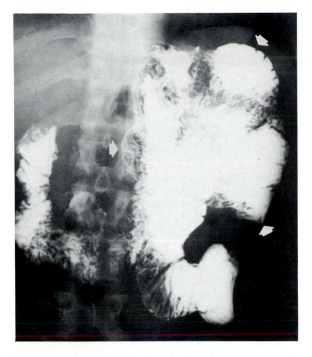

**Fig. 10–35. Retroanastomotic hernia.**
Upper GI series post-Billroth II shows the herniated efferent loop encapsulated in the left upper quadrant (arrows). The afferent loop with a duodenal diverticulum is also opacified with barium. (Courtesy of Gary G Ghahremani, MD, Evanston Hospital, Evanston, Ill.)

cramping abdominal pain and signs of a high small bowel obstruction. These nonspecific findings may be mistaken for stomal edema, dumping, or pancreatitis, and the correct diagnosis may be delayed until strangulation has developed.[10,11,55] This contributes to the reported mortality rate of 32% for surgically treated cases and almost 100% for untreated patients.[11]

Careful fluoroscopic evaluation discloses that the obstruction is situated not at the gastric stoma but more distally in either of the anastomotic limbs. Gradual opacification of the partially obstructed efferent loop shows its abnormal position just lateral and posterior to the gastrojejunostomy (Fig. 10–35). Some degree of dilatation and stasis is usually associated.

# References

1. Balthazar EJ: Intestinal malrotation in adults: Roentgenographic assessment with emphasis on isolated complete and partial nonrotations. AJR 126: 358–367, 1976

2. Wang CA, Welch CE: Anomalies of intestinal rotation in adolescents and adults. Surgery 54: 839–855, 1963

3. Gale ME, Gerzof SG, Kiser LC, et al: CT appearance of afferent loop obstruction. AJR 138: 1085–1088, 1982

4. Jaramillo D, Raval B: CT diagnosis of primary small-bowel volvulus. AJR 147: 941–942, 1986

5. Lieberman JM, Haaga JR: Case report: Duodenal malrotation. J Comp Assist Tomogr 6(5): 1019–1020, 1982

6. Jones TW: Paraduodenal hernia and hernias of the foramen of Winslow. In Hernia. Edited by IM Nyhus, HN Harkins. JB Lippincott, Philadelphia, 1964 pp 577–601

7. Mueller EC: Congenital internal hernia. Am J Surg 97: 201–204, 1959

8. Pennell TC, Shaffner LS: Congenital internal hernia. Surg Clin N Am 51: 1355–1359, 1971

9. Zimmerman LM, Laufman H: Intra-abdominal hernias due to developmental and rotational anomalies. Ann Surg 138: 82–91, 1953

10. Hardy JD: Problems associated with gastric surgery: Review of 604 consecutive patients with annotation. Am J Surg 108: 699–716, 1964

11. Markowitz AM, Retroanastomotic hernia. In Hernia. Edited by IM Nyhus, HN Harkins. JB Lippincott, Philadelphia, 1964, pp 607–616

12. Mock CJ, Mock HE Jr: Strangulated internal hernia associated with trauma. Arch Surg 77: 881–886, 1958

13. Winterscheid LC: Mesenteric hernia. In Hernia. Edited by LM Nyhus, HN Harkins. JB Lippincott, Philadelphia, 1964, pp 602–605

14. Murphy DA: Internal hernias in infancy and childhood. Surgery 55: 311–315, 1964

15. Williams AJ: Roentgen diagnosis of intra-abdominal hernia. An evaluation of the roentgen findings. Radiology 59: 817–825, 1952

16. Ghahremani GG, Meyers MA: Internal abdominal hernias. Curr Probl Radiol 5: 1–30, 1975

17. Meyers MA: Paraduodenal hernias. Radiologic and arteriographic diagnosis. Radiology 95: 29–37, 1970

18. Bertelsen S, Christiansen J: Internal hernia through mesenteric and mesocolic defects. A review of the literature and a report of two cases. Acta Chir Scand 133: 426–428, 1967

19. Nathan H: Internal hernia. J Int Coll Surg 34: 563–571, 1960

20. Parsons PB: Paraduodenal hernia. AJR 69: 563–589, 1953

21. Hansmann GH, Morton SA: Intra-abdominal hernia. Report of a case and review of the literature. Arch Surg 39: 973–986, 1939

22. Berens JJ: Small internal hernias in the paraduodenal area. Arch Surg 86: 726–732, 1963

23. Meyers MA: Arteriographic diagnosis of internal
    (left paraduodenal) hernia. Radiology 92: 1035–
    1037, 1969
24. Callander CL, Rusk GY, Nemir A: Mechanism,
    symptoms, and treatment of hernia into descend-
    ing mesocolon (left duodenal hernia); plea for
    change in nomenclature. Surg Gynecol Obstet 60:
    1052–1071, 1935
25. Roberts WH, Dalgleish AE: Internal hernia of
    embryological origin. Anat Rec 155: 279–285,
    1966
26. Moynihan BGA: On Retroperitoneal Hernia.
    Chapter 2: Duodenal folds and fossae. Bailliere,
    Tindall and Cox, London, 1889, pp 19–70
27. Landzert: Über die hernie Retroperitonealis
    (Treitz) und ihre Beziehungen zur Fossa
    duodeno-jejunalis. St Petersb Med Ztschr, MF 2:
    306–350, 1871
28. Waldeyer W: Hernia retroperitonealis, nebst Ber-
    merkungen zur Anatomie des Peritoneums. Arch
    Path Anat 60: 66–92, 1874
29. Filtzer H, Sedgewick CE: Strangulated para-
    duodenal hernia. Report of a case. Surg Clin N
    Am 53: 371–374, 1973
30. Freund H, Berlatzky Y: Small paraduodenal her-
    nias. Arch Surg 112: 1180–1183, 1977
31. Mayo CW, Stalker LK, Miller JM: Intra-abdomi-
    nal hernia. Review of 39 cases in which treatment
    was surgical. Ann Surg 114: 875–885, 1941
32. Ghahremani GG, Meyers MA: Hernias. Chapter
    7 in Surgical Radiology. Edited by JG Teplick,
    ME Haskin. WB Saunders, Philadelphia, 1981
33. Lechner G, Gebhardt HD: Rechtseitäge para-
    duodenale Hernie. Fortschr Roentgenstr 105:
    904–907, 1966
34. Day DL, Drake DG, Leonard AS, et al: CT find-
    ings in left paraduodenal herniae. Gastrointest
    Radiol 13(1): 27–29, 1988
35. Passas V, Karavias D, Grilias D, et al: Computed
    tomography of left paraduodenal hernia. J Comp
    Assist Tomogr 10(3): 542–543, 1986
36. Erskine JM: Hernia through the foramen of
    Winslow. Surg Gynecol Obstet 125: 1093–1109,
    1967
37. Dardik H, Cowen R: Herniation of the gallblad-
    der through the epiploic foramen into the lesser
    sac. Ann Surg 165: 644–646, 1967
38. Vint WA: Herniation of the gallbladder through
    the epiploic foramen into the lesser sac: Radio-
    logic diagnosis. Radiology 86: 1035–1040, 1966
39. Hollenberg MS: Radiographic diagnosis of her-
    nia into the lesser peritoneal sac through the fora-
    men of Winslow. Report of a case. Surgery 18:
    498–502, 1945
40. Khilnani MT, Lautkin A, Wolf BS: Internal her-
    nia through the foramen of Winslow. J Mount
    Sinai Hosp 26: 188–193, 1959
40a. Popky GL, Lapayowker MS: Persistent descend-
    ing mesocolon. Radiology 86: 327–331, 1966
41. Henisz A, Matesanz J, Westcott JL: Cecal hernia-
    tion through the foramen of Winslow. Radiology
    112: 575–578, 1974
42. Cimmino CV: Lesser sac hernia via the foramen
    of Winslow. A case report. Radiology 60: 57–59,
    1953
43. Stankey RM: Intestinal herniation through the
    foramen of Winslow. Radiology 89: 929–930,
    1967
44. Lefort H, Dax H, Vallet G: Herniation through
    the foramen of Winslow (roentgenologic and clin-
    ical considerations based on an analysis of 25
    cases). J Radiol 48: 157–166, 1967
45. Schwartz A, Feuchtwanger MM: Hernia through
    the foramen of Winslow. Isr J Med Sci 4: 117–
    121, 1968
46. Goldberger LE, Berk RN: Cecal hernia into lesser
    sac. Gastrointest Radiol 5: 169–172, 1980
47. Rooney JA, Carroll JP, Keeley JL: Internal her-
    nias due to defects in the meso-appendix and
    mesentery of small bowel, and probable Ivemark
    syndrome. Report of two cases. Ann Surg 157:
    254–258, 1963
48. Dalinka MK, Wunder JF, Wolfe RD: Internal
    hernia through the mesentery of a Meckel's di-
    verticulum. Radiology 95: 39–40, 1970
49. Cohen AM, Patel S: Arteriographic findings in
    congenital transmesenteric internal hernia. AJR
    133: 541–543, 1979
50. Kondi ES, Gallitano AL, Katz SJ: A new variant of
    intra-abdominal hernia. Ann Surg 181: 442–446,
    1975
51. Gallagher HW: Spontaneous herniation through
    the transverse mesocolon: A review of the litera-
    ture and the report of a case. Br J Surg 36: 300–
    305, 1949
52. Meyers MA, Whalen JP: Roentgen significance of
    the duodenocolic relationships. An anatomic ap-
    proach. AJR 117: 263–274, 1973
53. Carlisle BB, Killen DA: Spontaneous transverse
    mesocolic hernia with re-entry into the greater
    peritoneal cavity: Report of a case with review of
    the literature. Surgery 62: 268–273, 1967
54. Morton CB, Alrich EM, Hill LD: Internal hernia
    after gastrectomy. Ann Surg 141: 759–764,
    1955
55. Sabesta DG, Robson MC: Petersen's retroanas-
    tomotic hernia. Am J Surg 116: 450–453,
    1968

# 11 Pathways of Extrapelvic Spread of Disease

## General Introduction

Diseases arising from the pelvic contents may first manifest themselves by signs and symptoms remote from their source of origin. Gastrointestinal tract perforations, in particular, may dissect along anatomic planes of the pelvis to first present in the buttock, hip, thigh, and even the lower leg and the retroperitoneal space of the abdomen. Pain, mass, or crepitation at these sites may be very misleading since the origin of the underlying inflammatory condition or the neoplastic, traumatic, or foreign body perforation of the bowel within the pelvis often remains clinically occult. Radiologic evaluation may be crucial in redirecting the diagnostic and therapeutic approach as well as in documenting the extent of disease.

The most common extraabdominal extension of gastrointestinal tract perforations, beyond the development of ischiorectal abscesses, is to the buttocks, hips, and lower extremities. Of the cases in the literature reported as subcutaneous emphysema of the leg arising from intestinal perforations,[1,2] diverticulitis and appendicitis account for most of those resulting from infection. Carcinoma of the colon with perforation, uterine carcinoma, foreign body, and trauma to the rectum were other causes.

Most cases of extraperitoneal spread reported have created serious diagnostic problems with admitting diagnoses of thrombophlebitis, sciatica, gas gangrene, inguinal abscess, Spigelian hernia, and even fractured hip, until surgery or autopsy uncovered a definitive diagnosis. The clinical presentation is often pain in the hip or buttock.[1,3–7] with the development of crepitation, particularly in the thigh, incision may then display severe necrotizing fasciitis. It is often not until blunt dissection is then carried out along the femoral canal, beneath the inguinal ligament, that an extraperitoneal abscess is revealed as evidence of a more severe process extending from the pelvis.

The pathogenesis of subacute cellulitis and emphysema of gastrointestinal origin depends on four basic factors[8]: (a) perforation of the bowel, (b) an adequate pressure gradient between the lumen of the bowel and ultimately the subcutaneous space, (c) the anatomic site of perforation, and (d) infection.

The major mechanism of gas formation is not the gas-forming organisms in feces, but the pressure gradient between the lumen of the gut and surrounding tissue. Large pressure gradients are associated with vigorous peristaltic contractions.[9] Gas pressures in the intestinal lumen may rise to more than 60 cm $H_2O$ during peristalsis, while soft-tissue tension is usually about 5 cm $H_2O$. The intraabdominal pressure may be greatly increased by the contraction of the diaphragmatic and abdominal muscles. This increased pressure is transmitted to the contents of the intestinal tract and promotes their evacuation, especially at sites of perforation when the sphincters are intact.[9,10] This mechanism, enhanced by bacterial gas formation, accounts for the rapidity of its accumulation.

The anatomic site of perforation largely determines the pathway of spread of the sinus tract to the subcutaneous position. The usual route of extravasation from the bowel is directly through a pathologic defect in the parietal peri-

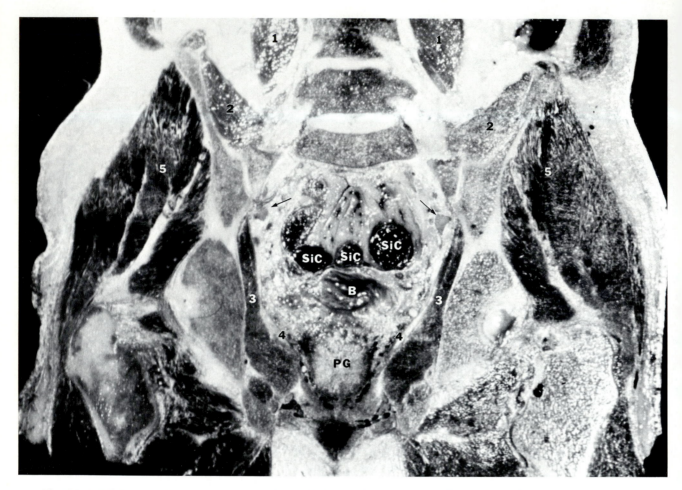

**Fig. 11–1. Midocoronal anatomic section through the pelvis at the level of the urinary bladder** (B), **prostate gland** (PG), **and loops of sigmoid colon** (SiC).
The course and relationships of the psoas major (1), iliacus (2), obturator internus (3), levator ani (4), and gluteal muscles (5) are shown. These are invested by fascia.

The superior gluteal vessels (arrows) pass out of the pelvis at the level of the greater sciatic foramina. (Courtesy of Manuel Viamonte Jr, MD, Mt. Sinai Hospital, Miami Beach, Fla. From Meyers and Goodman[1])

toneum of fascia contiguous with this defect into the intermuscular planes and subcutaneous spaces. Solid parenchymatous organs and serous membranes have a relatively great resistance to the diffusion of gases, whereas loose areolar and fascial structures readily allow the passage of gas.

Cases of perforated diverticulitis or carcinoma of the sigmoid or descending colon usually present in the left leg or buttock, and appendicitis or perforation of the cecum in the right leg and buttock. Because of variations in position and length of the appendix and in redundancy of the sigmoid, perforations from these sites may extend to the side opposite to

that ordinarily expected. Traumatic or neoplastic perforation of the rectum may present in either or both buttocks and legs. Spread from the pelvis may occur also into the abdominal wall and upward as an extraperitoneal abscess.[2,11–13]

The most common offending organism is *E. coli*. Occasionally, cultures isolate *Clostridium welchii*, *Aerobacter aerogenes*, and *Proteus*.[3,5,6,11,13]

Surgical findings have not often localized the particular pathway of spread in the presence of a pelvic abscess with frequent necrotizing dissection toward the inguinal region, perineum, thigh and hip joint, buttock, and paravertebral gutter.[5,11]

Meyers and Goodman have established the

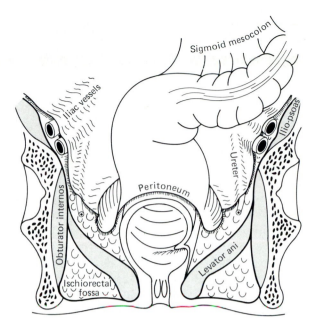

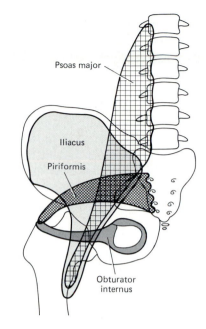

**Fig. 11–2. Posterior coronal section at level of the rectum showing planes of pelvic fascia** (bold lines). The endopelvic fascia covers the major muscles of the pelvis. The internal iliac arteries lie superficial to the fascia and then continue within tunneled extensions as they pass to the gluteal region. (From Meyers and Goodman[1])

**Fig. 11–3. Extrapelvic insertions of abdominal and pelvic muscles.**
The iliopsoas muscle group inserts medially on the lesser trochanter of the femur, and the piriformis and obturator internus insert laterally on the greater trochanter. (From Meyers and Goodman[1])

correlation between the anatomic pathways and the radiologic documentation of the extrapelvic spread of disease.[1] The insertions of the iliopsoas, piriformis, and obturator internus muscles, within their fascial investments, and the ensheathed penetrations of the superior gluteal arteries provide avenues of dissection to the buttocks, hips, and thighs.

# Anatomic Considerations

Figure 11–1 is an anatomic section showing the relationships of the major muscles of the pelvis. The levator ani and coccygeus muscles form the floor of the pelvis (pelvic diaphragm). This is the most inferior portion of the body wall and closes the abdominopelvic cavity. The obturator internus and the piriformis muscles originate within the pelvis and thus form part of the pelvic wall, but they are really muscles of the lower limbs.

The endopelvic fascia is the internal investing fascia of the pelvis. Its parietal layer (Fig. 11–2)

covers the levator ani, coccygeus, and the intrapelvic portions of the obturator internus and piriformis muscles. It is directly continuous above with the transversalis (endoabdominal) fascia lining the abdominal cavity. The visceral layer of the endopelvic fascia covers the urinary bladder, lower third of the ureters, uterus, vagina, and the rectum.

Four of the pelvic muscles have important extrapelvic insertions. These are illustrated in Figure 11–3:

1. The psoas major originates from the transverse processes and bodies of the lumbar vertebrae and inserts on the lesser trochanter of the femur.
2. The iliacus originates primarily from the upper two thirds of the iliac fossa and the ala of the sacrum and inserts with the tendon of the psoas major on the lesser trochanter of the femur. In its common insertion, it comprises the iliopsoas muscle group.
3. The piriformis originates from the sacrum and the margin of the greater sciatic foramen

and inserts on the lesser trochanter of the femur.

4. The obturator internus originates from the margins of the obturator foramen and inserts on the greater trochanter of the femur.

It is also important to recognize that the pelvic blood vessels lie in front of the pelvic fascia, i.e., superficial to the parietal layer of the endopelvic fascia. The superior and inferior gluteal branches of the internal iliac arteries passing out of the pelvis (Fig. 11–1) must perforate the fascia and carry extensions of the fascia with them to the gluteal region. For example, the fascia of the piriformis is prolonged outward through the greater sciatic foramen and joins the gluteal fascia. The internal iliac vessels and their branches lie in the subperitoneal tissue in front of the fascia, and the branches to the gluteal region, particularly the superior gluteal artery (the largest branch of the hypogastric artery), emerge in special sheaths of this tissue, paralleling the border of the piriformis, to reach and supply the gluteus muscles.

In this way, the fascial investments of the iliopsoas, piriformis, and obturator internus muscles and the fascial sheaths of the superior gluteal arteries provide anatomic pathways to the buttocks, hips, and thighs. Superiorly, the pelvic tissues above the levator ani and coccygeus muscles are continuous with the extraperitoneal portion of the abdomen.

# Radiologic Findings

Radiologic findings may first identify the presence, extent, and location of the primary process. Subcutaneous emphysema presents as gas in the fascial planes between the muscles and interstitial tissues, in contrast to gas gangrene where the gas lies within the muscles. In the hip, it may first appear about the greater or lesser trochanter.[1,4,7,13] The first site of appearance or area of maximum development of cellulitis or subcutaneous emphysema should indicate the appropriate anatomic level and likely nature of perforation of the bowel. Radiologic studies may then confirm the cause and anatomic pathway of spread. Computed tomography may be particularly useful in this regard.[14]

Figure 11–4 illustrates gluteal spread from a traumatic perforation of the rectum occasioned by a barium enema study. Dissection from the pelvis toward the gluteal area is strikingly illustrated in this case by the extravasated contrast agent tracking within the fascial extension of the superior gluteal artery through the greater sciatic foramen. Indeed, the vessel is shown as a tubular filling defect within its opacified endopelvic sheath. Tenderness in the buttock was a consequence of this anatomic extension.

Figure 11–5 illustrates a similar pathway in an instance of sigmoid diverticulitis perforating to the buttock, in a patient presenting with fever and vague pain in the right buttock. Perforation of the sigmoid colon in this case is directed along the extension of the superior gluteal artery through the greater sciatic foramen to the right buttock. The initial symptom of pain in this site heralded the progression to a prominent gluteal abscess.

Figure 11–6 illustrates extension within the fascial investment of the piriformis muscle from perforating sigmoid diverticulitis in a patient presenting with fever and pain in the left hip. Loculated extravasation from this area along the plane of the piriformis muscle extended to the left buttock and hip.

Figure 11–7 illustrates an instance of the clinical and radiographic presentation of septic arthritis of the hip complicating an underlying sigmoid diverticulitis. This may be initially very misleading in the absence of soft-tissue gas.[15]

Figure 11–8 demonstrates clinically occult extrapelvic spread in a case of appendicitis in a patient presenting with fever and right hip pain and tenderness. Necrotic cellulitis and interstitial emphysema of the right thigh in this patient progressed via the iliopsoas muscle group from a perforated appendicitis that was not diagnosed antemortem.

Figure 11–9 reveals extension of intrapelvic malignancy into the thigh along the course of the obturator internus muscle. The outlets provided by the muscles and lymphatics in their fascial investments through the foramina may constitute anatomic pathways for the extrapelvic spread of carcinomas and lymphomas.[16,17]

Figure 11–10 illustrates that, superiorly, extension from the subperitoneal pelvic tissues preferentially seeks out the posterior pararenal

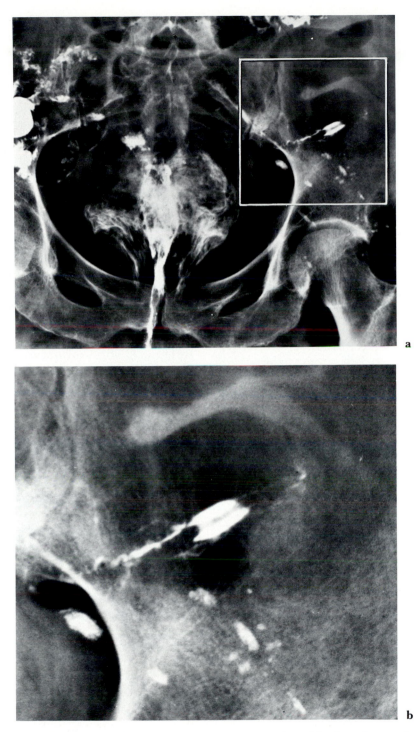

**Fig. 11–4. Rectal extravasation complicating a barium enema study, with gluteal spread.**
(**a**) Postevacuation film. Contrast agent has infiltrated the intramural and extrarectal pelvic tissues.
(**b**) Magnification of area outlined in **a** demonstrates extravasation within the tunneled fascial sheath of the superior gluteal artery progressing through the greater sciatic foramen toward the buttock.
(From Meyers and Goodman[1])

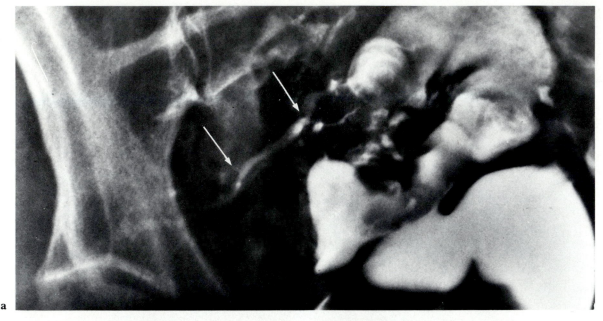

a

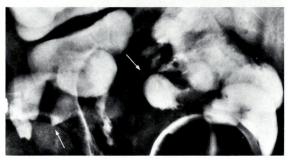

b

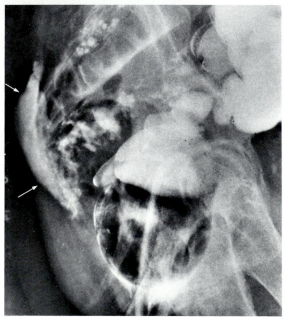

c

**Fig. 11–5. Sigmoid diverticulitis perforating to the right buttock.**

(**a**) Sinus tract (arrows) leads from a site of inflammatory narrowing in the sigmoid colon along the course of the superior gluteal artery to the right buttock.

(**b** and **c**) Ten days later, a follow-up study shows that the sinus tract remains evident, and there is now a large abscess cavity (arrows) deep in the gluteal muscle.

(From Meyers and Goodman[1])

**Fig. 11–7. Septic arthritis of the left hip secondary to sigmoid diverticulitis.**

(**a**) Destruction of the hip joint due to septic arthritis.

(**b**) Barium enema study shows segmental narrowing of the sigmoid colon due to acute diverticulitis. Barium has entered the hip joint through a fistulous communication.

(From Smith et al[17a])

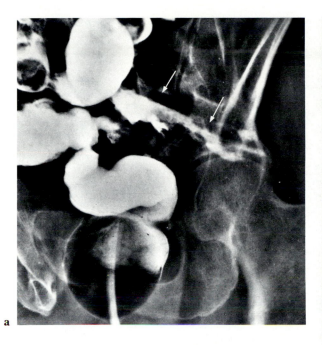

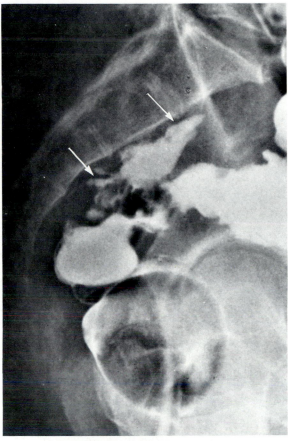

**Fig. 11–6. Sigmoid diverticulitis perforating to the left buttock and hip.**
Oblique (**a**) and lateral (**b**) projections of barium enema study demonstrate extension from inflammatory narrowing of the distal sigmoid colon along the course of the piriformis muscle (arrows).
(From Meyers and Goodman[1])

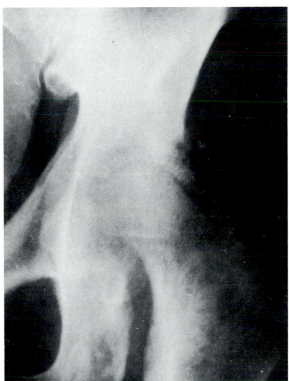

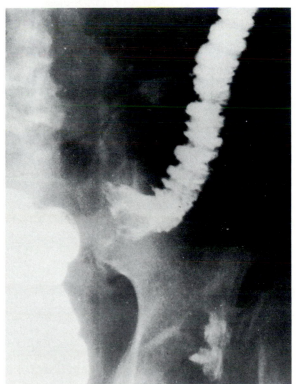

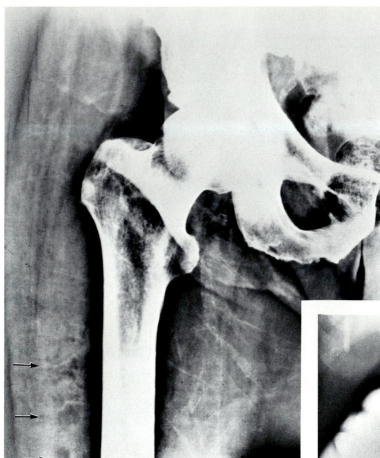

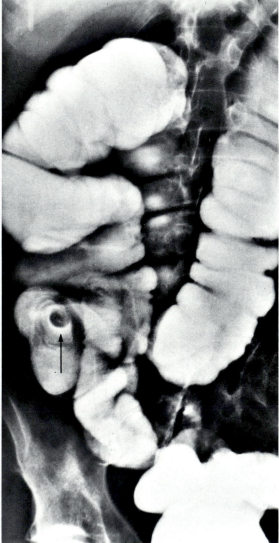

**Fig. 11–8. Appendicitis perforating to the right thigh.**

(**a**) Loculated intersitial gas lateral to the right femur (arrows). Aspiration cultured *E. coli.*

(**b**) Barium enema study demonstrates nonopacification of the appendix with a prominent defect near its confluence with the caput cecum (arrow), despite reflux obtained into the terminal ileum. These findings were proved due to perforated appendicitis.

(From Meyers and Goodman[1])

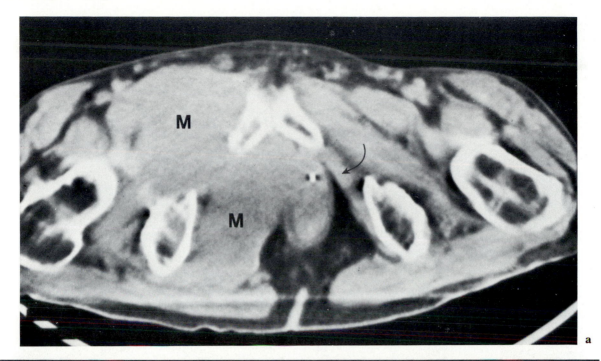

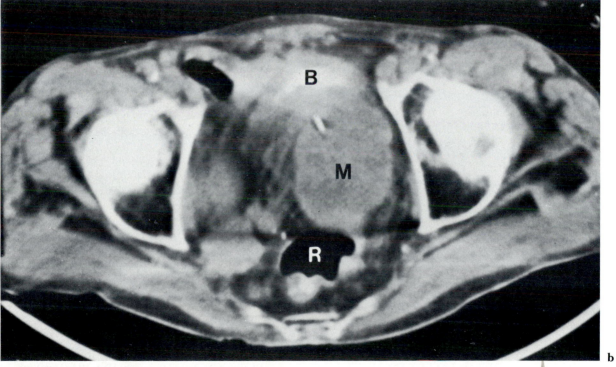

**Fig. 11–9. Recurrence of carcinoma of the colon extending through the obturator foramen to the thigh.**
(a) CT scan at the level of the symphysis pubis demonstrates the recurrent mass (M) extending from the pelvis through the obturator foramen on the right to the thigh.

The normal obturator internus muscle is seen on the left (curved arrow).

(b) At a higher level, the mass continues to the ischiorectal fossa, displacing the rectum (R) to the left and lying between the rectum and the urinary bladder (B).

compartment of the extraperitoneal region of the abdomen.[1,18–21] The characteristic features allow precise radiologic localization, as detailed in Chapter 4.

# References

1. Meyers MA, Goodman KJ: Pathways of extrapelvic spread of disease: Anatomic-radiologic correlation. AJR 125: 900–909, 1975
2. Edwards JD, Eckhauser FE: Retroperitoneal perforation of the appendix presenting as subcutaneous emphysema of the thigh. Dis Colon Rectum 29(7): 456–458, 1986
3. Fiss TW Jr, Cigtay OS, Miele AJ, et al: Perforated viscus presenting with gas in the soft tissues (subcutaneous emphysema). AJR 125: 226–233, 1975
4. Korsten J, Mattey WE, Bastidas J, et al: Subcutaneous emphysema of the thigh secondary to ruptured diverticulum of the ascending colon. Radiology 106: 555–556, 1973
5. Linscheid RI, Kelly PJ, Symmonds RE: Emphysematous cellulitis of the hip and thigh resulting from enteric fistula. J Bone J Surg 45: 1691–1697, 1963
6. Mzabi R, Himal HS, MacLean LD: Gas gangrene of the extremity: The presenting clinical picture in perforating carcinoma of the caecum. Br J Surg 62: 373–374, 1975
7. Pickels RF, Karmody AM, Tspogas MJ, et al: Subcutaneous emphysema of the lower extremity of gastrointestinal origin: Report of a case. Dis Colon Rectum 17: 82–86, 1974
8. Oetting HK, Kramer NE, Branch WE: Subcutaneous emphysema of gastrointestinal origin. Am J Med 19: 872–886, 1955
9. Quigley JP, Brody DA: A physiologic and clinical consideration of pressures developed in the digestive tract. Am J Med 13: 73–81, 1952
10. Burt CV: Pneumatic rupture of intestinal canal with experimental data showing mechanism of perforation and pressure required. Arch Surg 22: 875–902, 1931
11. Ainsworth J: Emphysema of the leg following perforation of the pelvic colon or rectum. Br J Radiol 32: 54–55, 1959
12. Altemeier WA, Alexander JW: Retroperitoneal abscess. Arch Sug 83: 512–524, 1961
13. Shaffer RD: Subcutaneous emphysema of the leg secondary to toothpick ingestion. Arch Surg 99: 542–545, 1969
14. Meshkov SL, Seltzer SE, Finberg HJ: CT detection of intraabdominal disease in patients with lower extremity signs and symptoms. J Comp Assist Tomogr 6(3): 497–501, 1982

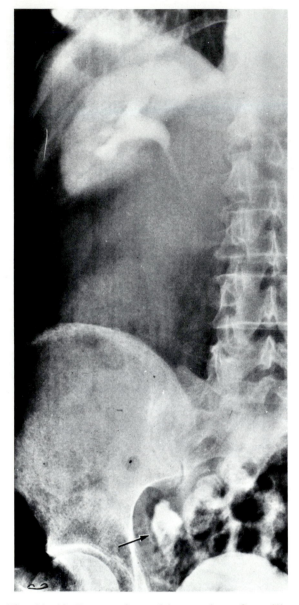

**Fig. 11–10. Extraperitoneal hemorrhage from iliac artery.**
Difficulty in passing the catheter through the iliac artery during attempted cardiac catheterization was encountered. Contrast agent was introduced to evaluate the cause of the difficulty, and this demonstrated local extravasation. Right lower quadrant guarding and tenderness developed. Delayed film demonstrates persistent localized extravasation (arrow) from the right external iliac artery.

A soft-tissue mass representing a large amount of blood now occupies the right abdomen. This displaces the lower pole of the kidney laterally, obstructs the ureter, and obliterates the lateral edge of the psoas muscle and the flank stripe. These features localize the hematoma to the extraperitoneal posterior pararenal compartment. (From Meyers and Goodman[1])

15. Smith WS, Ward RM: Septic arthritis of the hip complicating perforation of abdominal organs. JAMA 195: 170–172, 1966
16. Abratt RP, Pontin AR, Roman TE, et al: Tumour spread through the obturator foramen. Br J Radiol 58: 673–674, 1985
17. Rao BK, Lange TA, Hafez GR, et al: Extension of recurrent rectal carcinoma through sciatic foramen: Diagnosis by computed tomography. Comp Radiol 6: 193–197, 1982
17a. Smith HJ, Berk RN, Janes JO, et al: Unusual fistulae due to colonic diverticulitis. Gastrointest Radiol 2: 387–392, 1978
18. Meyers MA: Acute extraperitoneal infection. Semin Roentgenol 8: 445–464, 1973
19. Meyers MA: Radiologic features of the spread and localization of extraperitoneal gas and their relationship to its source: An anatomical approach. Radiology 111: 17–26, 1974
20. Meyers MA, Whalen JP, Peelle K, et al: Radiologic features of extraperitoneal effusions: An anatomic approach. Radiology 104: 249–257, 1972
21. Illescas FF, Baker ME, McCann R, et al: CT evaluation of retroperitoneal hemorrhage associated with femoral arteriography. AJR 146: 1289–1292, 1986

# 12 Dynamics of Plain-Film Analysis of the Abdomen

## General Introduction

The value of plain-film diagnosis in *acute* abdominal conditions is unquestioned. The visceral gas pattern is studied routinely in patients presenting clinical evidence of intestinal obstruction, perforation of a viscus, or an intra-abdominal mass. Little appreciated and often neglected, however, are the diagnostic potentialities of abdominal films in more chronic and clinically occult conditions.[1,2]

Accurate plain-film analysis of the abdomen is one of the most difficult challenges of diagnostic radiology. While it is classically presented as the introduction to radiology of the abdomen in textbooks, courses, and student seminars, long experience with contrast studies is required to establish criteria and visual sensitivity. Since abdominal symptoms are commonly nonspecific, there are many clinical instances in which the site of primary disease is not clear originally. Radiologic investigation is often initiated by a study focusing attention on another organ or body system, but including plain-film visualization of portions of the gastrointestinal tract. Abnormal findings peripheral to the anticipated area of interest may therefore be of considerable importance in directing attention immediately to the true primary site of disease. This diagnostic serendipity can be increased by an understanding of the factors involved. Although the diagnostic potential of the plain film of the abdomen can be fully realized only after familiarity with the appearance of organic abnormalities on contrast studies, an understanding of the dynamics of visual perception can be usefully applied to the analysis of the plain film so that pitfalls can be avoided and diagnostic pickups made.[1]

## Visual and Anatomic Factors

Recognition of significant abnormalities in the alimentary tract without the use of contrast media is dependent upon two basic factors: (1) visual factors and (2) anatomic and physical factors.

## Visual Factors: Perception of the Roentgen Image

Visual search is the first step in reading a radiograph. At the luminance available for reading an abdominal x-ray, photopic vision is employed. This allows for the greatest visual acuity when the image is focused on the fovea centralis. However, this is a relatively small area due to the fact that the cones, which are responsible for visual acuity, are concentrated at the fovea, especially at its center, and accounts for the rapid decline in acuity just a few degrees from the fovea centralis. Of necessity, then, peripheral vision is used as the initial step in reading a radiograph. Use of peripheral vision allows for a considerably larger, although not as acute, field of vision in which to select possible abnormal areas from numerous areas of suboptimal quality images projected on the retina. There is a direct relationship between visual field size and the time required to locate a target.[3] After an object of possible interest is located, the eye then moves to a position that focuses the fovea centralis on this point. In this position detailed information can be obtained.

After an area of interest is identified, the eye moves to another area of interest.[4,5] Each movement, known as a saccade, allows for the fovea centralis to fix on a new point of interest. Typically there are two to three saccadic movements per second. The actual visual fixations occupy 90% of viewing time and the saccadic movements 10%. The normal human eye, using photopic vision, can resolve a visual angle of only 2.0°. Translated to reading a 14 × 17 in. film of the abdomen, this means that at 30 in. detailed vision is equal to a circle of 1 in. in diameter, or that 300 separate eye fixations are necessary to cover the entire film.[6]

Visual fixations tend to cluster around angles and sharp curves.[4,5] In addition, if a contour is unpredictable or unusual, i.e., it changes direction irregularly and rapidly, visual fixation also will cluster at these points. Wide individual variations in regard to search patterns by radiologists are influenced by prior knowledge.[6,7]

In addition to topographic changes, other factors such as contrast, size, and shape are important. A target of relatively high contrast will be rapidly detected by peripheral vision. Also, a single high-contrast target that occupies an empty field is detected easily and almost immediately fixated.[8] Similar items of the same shape and size take a prolonged time to detect if the contrast is low.[9] Size and luminance also have been shown to affect eye fixation.[10]

It can be concluded that the brain has chosen certain informative details in order to remember or recognize an object. This internal perception within the brain can then take place either by the serial recognition or by the one-step holistic process. Recent evidence, especially in regard to visual perception, tends to support the step-by-step theory. Visual perception and internal perception are not mechanical recordings of elements, but working together are the means for grasping significant structural patterns.[11] Examples of this are dramatically illustrated by figure–ground reversal or multistability in perception[12] (Fig. 12–1). How one image superimposed upon another or projected within

another is appreciated visually is determined by which is seen as the figure and which is perceived as the background. The factors that influence the perception of shape in the basic figure–ground relationship of any picture have been extensively studied,[13–16] and are directly applicable to plain-film analysis of the abdomen. These laws of visual organization involve area, closedness, symmetry, and continuity. The smaller a closed region, the more an area has closed contours; the more symmetrical a closed region, the more it tends to be seen as a figure. It is often these features that permit the identification of an abnormality discriminated from the background of normalcy within an abdominal radiograph.

The point of basic interest in multistable images that spontaneously alternate, as in Figure 12–1, is that one line can have two shapes. A simple curved line is convex on one side but concave on the other. The perceptual representation of a contour is specific to which side is regarded as primary. This achieves added significance when one regards the internal representation or memory of an object as a step-by-step process.

It must also be appreciated, however, that expectations that the reader brings to a film may be misleading. This has been demonstrated by psychologists by a series of drawings with subtle progressive differences until the last panel depicts and illustration radically different from the first (Fig. 12–2). The recognizable point of transition where the image shifts in the viewer's perception is different, depending whether the viewer traces the series from left to right or backward. This illustrates that preconditioning—in other words, the concepts of expectation, prior knowledge, and experience—determine in large measure visual perceptions. "Perception depends on learning. It is not that (the radiologist) will see only what he expects to see, but that he will also see what contradicts his expectations."[17] The influence of prior knowledge aids the radiologist not only to fixate on important areas of a radiograph, but to search or scan other areas to confirm or refute his memory expectation. The limitations to recent computational theories of perception that integrate work in neurophysiology, psychology, and artificial intelligence[18] testify to the astonishing complexity and sophistication of human vision.

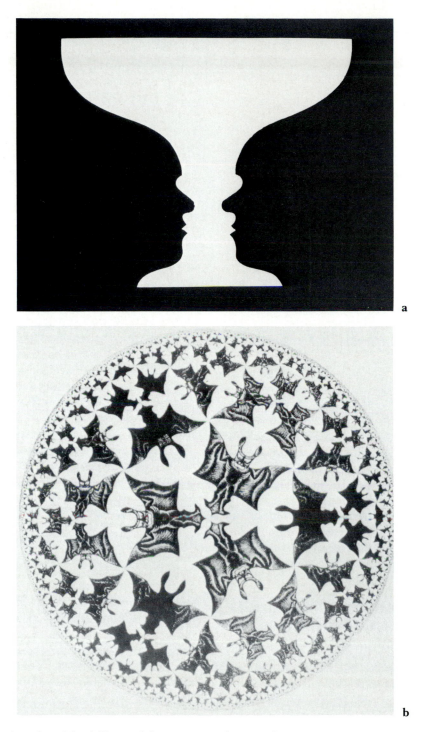

**Fig. 12–1. Examples of multistability and figure–ground reversal.**
(**a**) The white area can be viewed as a goblet or the black area as the silhouettes of two profiles. Both images, however, cannot be perceived simultaneously.
(**b**) The black images can be seen as devils or the white outlines as angels. (From M. Escher)

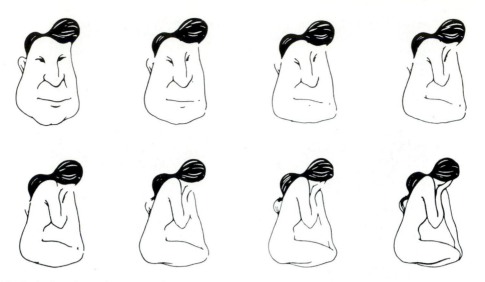

**Fig. 12–2. A drawing of a man's face subtly changes to the outline of a young female.**
The transition point is dependent not only on subjective variations but on the sequence followed.

## *Anatomic and Physical Factors*

The second basic factor is a knowledge of normal anatomic relationships and variants and the effect of physical, physiologic, and pathologic processes. Fundamental considerations detailed in other chapters include variations in positions of structures, the relationships maintained and bounded by mesenteric attachments, the distribution of intra- and extraperitoneal fat providing the lucent interfaces of organ and viscus contours, and the governance of the configuration of the hollow viscera, not only by anatomic and physiologic specific characteristics, but also by general physical laws.

## Classification of Abdominal Plain-Film Abnormalities

The classification in Table 12-1 is based on the fact that the initial detection of an abnormality in the scanning of a radiograph is dependent on

**Table 12–1.** Classification of significant abnormalities in plain films of the abdomen based on visual search patterns.

| *Topographic* | *Contrast* |
|---|---|
| Abnormal location | Increased density |
| Abnormal orientation | Increased lucency |
| Loss of normal finding | |
| Contour defect (acute angles; sharp, unusual curves) | |

optic fixations, attracted by topographic alterations in direction and contrast differences. Targets with certain characteristics, such as sharp angles and contours, high contrast, and unexpected orientation, are often rapidly detected. In this context, the term "plain film" includes instances without contrast opacification of the alimentary tract. The area of abnormality may be included incidentally in other investigations, including chest films, intravenous urography, and abdominal arteriography.

## Unusual Location

Recognition of the abnormal location of a shadow implies, of course, familiarity with the normal position of the structures of the abdomen visualized in a plain film. Once the observer has acquired this basic information, visual search then rapidly uncovers the presence of the unexpected location of a well-defined structure.

## *Normal Variants and Congenital Abnormalities*

There are a few anatomic variants and benign congenital abnormalities that may be mistaken for pathologic conditions. The most misleading of these include the following:

**Fig. 12–3. Hepatodiaphragmatic interposition of the colon.**
The abnormally located hepatic flexure is recognized by its haustral markings. (From Meyers and Oliphant[1])

———————————————————————▷

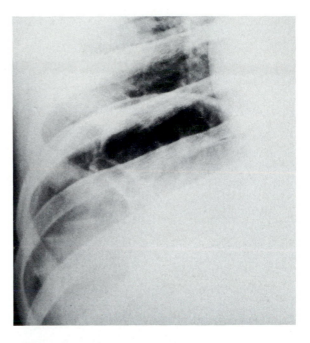

1. *Hepatodiaphragmatic interposition of the colon (Chilaiditi's syndrome).* As a variant of rotation of the gut, the hepatic flexure of the colon may be insinuated between the liver and the diaphragm,[19] simulating the presence of a right subphrenic abscess. Identification of the characteristic haustral markings, however, establishes the presence of this interposition (Fig. 12–3).
2. *Gas within an ascending subhepatic appendix.* This may mimic air within the common bile duct[20] or a localized abscess within Morison's pouch (the right posterior subhepatic space). The characteristic tubular collection of radiolucency is oriented upward and to the left and is associated with a high cecum (Fig. 12–4).

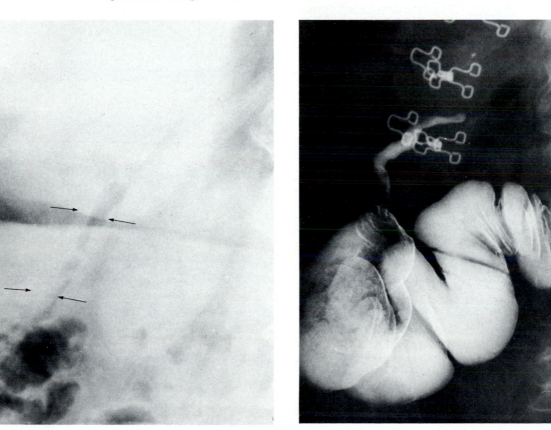

a                                                                                          b

**Fig. 12–4. Ascending subhepatic appendix.**
(**a**) Plain film. Tubular radiolucency (arrows) is directed superiorly and medially beneath the edge of the liver, anterior to the right kidney.
(**b**) Barium enema study verifies the position of the appendix and its association with a mobile undescended cecum.
(From Meyers and Oliphant[1])

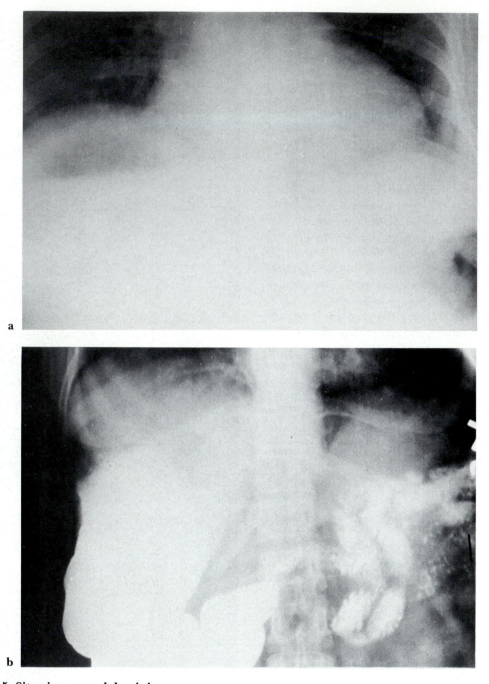

**Fig. 12–5. Situs inversus abdominis.**
(**a**) Erect plain film. Air–fluid level beneath right diaphragm. No gastric bubble beneath left diaphragm. The heart is not rotated.
(**b**) Upper GI series verifies the condition.
(From Meyers and Oliphant[1])

3. *Situs inversus abdominis.* This may be very misleading on plain films unless the complex of
findings is recognized. The air–fluid level beneath the right diaphragm on erect films (Fig.
12–5a) may be easily mistaken for a subphrenic
abscess. Absence of associated pulmonary basilar or pleural changes, and particularly of an
identifiable gastric air bubble on the left, leads
to a confirmatory upper GI series (Fig. 12–5b).

## Ulcers and Diverticula

These abnormalities may be revealed on plain
films as luminal gas continuing beyond the projected mucosal contour of a viscus. While this
does present an unusual radiolucency, it is primarily its unexpected location that attracts visual search.

Most common in this category is a lesser curvature gastric ulcer. Benign ulcers of the stomach often trap gas, and the majority occur along
the lesser curvature, which is presented in profile in the AP or PA projections (Fig. 12–6). I
have noted them on plain films ranging in size
from 2 mm to 5 cm. If the ulcer is penetrating
into the pancreas, it is an occasional diagnostic
"pickup" in a lumbosacral spine series obtained
for back pain.

Diverticula of the bowel also may trap gas and
present a misleading appearance until their true

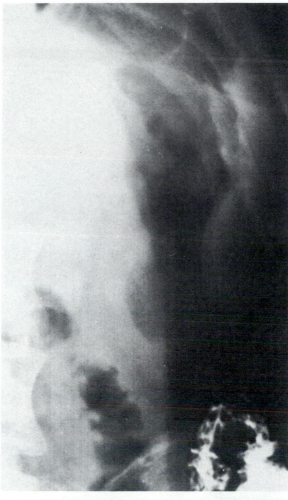

a

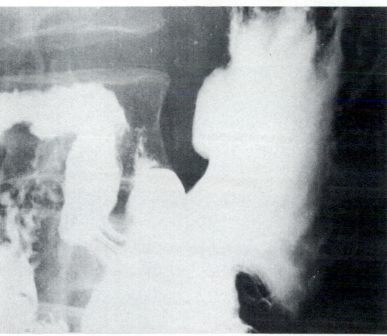

**Fig. 12–6. Large benign ulcer
of the lesser curvature of the
stomach.**
(a) Plain film. A collection of
gastric luminal gas projects beyond the mucosal contour.
(b) Upper GI series confirms
the diagnostic criteria.
(From Meyers and Oliphant[1])

b

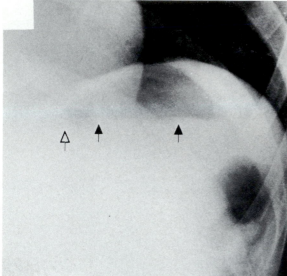

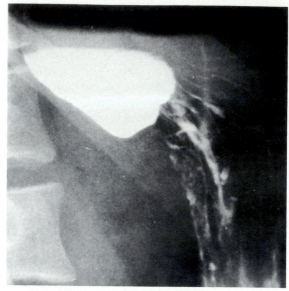

△

**Fig. 12–7. Gastric diverticulum.**
(**a**) On erect chest film there are two air–fluid levels. They are of different sizes and planes.
(**b**) Confirmatory upper GI series.
(From Meyers and Oliphant[1])

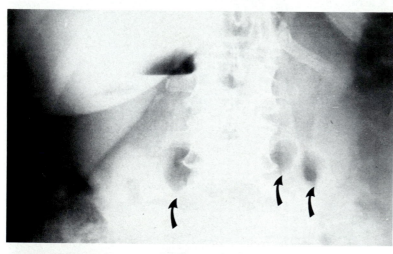

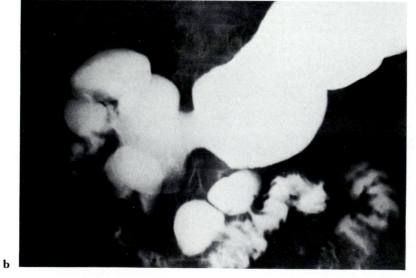

◁

**Fig. 12–8. (a** and **b) Multiple diverticula of the duodenal loop** present as confined collections of gas (arrows) without mucosal characteristics in the region of L2.
(From Meyers and Oliphant[1])

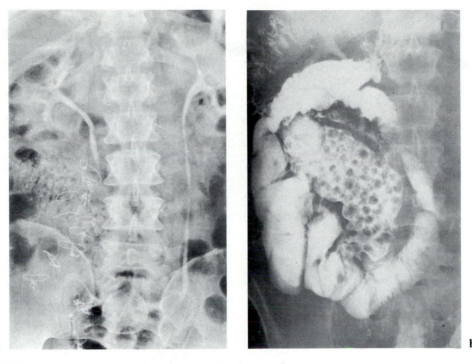

a                                                                                                                        b

**Fig. 12–9. Meckel's diverticulum containing watermelon seeds.**
(**a**) Mottled lucencies resembling an abscess are seen in the right abdomen.
(**b**) Barium studies document multiple filling defects secondary to ingested seeds within a large Meckel's diverticulum.

nature is revealed. Figure 12–7a illustrates a small air–fluid collection medial to the gastric fundus. The two air–fluid levels are not on the same plane, indicating that if communication exists, it is not widely patent. It appears that the small neck of the gastric diverticulum in this case (Fig. 12–7b) prevents equalization of the hydrostatic pressures.

Diverticulosis of the small bowel (Figs. 12–8 and 12–9) and of the colon (Fig. 12–10) can be confused with intra- or extraperitoneal abscesses.

## Abnormal Orientation

Visual search is attracted by the curves and angles of abnormally oriented images. Anatomic symmetry often is distorted. The visual forces of tension are represented in the radiograph by unpredictable direction, unbalanced grouping, or convergence (Fig. 12–11).

## Loss of Normal Outlines

The most subtle abnormality to detect is loss of a normal finding on the plain film. The usual visual forces attracting eye fixations are not present in such instances. Rather, disciplined checking of the normal images along the lines of a careful inventory is necessary. The soft-tissue outlines in the abdomen normally seen include particularly the hepatic and splenic angles, the flank stripes, and the lateral margins of the psoas muscles. A significant disease process in the abdomen may be revealed only by effacement or segmental loss of a normal shadow.

## Contour Defect

The outline of a normally pliable gas-containing viscus generally is characterized by symmetry and a gradual transition in size and contour.

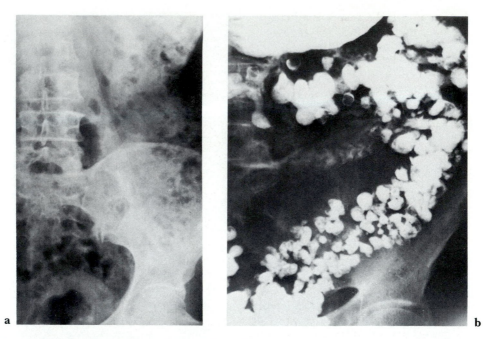

**Fig. 12–10. (a and b) Massive diverticulosis of the colon** presents as mottled collections of a gas mimicking abscess formation. Their relationship to the colon is difficult to ascertain on the plain film. (From Meyers and Oliphant[1])

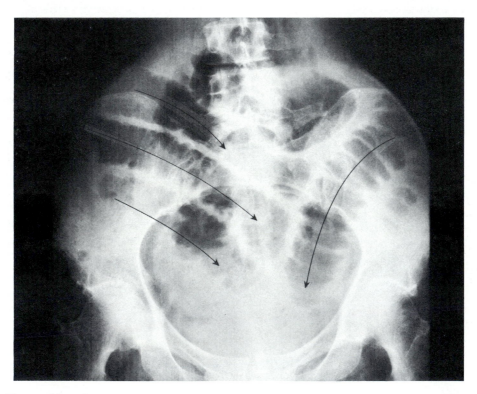

**Fig. 12–11. Femoral hernia.**
The normal orientation of small bowel loops is lost as they are drawn toward a point of convergence at the left femoral ring. (From Meyers and Oliphant[1])

**Fig. 12–12. Leiomyoma of the gastric fundus.**
On barium enema study a conspicuous, smooth spherical mass projects within the stomach. (From Meyers and Oliphant[1])

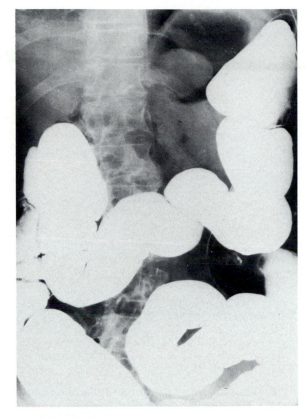

**Fig. 12–13. Ileocolic intussusception.**
(**a**) IVP demonstrates large mass within the transverse colon, presenting a rounded outline distally with abrupt angles to luminal contour (*arrows*).
(**b**) Barium enema verifies the intussusception with typical coil-spring folds.

This plain-film abnormality is also an excellent example of multistability. The border of the image is formed, but the mind must discriminate between perceiving it as part of the figure or the ground. If the contour of the mass is first viewed as a concave line, the eye follows it distally toward the normal distal transverse colon and is led astray. On the other hand, if the contour is perceived as a convex line, scanning then proceeds proximally and recognition of the full features of the lesion is obtained.
(From Meyers and Oliphant[1])

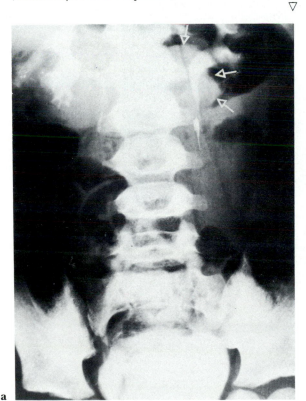

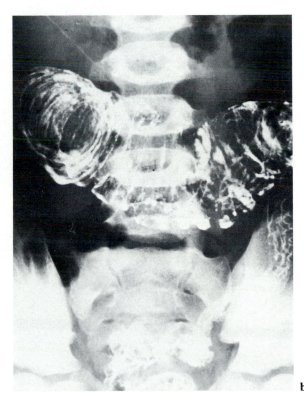

a

b

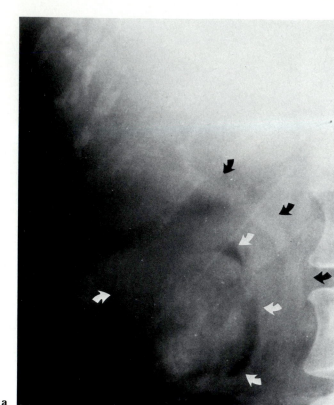

**Fig. 12–14. Prolapsed gastric leiomyoma within the duodenal bulb.**

(**a**) Intravenous cholangiography shows a large mass within the duodenal bulb, enlarging it and almost completely obliterating the lumen. This is revealed by the very thin rim of air surrounding it (white arrows). Some calcifications are present within the mass. Its position within the duodenal bulb is further confirmed by its relationship to the common bile duct, displacing it posteriorly and medially (black arrows).

(**b**) The findings are confirmed in the upper GI series, which further shows its pedunculated origin from the gastric antrum. Note the widened pyloric channel.

(From Meyers and Oliphant[1])

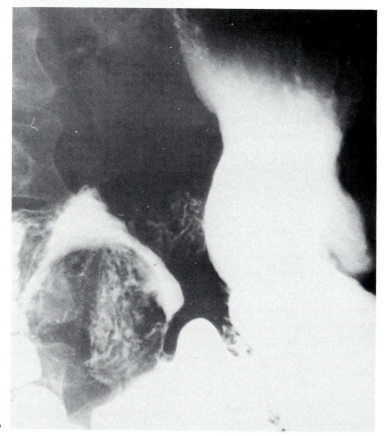

**Fig. 12–15. Intestinal *Ascaris lumbricoides*.**
On IVP, there is a conspicuous, elongated soft-tissue mass within the lumen of a distal ileal loop (arrows). Its contours are sharply outlined. (From Meyers and Oliphant[1])

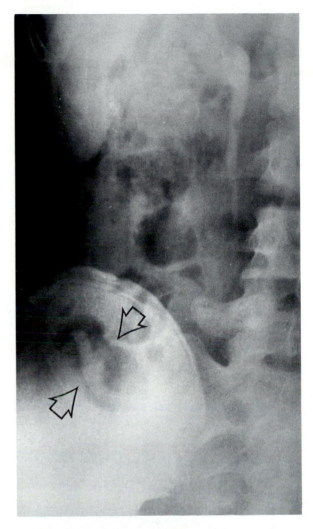

Visual fixations in a search pattern of an abdominal film are drawn to acute angles and sharp, unusual curves. These alterations involving intestinal contour should be searched for and not overlooked in an attempt to "see through" the "superimposed" bowel.

The contour of luminal gas may be altered in a variety of patterns. Most striking is a prominent intraluminal filling defect that produces a sharp angle in the luminal contour (Fig. 12–12).

Figure 12–13a illustrates an intravenous urogram obtained in a child with colicky abdominal pains. Incidental to study of the urinary system, acute contour angles of a prominent rounded density were noted projecting within the distal transverse colon, and this was then observed to represent actually the distal end of a large sausage-shaped mass. Barium enema (Fig. 12–13b) confirmed the presence of an ileocolic intussusception.

Figure 12–14a is an intravenous cholangiogram obtained in a patient with the clinical diagnosis of acute biliary colic. A prominent mass enlarging the contour of the duodenal bulb was noted, leading to an upper GI series (Fig. 12–14b). At surgery, a gastric leiomyoma that had prolapsed across the pylorus and impacted within the duodenal bulb was removed.

Figures 12–15 and 12–16 depict a filiform body with gentle curves within a gas-filled small bowel loop, representing *Ascaris*. This illustrates the dynamic visual principle that if a smaller shadow falls within a larger image of contrasting density, its visualization is greatly enhanced if it is sharply outlined.

These same fundamental contour defects, ranging from subtle to gross, may reveal readily the presence of malignancy when a plain film of the abdomen is scanned, whether the neoplasm is polypoid (Fig. 12–17a and b), annular (Fig. 12–17c–e), scirrhous (Fig. 12–17f) or ulcerated (Fig. 12–17g).

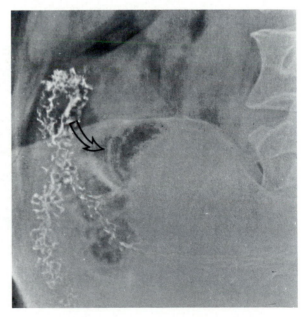

**Fig. 12–16. Intestinal *Ascaris lumbricoides*.**
A filiform body is outlined within a gas-filled small bowel loop overlying the ilium (arrow).

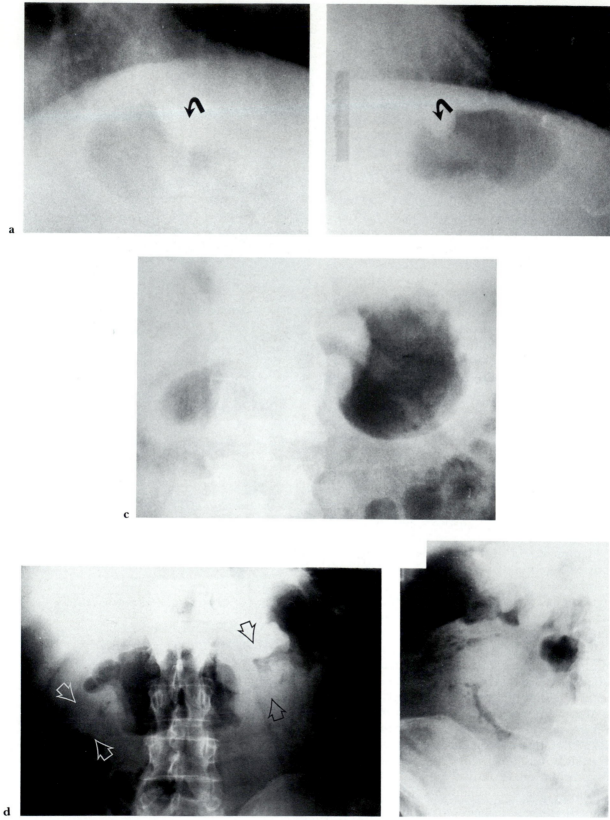

**12–17**

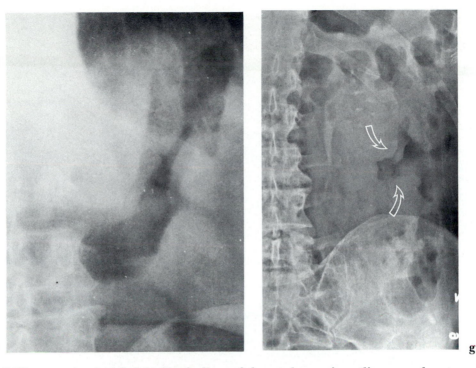

f                                                                                g

**Fig. 12–17. Different examples of plain-film findings of abrupt changes in outline secondary to malignancy.**
Note that it is basically the acute angles in contour that attract visual attention.
(**a**) Carcinoma of the gastric fundus. Angled defect (arrow) of superior and lateral contour.
(**b**) Carcinoma of gastric fundus. Angled polypoid contour defect of superior wall (arrow).
(**c**) Carcinoma of body and antrum of stomach. Shelflike abrupt change in contour with narrowed antral lumen ("apple-core" lesion).
(**d**) Double primary carcinomas of the transverse colon. Two "apple-core" lesions (arrows).
(**e**) Fungating polypoid carcinoma of the cecum. Irregularly narrowed lumen with multiple limited extensions into large soft-tissue mass.
(**f**) Lymphosarcoma of stomach. Abrupt transitions in luminal contour and individual rugae, with appearance of rigidity.
(**g**) Ulcerated leiomyosarcoma of small bowel (arrow).
(From Meyers and Oliphant[1])

Contour defects may be associated with other plain-film abnormalities to enable precise identification (Fig. 12–18).

The variety of basic pathologic lesions that may be identified include inflammatory (Fig. 12–19), ischemic (Fig. 12–20), and chronic ulcerative (Fig. 12–21) processes as well as diffuse malignancy (Fig. 12–22). The type of contour defect can be correlated with such factors as length and distribution to arrive at a reasonable diagnosis on the plain film alone. Indeed, while a gastrointestinal contrast study is necessary to document the abnormality, many of the features often are not better illustrated.

# Increased Contrast Density

The perception of increased contrast is related not only to the differential density, but also to the size, associated angles, and sharpness of outline. Most cases involve the presence of abnormal calcifications. Their variety and differential diagnosis have been extensively detailed.[21]

Abnormal densities range from the readily apparent to the extremely subtle. Figure 12–23 was obtained from a patient who had had multiple operations, the most recent for intestinal obstruction with lysis of adhesions. Continued ab-

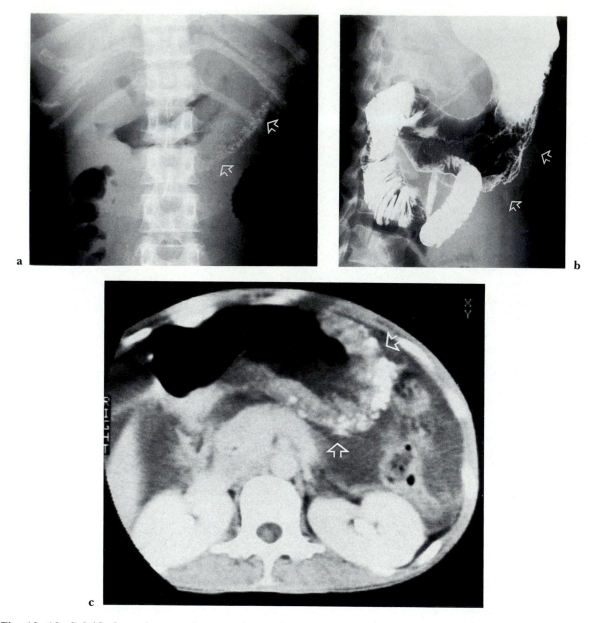

**Fig. 12–18. Calcified mucin-secreting gastric carcinoma.**
(**a**) Plain film shows sharp contour abnormalities and filling defects. Increased contrast density provided by the calcifications paralleling the distorted lumen indicates marked thickening of the gastric wall (arrows). (**b** and **c**) Upper GI series and CT confirm the plain-film observations.

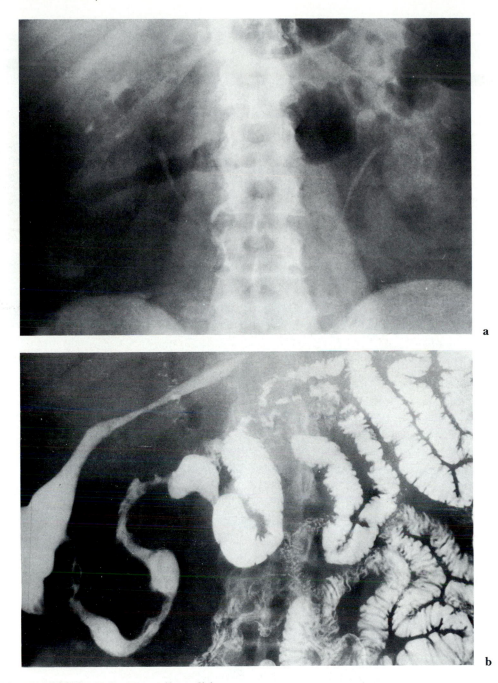

a

b

**Fig. 12–19. (a and b) Granulomatous ileocolitis.**
Long stricture of right colon, with transition to normal-appearing haustral contour at mid-transverse colon.
(From Meyers and Oliphant[1])

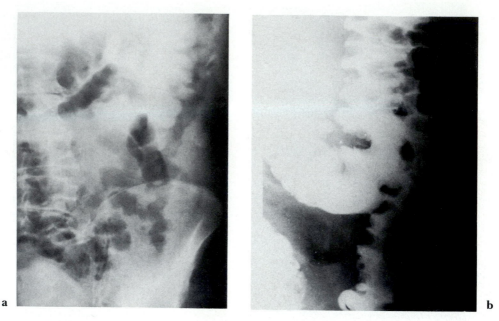

**Fig. 12–20. Ischemic colitis.**
(a) Plain film shows multiple scalloped contours of distal transverse colon, splenic flexure, and descending colon.
(b) Barium enema verifies the characteristic "thumbprinting" produced by the submucosal hematomas.
(From Meyers and Oliphant[1])

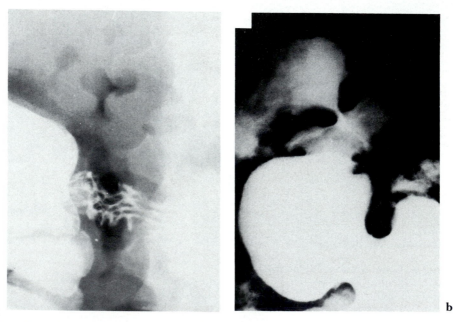

**Fig. 12–21. Cloverleaf deformity of duodenal bulb.**
(a) Stellate collection of gas superior to hepatic flexure on barium enema study.
(b) Chronic pseudodiverticular deformity of bulb is confirmed on upper GI series.
(From Meyers and Oliphant[1])

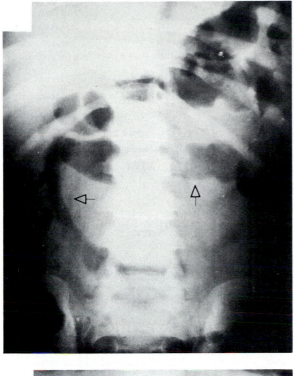

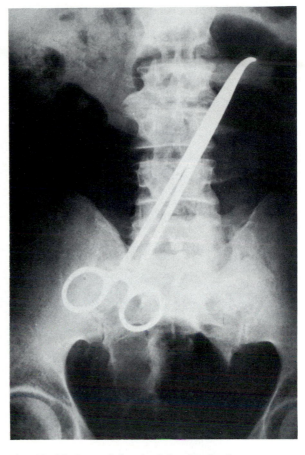

**Fig. 12–23. Intraabdominal foreign body.**
The extreme density, sharp contour, and familiar outline make the retained hemostat readily recognizable. (From Meyers and Oliphant[1])

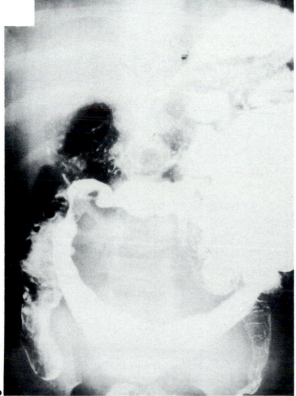

**Fig. 12–22. Lymphosarcoma of small bowel.**
(**a**) Plain film reveals fixed, angulated, dilated small bowel loop with no mucosal markings (*arrows*).
(**b**) Small bowel series confirms the presence of aneurysmal dilatation secondary to gross ulceration, associated with a mass.
(From Meyers and Oliphant[1])

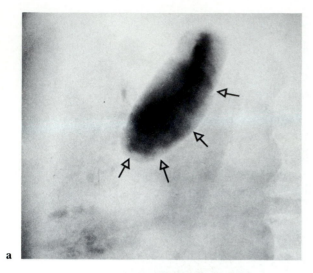

a

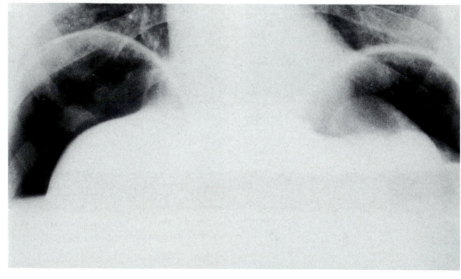

b

**Fig. 12–24. Free intraperitoneal air.**
(**a**) Supine. Although no increased lucency is directly apparent, it is revealed by the visualized density of the wall of a small bowel loop. This presents as a subtle white line around the gas-containing lumen (*arrows*).
(**b**) Erect film documents considerable free air.
 At surgery, a perforated duodenal ulcer was found.
(From Meyers and Oliphant[1])

dominal symptomatology led to a plain film of the abdomen that revealed a retained hemostat.

 Among the most subtle examples of increased contrast density are instances of free intraperitoneal gas. Figure 12–24a represents a portion of a supine projection obtained as a preliminary film to an intravenous urogram for the evaluation of abdominal pain. The ability to visualize the wall thickness of an intestinal loop is strong evidence of the presence of free intraperitoneal gas, contrasting the soft tissue of the wall against the intraluminal gas ("bas-relief" sign). It is noteworthy that no gross overall lucency is directly apparent, although an erect film (Fig. 12–24b) confirms the presence of free air.

 In other cases of free air, its increased lucency may also not be readily appreciable directly but rather it is the visualization of structures occasioned by their relatively increased contrast density that establishes the diagnosis (Fig. 12–25).

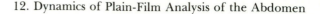

**Fig. 12–27. Pneumatosis cystoides intestinalis.**
(**a**) Plain film shows a pattern of circumscribed, gently arcuate radiolucencies projecting over the ilium.
(**b**) Contrast study documents both linear and spherical intramural collections of gas are present in the cecum and ascending colon.
(From Meyers and Oliphant[1])

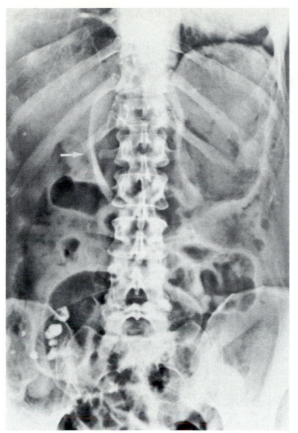

12–25

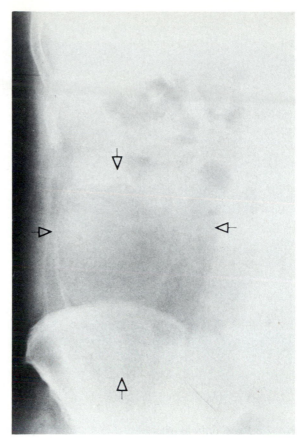

12–26

**Fig. 12–25. Free intraperitoneal air.**
Supine view shows visualization of falciform ligament
(arrow).

**Fig. 12–26. Extraperitoneal liposarcoma.**
A large lucent mass (*arrows*) displaces the kidney. For
its size the radiolucency is not striking but its well-
defined borders add to its recognition. (From Meyers
and Oliphant[1])

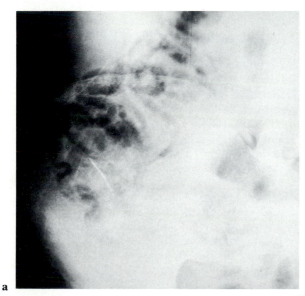

a

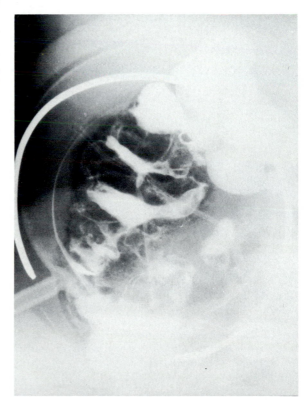

b

12–27

481

# Increased Radiolucency

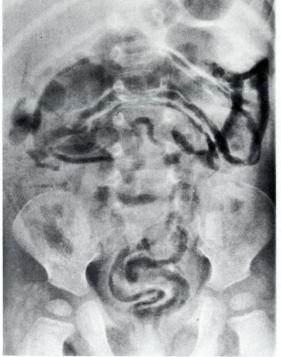

Increased lucency is generally more difficult to appreciate on plain films than is increased density. The radiolucency may blend with fatty or intestinal gas shadows and may not present high contrast against soft-tissue water density (Fig. 12–26). Furthermore, many of the pathologically increased radiolucencies are not associated with sharp angles that would heighten their visual perception. Examples of this include the mottled nature of extraperitoneal gas and abscesses, many intraperitoneal and parenchymatous abscesses, and ovarian dermoids. Even if the lucent shadows are gently arcuate, they may be conspicuous, particularly if they are parallel to other normal radiolucencies. This is seen in instances of intramural gas heightened by their close association with the contour of intraluminal gas (Figs. 12–27 through 12–29).

**Fig. 12–28. Pneumatosis coli.**
Conspicuous intramural gas is present throughout the left colon.

# References

1. Meyers MA, Oliphant M: Pitfalls and pickups in plain-film diagnosis of the abdomen. Current Problems in Radiology. Year Book Medical Publishers, Chicago, Vol. IV, No. 2, 1–37, March–April, 1974
2. Wolf BS, Khilnani MT, Lautkin A: Diagnostic Roentgenology of the Digestive Tract without Contrast Media. Grune & Stratton, New York, 1960
3. Johnston D: Search performance as a function of peripheral acuity. Hum Factors 7: 527–535, 1965
4. Noton D, Stark L: Scan paths in eye movements during pattern reception, Science 171: 308–311, 1971
5. Noton D, Stark L: Eye movements and visual perception. Sci Am 224: 34, 1971
6. Llewellyn TE, Landown EL: Visual search patterns in radiologists in training. Radiology 81: 288–292, 1963
7. Kundel HL, Wright DJ: The influence of prior knowledge on visual search strategies during viewing of chest radiographs. Radiology 93: 315–320, 1969
8. Lusted LB: Applications of signal detectability theory. In Symposium on Perception of the Roentgen Image. Radiol Clin N Am 7: 435–445, 1969
9. Thomas EL: Search behavior. Radiol Clin N Am 7: 403–417, 1969

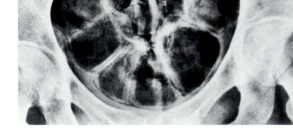

**Fig. 12–29. Necrotizing enterocolitis.**
In this adult with systemic lupus erythematosis, intramural radiolucencies parallel the contour of intraluminal colonic gas.

10. Steinman RM: Effect of target size, luminance, and color on monocular fixation. J Opt Soc Am 55: 1158–1165, 1965

11. Arnheim R: Art and Visual Perception. A Psychology of the Creative Eye. University of California Press, Berkeley, 1971

12. Attneave F: Multistability in perception. Sci Am 225: 62, 1971

13. Cornsweet TN: Visual Perception. Academic Press, New York, 1970

14. Dodwell PC: Visual Pattern Recognition. Holt, Rhinehart & Winston, New York, 1970

15. Koffka K: Principles of Gestalt Psychology. Harcourt, Brace, New York, 1935

16. Wertheimer M: Principles of perceptual organization. Readings in Perception. Edited by D Beardslee, M. Wertheimer, Van Nostrand, Princeton, N.J., pp 115–135, 1958

17. Hebb DO, Favreau O: The mechanism of perception. In Symposium on Perception of the Roentgen Image. Radiol Clin N Am 7: 393–401, 1969

18. Marr D: Vision: A Computational Investigation into the Human Representation and Processing of Visual Information. W. H. Freeman and Co., San Francisco, 1982

19. Chilaiditi D: Zur Frage der Hepatoptose und Ptose im Allgemeinen im Anschlub an drei Falle von temporarer partieller Leberverlagerung. Fortschr Geb Roentgenstr 16: 173–208, 1910–1911

20. Reilly HF Jr, Mosenthal W, Dyke JR: Normal gas-filled appendix simulating biliary-free air in a case of acute cholecystitis. Radiology 89: 931–932, 1967

21. McAfee JG, Donner MW: Differential diagnosis of calcifications encountered in abdominal radiographs, Am J Med Sci 243: 609–650, 1962

# Index